# Vaccine Adjuvants

# Infectious Disease

SERIES EDITOR: *Vassil St. Georgiev*
*National Institute of Allergy and Infectious Diseases*
*National Institutes of Health*

# Vaccine Adjuvants

*Immunological and Clinical Principles*

Edited by

## Charles J. Hackett, PhD

*Division of Allergy, Immunology, and Transplantation*
*National Institute of Allergy and Infectious Diseases, NIH*
*Bethesda, MD*

## Donald A. Harn, Jr., PhD

*Department of Immunology and Infectious Disease,*
*Harvard School of Public Health*
*Boston, MA*

HUMANA PRESS ✳ TOTOWA, NEW JERSEY

Production Editor: Melissa Caravella

Cover design by Patricia F. Cleary

This publication is printed on acid-free paper. ∞
ANSI Z39.48-1984 (American National Standards Institute) Permanence of Paper for Printed Library Materials.

For additional copies, pricing for bulk purchases, and/or information about other Humana titles, contact Humana at the above address or at any of the following numbers: Tel.: 973-256-1699; Fax: 973-256-8341; E-mail: orders@humanapr.com; or visit our Website: www.humanapress.com

Printed in the United States of America. 10 9 8 7 6 5 4 3 2 1
eISBN 1-59259-970-2

Library of Congress Cataloging-in-Publication Data

Vaccine adjuvants : immunological and clinical principles / edited by Charles J. Hackett
  and Donald A. Harn.
      p. ; cm. -- (Infectious disease)
  Includes bibliographical references and index.
  ISBN 0-89603-892-0 (alk. paper)
    1. Immunological adjuvants. 2. Vaccines. I. Hackett, Charles J., 1947-. II. Harn, Donald
A. III. Infectious disease (Totowa, N.J.)
  [DNLM: 1. Vaccines--immunology. 2. Adjuvants, Immunologic. QW 805 V1153 2006]
  QR187.3.V32 2006
  615'.372--dc22
                                                                                            2005046100

# Preface

Modern vaccines increasingly rely on administration with additional substances—adjuvants—in order to stimulate effective immune responses. Although the concept of adjuvants has been recognized for at least 80 years, their mechanism of action has been only partially understood, and the pathway to rational design of safe and effective adjuvants has been unclear. There have been few principles to guide adjuvant research, relying largely on increasing antigen uptake by macrophages and based heavily on empirical approaches.

However, by the mid- to late-1990s, major advances in basic immunology forever changed the strategies for discovery, design, development, and use of vaccine adjuvants. First, discoveries of receptors that rapidly signal the presence of invading viruses, bacteria, and parasites pinpointed the innate immune system as the target of adjuvants. That is, adjuvants serve an absolutely essential function for the development of B- and T-cell responses by triggering antigen-presenting cells, in particular dendritic cells, to upregulate co-stimulatory molecules, to process and present antigens, migrate to lymph nodes, and secrete cytokines that trigger appropriate Th1 (cell-mediated) or Th2 (antibody-dominated) responses. The concept that adjuvants trigger innate immune receptors that are hard-wired to detect microbial molecules underlies all of the chapters in this volume. Microbial molecules include bacterial cell wall compounds, viral and bacterial nucleic acids, parasite sugars, and proteins and lipoproteins that are generally essential components of pathogens. In addition, there are increasingly refined technologies available to monitor the immune system in response to infection, including "chip" analyses of gene expression, proteomic approaches, and peptide-major histocompatibility complex tetramers to monitor antigen-specific T cells. Together, these advances raised the exciting prospect not only for the development of safer and more effective adjuvants to trigger powerful immune responses, but also to design adjuvants that manipulate the direction of the immune response to yield Th1, Th2, cytotoxic T cell, or combinations of desired responses.

*Vaccine Adjuvants* comprises a highly select group of chapters that detail major research areas in this new era of adjuvant discovery, design, development, and use. Articles include a focus on specific receptor–ligand interactions, including the molecular features needed for a compound to possess adjuvant activity. The critical interface zone between the innate and adaptive immune systems is analyzed to show how adjuvants exert their effects on T- and B-cell activation.

*Vaccine Adjuvants: Immunological and Clinical Principles* also addresses why there is a need for developing a variety of distinct adjuvants. In the future, no single adjuvant will fit all needs. Chapters detail specific properties and uses of such diverse adjuvants as modified bacterial toxins, synthetic mimetics of bacterial cell wall lipids, parasite sugar moieties, plant saponins, microparticles, and CpG-containing nucleic acids. This developing repertoire is contributing toward eventually having an arsenal of such compounds that can function specifically to direct immunity to Th1 or Th2 responses, that can work optimally in the gut, lung, skin, or other desired route of vaccination, and which potentially may be optimized for distinct age groups or individuals with different needs. For example, as we gain insight into the genetic makeup of different human populations and the genetic influences on immune responses, it may be possible to tailor adjuvants to specific genotypes to yield optimally safe and effective responses. These chapters address key areas that underpin a new era of research that will lead to the rational design of new adjuvants and a new set of principles for their use.

*Charles J. Hackett, PhD*
*Donald A. Harn, Jr., PhD*

# Contents

# Contributors

ANSHU AGRAWAL, PhD • *Department of Pathology, Emory Vaccine Center, Emory University, Atlanta, GA*

SUDHANSHU AGRAWAL, *Department of Pathology, Emory Vaccine Center, Emory University, Atlanta, GA*

SHIZUO AKIRA, MD, PhD • *Department of Host Defense, Research Institute for Medical Diseases, Osaka University and CREST, Osaka, Japan*

IGOR C. ALMEIDA, PhD • *Department of Parasitology, University of São Paulo, São Paulo, Brazil*

CHRISTINE ANDERSON, MS • *BSL-3 Animal and Tissue Culture Core Laboratory, Harvard Medical School, Boston, MA*

GEORGE M. BAHR, FRCPath, PhD • *Department of Microbiology and Immunology, Balamand University Medical School, Koura, Lebanon*

JORY BALDRIDGE, PhD • *Discovery Research, Corixa Corporation, Hamilton, MT*

BRUCE BEUTLER, MD • *Department of Immunology, Scripps Research Institute, La Jolla, CA*

MARCO A. CAMPOS, PhD • *Department of Biochemistry and Immunology, Federal University of Minas Gerais, Centro de Pesquisas Rene Rachou, Fundacao Oswaldo Cruz, Belo Horizonte, Brazil*

MICHELE CARTER, MS • *Department of Immunology and Infectious Diseases, Harvard School of Public Health, Boston, MA*

CHRISTOPHER CLUFF, DVM, PhD • *Discovery Research, Corixa Corporation, Hamilton, MT*

JULIE M. CURTSINGER, PhD • *Department of Laboratory Medicine and Pathology, Center for Immunology, University of Minnesota, Minneapolis, MN*

AKRAM DA'DARA, PhD • *Department of Immunology and Infectious Diseases, Harvard School of Public Health, Boston, MA*

HEATHER L. DAVIS, PhD • *Pharmacology Research and Development, Coley Pharmaceutical Group, Ottawa, Ontario, Canada*

KIMBERLY DENIS-MIZE, PhD • *Research and Development, Chiron Corporation, Emeryville, CA*

STEPHANIE DILLON, PhD • *Department of Pathology, Emory Vaccine Center, Emory University, Atlanta, GA*

JOHN J. DONNELLY, PhD • *Research and Development, Chiron Corporation, Emeryville, CA*

*ix*

RICARDO T. GAZZINELLI, DVM, PhD • *Department of Biochemistry and Immunology, Federal University of Minas Gerais, Centro de Pesquisas Rene Rachou, Fundacao Oswaldo Cruz, Belo Horizonte, Brazil*

CHARLES J. HACKETT, PhD • *Division of Allergy, Immunology, and Transplantation, National Institute of Allergy and Infectious Diseases, NIH, Bethesda, MD*

DONALD A. HARN, JR., PhD • *Department of Immunology and Infectious Diseases, Harvard School of Public Health, Boston, MA*

HIROAKI HEMMI, PhD • *Department of Host Defense, Research Institute for Medical Diseases, Osaka University and CREST, Osaka, Japan*

ROBERT HERSHBERG, MD, PhD • *Dendreon Corporation, Seattle, WA*

MARC JENKINS, PhD • *Department of Microbiology, Center for Immunology, University of Minnesota, Minneapolis, MN*

DAVID JOHNSON, PhD • *Discovery Research, Corixa Corporation, Hamilton, MT*

CHARLOTTE READ KENSIL, PhD • *Research and Development, Antigenics Inc., Lexington, MA*

ARTHUR M. KRIEG, MD • *Research and Development, Coley Pharmaceutical Group, Wellesley, MA*

ED C. LAVELLE, PhD • *Adjuvant Research Group, School of Biochemistry and Immunology, Trinity College Dublin, Dublin, Ireland*

OLIVE LEAVY, BSc • *Immune Regulation Research Group, Department of Biochemistry, Trinity.College Dublin, Dublin, Ireland*

GUI LIU, PhD • *Research and Development, Antigenics Inc., Lexington, MA*

MATTHEW F. MESCHER, PhD • *Center for Immunology, Department of Laboratory Medicine and Pathology, University of Minnesota, Minneapolis, MN*

KINGSTON H. G. MILLS, PhD • *Immune Regulation Research Group, School of Biochemistry and Immunology, Trinity College Dublin, Dublin, Ireland*

KENT MYERS, PhD • *Process Sciences, Corixa Corporation, Hamilton, MT*

GIOACCHINO NATOLI, MD • *Institute for Research in Biomedicine, Bellinzona, Switzerland*

KAZUNORI NISHIZAKI, PhD • *Department of Otolaryngology, Okayama University Medical School, Okayama, Japan*

DEREK T. O'HAGAN, PhD • *Research and Development, Chiron Corporation, Emeryville, CA*

MITSUHIRO OKANO, MD, PhD • *Department of Otolaryngology, Okayama University Medical School, Okayama, Japan*

DAVID PERSING, MD, PhD • *Discovery Research, Corixa Corporation, Seattle, WA*

BALI PULENDRAN, PhD • *Department of Pathology, Emory Vaccine Center, Emory University, Atlanta, GA*

CATHERINE ROPERT, PhD • *Centro de Pesquisas Rene Rachou, Fundacao Oswaldo Cruz, Belo Horizonte, Brazil*

JOÃO S. SILVA, PhD • *Department of Biochemistry and Immunology, University of São Paulo, São Paulo, Brazil*

MANMOHAN SINGH, PhD • *Research and Development, Chiron Corporation, Emeryville, CA*

JAMES STOREY, MS • *Research and Development, Antigenics Inc., Lexington, MA*

KIYOSHI TAKEDA, MD • *Department of Host Defense, Research Institute for Medical Diseases, Osaka University and CREST, Osaka, Japan*

PAUL THOMAS, PhD • *Department of Immunology, St. Jude's Children's Research Hospital, Memphis, TN*

JEFFREY B. ULMER, PhD • *Research and Development, Chiron Corporation, Emeryville, CA*

# 1

# Microbial Pathogenesis and the Discovery of Toll-Like Receptor Function

## Bruce Beutler

## INTRODUCTION

It has been known for many decades that specific molecules of microbial origin (lipoteichoic acid, bacterial lipopeptides, lipopolysaccharide [LPS], deoxyribonucleic acid [DNA], ribonucleic acid [RNA], and other conserved molecules) are endowed with adjuvant activity. The receptors for these molecules are the mammalian Toll-like receptors (TLRs), and they provide awareness of microbial infection. Not surprisingly, they also mediate adjuvant effects. However, they are not required for adaptive immune responses *per se*. TLRs lead to upregulation of costimulatory molecules by eliciting the production of type I interferon. However, entirely different pathways are responsible for many adaptive immune phenomena, including allograft rejection, which occurs in the absence of any TLR-mediated sensing activity.

## THE PRIMARY OBSERVATIONS: MICROBIAL TOXICITY AND THE STORY OF "ENDOTOXIN"

In most instances, scientific discovery occurs as the result of sustained inquiry into a puzzle of nature. The discovery of the TLRs and their function provides one such example: one that addressed a long-standing puzzle. The question that was asked was nothing less than "Why are microbes injurious to the host?" Or it might have been phrased, "How does the host 'know' when an infection is present?" Both questions have been answered in large part by the determination of just what the TLRs are and what they do.

The "toxicity" of localized infections has been recognized since antiquity. The search for precisely what is toxic within a nidus of infection began even before the link between microbes and infection was established, with the investigations of von Haller *(1,2)*, Magendie *(1,2)*, von Bergmann *(3,4)*, and Panum

From: *Vaccine Adjuvants: Immunological and Clinical Principles*
Edited by: C. J. Hackett and D. A. Harn, Jr. © Humana Press Inc., Totowa, NJ

*(5)*. At the dawn of the postmicrobial era, a directed search for microbial toxins began in earnest. One of the first toxins to be identified was "endotoxin," so called by Pfeiffer, a student of Koch, to distinguish it from the proteinaceous "exotoxins" already identified by Brieger *(1,2)*. Pfeiffer isolated endotoxin from cultures of *Vibrio cholerae*, using its lethal effect in animals as an assay endpoint *(6)*. Although he began his work with Gram-negative organisms, he later mistakenly attributed the lethal effect of preparations from Gram-positive organisms to the same heat-stable, alcohol-insoluble substance. This, in light of modern understanding, was perhaps the first indication that numerous molecules of microbial origin elicit similar signals, by activating structurally related (but distinct) host receptors.

Because endotoxin was abundant, stable, and able to mimic much of what an authentic infection could do to the host (i.e., provoke fever, shock, and tissue damage), it assumed central importance in the quest to understand how microbes harm the host. The molecular structure of endotoxin was probed by many workers, and by the 1940s, its LPS composition was apparent *(7,8)*. It was later deduced that the toxic center of an LPS molecule was the lipid moiety *(9)*, and the exact structure of the "lipid" component of an LPS molecule was first solved in the 1970s *(10)*.

Pfeiffer himself never appreciated that endotoxin (LPS) was the principal glycolipid constituent of the outer leaflet of the outer membrane of the Gram-negative bacterium, and it fell to later workers (Osborn and Nikaido, among others) to establish this *(11–15)*. In parallel with these analyses of endotoxin, the physicochemical structure of other microbial components proceeded, and it was apparent that numerous components of the microbe were endowed with toxicity, usually of a lesser magnitude than that of LPS.

### The Indirect Character of LPS Toxicity, and the Existence of a Solitary LPS Receptor

For many years, it was believed that LPS was capable of directly causing injury to mammalian cells and tissues. As an amphiphilic molecule, it might, perhaps, damage cell membranes, or exert an ionophoric effect. However, several facts spoke in favor of a specific mechanism of LPS toxicity. First, LPS toxicity was very much species-dependent, and for the most part, limited to mammals (an effect in avian embryos notwithstanding) *(16)*. Second, LPS was not toxic to most mammalian cells in culture. Third, it was capable of causing fever when administered in minute doses. For this last reason, a "endogenous pyrogen" was believed to exist *(17,18)*, and by extension, all of the effects of LPS might prove to be mediated by endogenous factors.

A compelling discovery, made in 1965, gave support to the hypothesis that LPS must exert its effects through a single biochemical pathway, and presumably, through a single receptor. Mice of the C3H/HeJ substrain were observed to be highly resistant to the lethal effect of LPS *(19)*, and ultimately, it became clear that they were refractory to all biological effects of LPS. Later, animals of a second, unrelated strain (C57BL/10ScCr) were shown to be resistant to LPS as well *(20)*. In each instance, it was believed that a spontaneous mutation had become fixed in the colony, rendering homozygous animals resistant to LPS. Codominant, monogenic heritability of the C3H/HeJ lesion was demonstrated in 1974 *(21)*, and not long thereafter, the defect in the C57BL/10ScCr strain was shown to be allelic *(22)*. Hence, a single gene—widely believed to encode the LPS receptor—was required for LPS sensing. This gene was named *Lps*, and the defective allele of C3H/HeJ mice was termed $Lps^d$. The fact that a single mutation could abolish LPS sensing proved that the pathway for LPS detection was unduplicated.

Formal proof that host cells mediate endotoxicity came with the demonstration that isolated macrophages produced an endogenous toxin capable of mediating at least some of the effects of LPS *(23)*, and later, with the demonstration that host hematopoietic precursors determine susceptibility to the lethal effect of LPS *(24)*. Chimeras produced by irradiating C3H/HeJ were LPS-sensitive if reconstituted with hematopoietic progenitors of C3H/HeN—but not C3H/HeJ —donors.

*Cytokines (Including Tumor Necrosis Factor)*
*Mediate the Lethal Effect of LPS: A Convenient Endpoint to Follow*

Macrophages, which had been shown to mediate the lethal effect of LPS, had been known first and foremost for their innate immune function: they acted to engulf and destroy invasive pathogens. They were also known for their ability to present antigen to cells of the adaptive immune system. Now, it seemed, they produced factors that could mediate the lethal effect of LPS. How did they do so?

In 1985, mouse tumor necrosis factor (TNF) was purified to homogeneity for the first time, and was shown to be made in great abundance in response to LPS, constituting approx 2% of the secretory product of LPS activated macrophages *(25,26)*. Immediately thereafter, it was shown that TNF was toxic to mice, provoking shock and organ injury much as LPS did, the role of TNF in endotoxicity was carefully investigated. Passive immunization against TNF offered mice significant protection against subsequent challenge with LPS *(27)*. Later, knockout of the p55 TNF receptor was shown to offer protection as well *(28)*. Moreover, mice lacking the interferon-α/β receptor were resistant to LPS *(29)*, perhaps reflecting the synergy that exists between TNF and interferon-α/β in numerous biological systems. In no case was resistance as profound as that observed in C3H/HeJ mice. However, the case for cytokine mediation of endotoxic shock became firmly established.

Once viewed as an antineoplastic mediator, TNF was exposed as both "toxin and tonic." Named for its ability to kill tumors through a necrotizing process in vivo *(30)*, and fortuitously able to lyse tumor cells in vitro as well *(31)*, TNF suddenly assumed central importance as an endpoint in the quest to understand LPS signaling. It was known to be more than a marker of endotoxin action: it was verifiably important to the syndrome that ensued. Moreover, it was easy to measure, and produced only under conditions that approximated host infection. It emerged that the TNF promoter had NF-κB motifs that were required for transcriptional activation *(32)*. Additionally, a translational activation step, induced by LPS, was required to produce TNF protein *(33)*.

THE BENEFITS OF LPS SENSING

Although exotoxins are most probably "intended" as weapons, endotoxin has a clear structural role, and it is toxic because the host has evolved to recognize it as such. As previously mentioned, extreme endotoxicity is a "mammals only" phenomenon among vertebrates. Why has the host chosen to react so violently to a nearly ubiquitous microbial molecule? Evidently, LPS recognition permits mammals to deal more effectively with a small inoculum of many Gram-negative organisms, and a small inoculum is the type that they are most likely to encounter.

In 1980, it was shown that *Salmonella typhimurium* is far more lethal when administered intraperitoneally to C3H/HeJ mice (which cannot sense LPS) than to C3H/HeN mice (which are closely related, but LPS-responsive) *(34,35)*. Subsequently, it was shown that the same type of immunodeficiency applies in *Escherichia coli* urinary tract infections *(36)*, as in *Francisella tularensis* infection *(37)*. In several other Gram-negative infections as well, LPS sensing is beneficial, *provided that the inoculum is a small one.* It must be assumed that a very strong, localized response to LPS favors the systemic immune response. Probably both innate and adaptive immunity are abetted. On the other hand, a large inoculum of Gram-negative organisms may kill the host as the result of overwhelming cytokine release. But perhaps evolution has calculated that the host would die under such circumstances in any case.

## The Mystery of the Initial Events in LPS Signal Transduction

By 1990, it was known that LPS was conveyed to the macrophage plasma membrane by interaction with a plasma protein, termed lipopolysaccharide-binding protein *(38–40)*. Lipopolysaccharide-binding protein acted to transfer LPS to a surface receptor, identified as CD14 *(41)*. A glycosylphosphoinositol-tethered protein without any cytoplasmic domain, CD14 could not be expected to elicit a transmembrane signal. Moreover, CD14 was not encoded by the *Lps*, which was known to reside on mouse chromosome 4 *(42,43)*. Hence, a "missing" subunit of the receptor must exist: a subunit that might well be encoded by *Lps*.

Once a signal was initiated, it was shown that tyrosine kinase(s) *(44–48)*, and serine/threonine kinase(s) (including p38 MAP kinase, the classical MAP kinases, and the Jun kinases) were activated *(49–51)*. It was also clear that NF-κB translocation to the nucleus was required for TNF production to occur *(32)*. Gradually, attention began to focus on the receptor, which must initiate all of these events. Attempts to find additional components of the LPS receptor through pure biochemical or expression cloning methods were uniformly unsuccessful, and positional cloning methods were therefore used in many labs, with the goal of elucidating the *Lps* locus.

## Identification of TLR4 As Lps

In 1998, the *Lps* locus was identified by positional cloning *(52,53)*. In C3H/HeJ mice, the TLR4 cytoplasmic domain was modified by a point mutation (P712H) *(53)*, although in C57BL/10ScCr mice, the locus was removed within the confines of a 74 kb deletion *(53,54)*. In the control substrains C3H/HeN and C57BL/10ScSn, the gene was normal. Hence, integrity of the TLR4 protein was required for LPS sensing. Concurrent claims that TLR2 was the LPS receptor *(55,56)*, based on the overexpression of TLR2 in HEK 293 cells, were apparent artifacts, because TLR4 mutations caused total insensitivity to LPS (hence, there could not be two independent pathways for LPS signaling) and because gene targeting studies did not sustain claims regarding TLR2 *(57)*. Hence, TLR4 emerged as the only known membrane-spanning component of the LPS receptor.

TLR4 undergoes direct contact with LPS to transduce the LPS signal. This is evident from genetic complementation studies *(58,59)* and from direct binding studies *(60)*, both of which indicate that LPS actually "touches" the TLR4 protein. Complementation analyses have also indicated that MD-2, a small protein shown to be tightly associated with the TLR4 ectodomain *(61)*, has direct contact with LPS *(62)*. Hence, a complex that is at least trimolecular (involving CD14, MD-2, and TLR4) engages LPS and evokes a signal. Of course, there may be other components of the receptor complex yet unknown.

## The Function of Other TLRs

At the time the function of TLR4 was deduced by positional cloning, a total of five TLR paralogs were known to be expressed in mammals *(63–66)*. In due course, all of the other paralogs were cloned *(67–70)*, and a total of nine mouse TLRs and ten human TLRs are now known to exist. The fact that numerous molecules of microbial origin elicit responses similar to those provoked by LPS suggested that the other TLRs might serve to transduce other microbial signals. Evidence in support of this idea came first from the work of Underhill and associates *(71)*, who suggested that TLR2 might actually transduce signals from Gram-positive organisms. Later, Akira and colleagues showed that lipopeptides and peptidoglycan from Gram-positive bacteria signaled via TLR2 *(57)*. TLR5

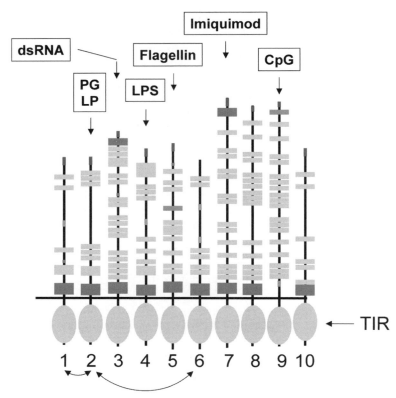

**Fig. 1.** Schematic illustration of the 10 human TLRs, highlighting domain structure (determined by simple modular architecture tool [SMART]). A conservative portrayal of specificity is shown. Although many molecules have been said to be recognized by TLR4, most claims are incorrect, and at present, the only molecule of microbial origin that clearly triggers a response is LPS. Peptidoglycan (PG) and lipopeptides (LP) trigger responses via TLR2. Imiquimod is a synthetic antiviral compound known to activate via TLR7. TLRs 1 and 2, and 6 and 2, engage in heterodimer formation. TIR motif constitutes the bulk of the cytoplasmic domain of each of the TLRs.

was implicated in the transduction of the flagellin signal *(72)*; TLR9 in transduction of the signals evoked by unmethylated DNA *(73)* (characteristic of all microbes). TLR3 appeared to carry the poly I:C response *(74)*. TLRs 1 and 6 are believed to form heteromeric complexes with TLR2, and to guide the specificity of the response *(75,76)*. Other TLRs (7, 8, and 10) have no known microbial specificity, although TLR7 responds to the drug imiquimod *(77)*, which exerts an antiviral effect (Fig. 1).

In *Drosophila*, eight of the nine Toll paralogs have no immune function, but rather, are concerned with development *(78)*. It is likely that these developmental functions are an evolutionary novelty. The TLRs have no developmental role in mammals, and the "Toll/Interleukin-1/Resistance" (TIR) domain, characteristic of all TLR family members and proteins of the IL-1 and IL-18 receptor family, has been primarily defensive in most of the proteins in which it has been observed, throughout the phylogenetic tree *(68)*.

## *DROSOPHILA* TOLL
## AND THE DISCOVERY OF MAMMALIAN TLRs

Toll, the namesake of the TLR paralogs in mammals, was first encountered in *Drosophila*. A forward genetic screen aimed at elucidating the signaling pathways that control dorsal–ventral polarity during embryogenesis revealed Toll as a maternal effect gene, required for the development of ventral structures *(79)*. A total of 12 genes were identified in the "Dorsal group" by mutagenesis. In addition to Toll, a protein ligand (Spätzle) and signaling proteins (Tube, Pelle, Cactus, and Dorsal) were required for ventralization.

The similarity between *Drosophila* Toll and a mammalian protein (the first of the two IL-1 receptor chains to be cloned) was noted in 1991 *(80)*. In subsequent years, the similarity between the IL-1 and Toll signaling pathways became obvious, as IRAK was a homolog of Pelle, and NF-κB and Dorsal were both Rel family members. It initially seemed curious that a fundamentally developmental pathway in the fruit fly would have homology to a fundamentally immune pathway in mammals.

The first mammalian TLR to be cloned, now known as TLR1 and originally dubbed "TIL," was identified in an EST library in 1994 *(63)*, as were all of the TLRs 1 through 6. Mapped to human chromosome 4 in 1996 *(64)*, TLR1 was believed to have a potential developmental role, in that it was even more similar to Toll than the IL-1 receptor. Contemporaneously, other Tolls were identified in Drosophila, all having effects on the development of the fly. Among these were such proteins as 18-wheeler (now Toll-2) and Tehao (now Toll-5). In all, nine members of the family are known to exist.

In 1996, Lemaitre and colleagues demonstrated that mutations of Toll or any of its downstream signaling proteins caused hyper-susceptibility to fungal infection *(81)*. Their work was predicated on the observation that Drosomycin, an antifungal protein produced by the fat body of the fly, was induced at the transcriptional level, and the Drosomycin gene had NF-κB-like motifs in its promoter: a fact previously observed in the case of the attacin and diptericin promoters as well *(82,83)*. The immune Toll signaling pathway makes use of a transcription factor distinct from that in the developmental pathway. Rutschmann and associates showed that Dif (one of three Rel-like proteins in the fly), rather than Dorsal (the developmental paralog) is required for immune defense *(84)*. In addition to providing antifungal immunity, the Toll pathway serves the recognition of Gram-positive bacteria *(85)*. A second pathway (Imd) serves recognition of Gram-negative bacteria and is ancestrally related to the TNF signaling pathway (Fig. 2).

The defensive function of Toll in adult flies prompted immediate speculation that TLRs might have defensive functions in mammals. Medzhitov and colleagues observed that "h-Toll" (later TLR4) could activate NF-κB when ligated on the surface of mammalian cells, and although unaware that TLR4 was the LPS receptor, suggested that the receptor might activate adaptive immunity *(65)*.

The precise role of TLR4 was revealed by the positional cloning of *Lps (52, 53)*. Later, gene knockout work confirmed the conclusions of the positional cloning *(86)*. Because LPS activates the expression of many proteins that are required for an adaptive immune response, and because LPS has a very well-studied adjuvant effect *(see* next section), TLR4 may be said to activate adaptive immunity. Of course, it also has many other effects besides this.

## THE ADJUVANT EFFECT OF LPS
## AND OTHER MICROBIAL MOLECULES

Within the maelstrom of an infectious lesion, a large number of cytokines are produced, serving to recruit inflammatory cells (including neutrophils, monocytes, and lymphocytes) from the blood, and to abet both the innate and the adaptive immune response to the infectious agent. In 1924, Lewis and Loomis first noted that tuberculous guinea pigs produced more antibodies than non-tuberculous guinea pigs when injected with antigens in aqueous solution (a phenomenon that they termed "allergic irritability" *(87,88)*. In 1928, Dienes and Schoenheit reported that a far more vigorous immune response developed when antigens were injected directly into tuberculous foci than into naïve animals. They subsequently found that heat-killed mycobacteria were capable of exerting the same effect, and that marked hypersensitivity to a protein antigen would follow secondary challenge *(89)*. In 1935, Hanks confirmed the observations of Dienes and Schoenheit, and reported that the "delayed" type of skin reaction to an antigen could not be transferred with serum, noting as well that the site and time of antigen injection could be separated from the site and time of mycobacterial infection, yet a strong adjuvant effect would be observed in

---

**Fig. 2.** *(Opposite page)* The LPS–TNF axis is mirrored in two microbial response pathways of the fly. The Toll pathway shows ancestral homology to the TLR signaling pathways; the *Imd* pathway shows ancestral homology to the two TNF signaling pathway, mediated by two distinct receptors. In mammals, TNF represents a "bridge" joining two key biochemical cascades, required for many aspects of inflammation. The existence of Lps2, a mammalian protein required for the "MyD88 independent" pathway of LPS signaling, has been disclosed by forward genetic methods.

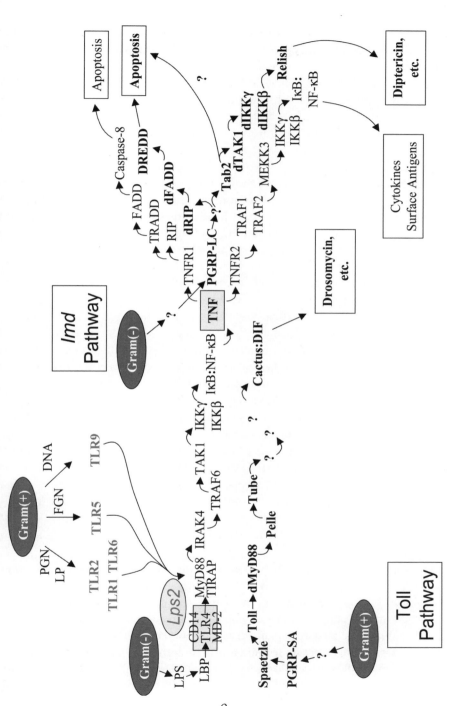

9

any case *(90)*: a finding that might now be explained on the basis of the fact that antibody production occurs within regional lymph nodes that drain the lesion. Freund *(91)* further noted that in tuberculous guinea pigs, endotoxin (culture filtrates of *Balantidium coli, Bacillus typhosus,* or meningococci) would elicit a Shwartzman-type reaction at the site of a tuberculin injection. Hence, the realization that factors of microbial origin could augment the immune response, and the fundamental similarity of many different microbial agents in their effects on the host, crystallized long ago.

Freund *(92–95)* and Saenz *(96–98)* experimented with the use of hydrophobic vehicles for admixture of tubercle bacilli with protein antigens. These analyses culminated with the 1942 demonstration, by Freund and McDermott, that proteins dissolved in a suspension of heat-killed mycobacteria and aqueous emulsion containing paraffin oil and a lanolin-like miscible fat markedly augmented the response to a protein antigen *(99)* (*see* ref. *100* for a detailed history).

Then as now, it was implicitly obvious that a vigorous immune response would result from the presentation of a given antigen in the context of an agent with which the immune system evolved to cope: that is, a bacterium. The prolonged and effective immune response to proteinaceous antigens of *Mycobacterium tuberculosis* (combined together as "tuberculin") was but one manifestation of this propensity. The addition of a hydrophobic medium clearly enhanced the adjuvant effect of killed mycobacteria, but the mycobacteria themselves were critically important to the preparation. Not only mycobacteria, but also other bacteria were found to have adjuvant effects *(101,102)*, and by the 1960s, LPS had been extensively examined for its adjuvant properties *(103,104)* and its ability to promote resistance to bacterial infection *(105)*. The fact that a relatively pure molecular species from microbes could elicit an adjuvant effect was intriguing, for the same reason that all of the effects of LPS were intriguing: a relatively uniform molecular species was exerting a strong biological response, yet the receptor remained undiscovered. Moreover, it was quite clear that only one receptor was involved. Skidmore and associates had shown by 1976 that the *Lps$^d$* mutation abolished the adjuvant effect of LPS *(106–111)*, in addition to its mitogenic effect.

Where practical application of the adjuvant effect of LPS was concerned, however, a problem was immediately apparent, in that LPS was too toxic for general use. It was determined in the 1960s that the toxic moiety of LPS was lipid A; the glycosyl moiety was essentially bereft of biological activity in general *(10)*. When the structure of lipid A was solved *(10)*, various partial structures and derivatives were examined in the thought that a less toxic alternative might be found. Monophosphoryl lipid A was extensively investigated for this purpose with some experimental successes *(112–116)*, as were LPS derivatives made by succinylating or phthalylinating the parent molecule *(117)*.

At the same time, other components of bacteria were implicated in the effect of Freund's adjuvant. Notably, bacterial nucleic acids *(118–122)* and "cord factor" (trehalose dimycolate) *(123,124)* were each found to promote the immune response to protein antigens. So, too, were polyA:U and peptidoglycan *(125–129)*. It is likely that other bacterial components are also important to the overall effect.

The fact that all of the adjuvant effects of bacteria seem to be mediated by TLRs is unsurprising seen in the context of the larger fact that these receptors recognize the presence of an infection in the first place. How, then, do they mediate the adjuvant effect of an infectious agent and the other effects (i.e., shock, fever, and systemic production of cytokines)? Several molecular events are undoubtedly important, although some may be seen as "markers" as much as they may be responsible for the final effect that is observed.

Production of TNF results from LPS activation of mononuclear cells, and this was taken as the most important endpoint to follow in the search for the LPS receptor, because TNF mediates the lethal effect of LPS, at least in large part *(27)*. TNF stimulates upregulation of both class I *(130)* and class II *(131)* major histocompatibility complex (MHC) antigens, which are required for antigen presentation wherever it may occur. The costimulatory B7.1 and B7.2 antigens are also upregulated by LPS *(132,133)*. LPS stimulates the production of both class I and class II interferons and IL-12. Interferon-γ and IL-12 direct Th0 lymphoid cells to differentiate toward the Th1 line. Whether directly or reflexively, LPS also induces the production of IL-4 and IL-10, which directs Th0 lymphoid cells to differentiate toward the Th2 line. LPS stimulates IL-1 production, which in turn stimulates T cells to make IL-2, an autocrine growth factor.

Hence, the adjuvant effects of LPS result from a very complex set of events that entail both the production of cytokines (which may act at short range or at a distance) and surface molecules. Most of the primary effects of LPS undoubtedly involve macrophages and dendritic cells, which are more sensitive to LPS than any other cells in the body. There is not yet good evidence of specificity, in the sense that some of these cells are responsive whereas others are not. However, the possibility exists, and with it, there is some hope that "subclasses" of antigen-presenting cells might exist—or might be fashioned—to shape the adaptive immune response that follows antigen presentation.

## EVOLUTION OF THE TLRs AMONG THE *VERTEBRATA*

Most (but not all) vertebrates exhibit adaptive immunity, although no invertebrates do. *Drosophila* have served as a superb model system in which to investigate innate immunity partly because of their advantages as a genetic system, and partly because they have nothing but innate immunity with which to defend themselves. Interestingly, Drosophila have nine Toll paralogs. But among them, only Toll-1 has an immune function *(78)*. Toll-9 of *Drosophila* is structurally similar to the 10 mammalian TLRs; TLRs 1 through 8 are far more different *(68)*. This suggests that the common ancestor of *Drosophila* and humans had at least two Toll-like proteins, descendants of which have remained intact to the present day.

In humans there are 10 TLR paralogs; in mice there are nine (TLR10 has become a degenerate pseudogene in mice). TLRs 1 and 6 diverged most recently: approx 130 MYA, according to the best estimates *(134)*. TLR10 diverged from the ancestor of these two paralogs approx 310 MYA. And TLR4 diverged approx 500 MYA. Yet orthologs of TLR4 have not been found in other vertebrate classes although their presence might be expected, and among vertebrates, only mammals are highly sensitive to LPS. In birds *(135)* and in reptiles *(136)*, two paralogs with strong similarity to TLR2 are known. In each instance, the duplication event that led to the TLR2-like paralogs was very recent: far more recent than the divergence of birds and reptiles themselves.

It would appear that some vertebrates depend far more heavily on TLRs than others do, and in mammals, expansion has exceeded that which has occurred in other vertebrate lines. However, so far as we know, only among invertebrates have the TLRs been diverted to serve developmental tasks. The specificities that TLRs serve have also probably varied with time. Witness the fact that LPS sensing is chiefly important among mammals. TLR4 has been retained to detect LPS in mammals.

## SIGNAL TRANSDUCTION FROM THE TLRs

In all instances, TLRs are endowed with TIR motifs, that are also observed in the IL-1 and IL-18 receptors, and in the antimicrobial resistance proteins of plants. This fact may be offered as evidence that the defensive role of the TLRs was ancestral, although the developmental function observed in *Drosophila* Tolls is more recent. The TIR domain is designed for heterotypic interaction with MyD88, a transducer of signals from all of the TLRs, except TLR3. MyD88, in turn, signals via death domain interactions to activate IRAK4 *(137)*, which interacts with TRAF-6. By an unclear mechanism, this leads to the activation of TAK-1, which phosphorylates IκB kinase, leading to NF-κB translocation to the nucleus, and transcriptional activation of genes concerned with the immune response. In the case of TLR4, a second TIR-bearing transducer (MAL, or TIRAP) is also activated *(138,139)*, and contributes to signaling as well (Fig. 2).

Though solidly based on gene knockout studies, this scheme must be viewed as minimalist, in the sense that many other proteins are known to be involved in LPS signaling, yet lack any clear connection to the receptor. Moreover, there is no satisfactory explanation for the differences in signals that emanate from different TLRs, such as TLR2 and TLR4 *(140,141)*. It is, therefore, probable that at least one (and perhaps several) other transducers engage the receptors themselves. As discussed below, a combination of forward and reverse genetic techniques have been used to identify these receptors.

## The IL-1 and IL-18 Signaling Axes

Both IL-1 and IL-18 are induced by LPS, and both cytokines signal via TIR-domain-bearing receptors. IL-1 and IL-18 receptors do not have leucine-rich repeats in their ectodomains; rather they are based on the immunoglobulin repeat fold. Although *Drosophila* had the opportunity to develop receptors of this form, there is no evidence of invertebrate repeats of this form. The IL-1 and IL-18 axes are fundamentally adaptive immune systems, and appear to have been diverging since the early days of vertebrate evolution. Each receptor signals in lymphoid cells, and each may be viewed as part of an amplification loop. The ST2 and SIGIRR receptors are of the same type, but their functions are less well understood.

## The TNF Signaling Pathway: Mammals and Drosophila

Although *Drosophila* have no TNF gene and no TNF receptor, they do have a signaling pathway that is remarkably similar to the TNF signaling pathway (Fig. 2). This is the *Imd* (immunodeficiency) pathway, which serves the detection of Gram-negative bacteria, and depends on a receptor that is a member of the peptidoglycan receptor protein family *(142)*. Perhaps through the assistance of a coreceptor yet to be identified, the *Imd* pathway is activated, involving signals that traverse RIP, FADD, and DREDD (equivalents of which are found in the TNFRI pathway) and Tab2, TAK1, IKKβ, and IKKγ (some representatives of which exist in the TNFR2 pathway). Hence, it may be inferred that the last common ancestor of *Drosophila* and mammals had an ancestral pathway, although it may only be guessed what receptor(s) this pathway might have served.

It will be recalled that in *Drosophila*, both the Toll signaling pathway (which serves the detection of Gram-positive bacteria and fungi) and the *Imd* pathway are required for effective antimicrobial defense. The situation in mammals is somewhat different, in that the two pathways persist, but are linked in tandem through the interposition of the cytokine TNF, which does not exist in flies (Fig. 2). The TLR4 signaling pathway, and indeed, all of the TLR pathways (as all of the pathways activate TNF synthesis) can be viewed as upstream executors of the TNF signaling pathway.

## LPS Tolerance

An important issue in LPS signaling concerns the downregulation that occurs once TLR4 has been activated. Known as LPS tolerance, this downregulation entails feedback inhibition may occur at many points in the signaling pathway,

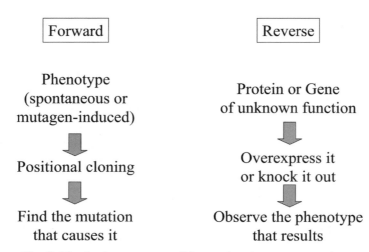

**Fig. 3.** The basic processes of forward and reverse genetics.

upstream of cytokine production and perhaps downstream as well. Hence, a primary challenge with LPS renders an animal refractory to further stimulation, at least for a time. This may be of importance both in the sense that a localized exposure to LPS is less likely to cause overwhelming sepsis, and in the sense that unfettered response to LPS might provoke an excessive adaptive immune response. It remains to be seen whether specific genetic lesions affect LPS tolerance, and if so, whether pharmacological approaches to LPS tolerance might be made, either with the intention of augmenting or blocking it.

It may also be noted that TNF tolerance occurs, and in the context of the tandem arrangement of LPS and TNF signaling pathways, this may be viewed as an added level of protection. In fact, TNF overproduction (when it occurs, for reasons unknown), can clearly cause autoimmune and/or inflammatory diseases such as Crohn's disease *(143)* and rheumatoid arthritis *(144)*. Both respond very well to TNF blockade.

## GENETICS, FORWARD GENETICS, AND THE UNFINISHED SEARCH FOR COMPONENTS OF THE LPS SIGNALING PATHWAY

"Forward genetics" (once merely known as "genetics") is a process by which genes are identified through analysis of phenotype. Reverse genetic methods begin with sequences of unknown function and work toward the definition of a phenotype (Fig. 3). The discovery of the LPS receptor-signaling subunit TLR4 was a forward genetic endeavor. TLR4 *(Lps)* was cloned by phenotype alone. The "core" elements of the TLR signal transduction pathways were subsequently deciphered by intuition and by reverse genetic methods. For example, the fact that MAL/TIRAP and MyD88 were both cytoplasmic proteins with TIR domains made it reasonable to believe that each might serve a transducing function. Such a function was established for MyD88 with respect to the IL-1 and IL-18 receptors early on *(145)*, before the ligands of the TLRs were known, and then generalized to encompass them. The connection between IRAK (later IRAK4) and MyD88 seemed logical, based on the fact that IRAK is activated by IL-1, and on the fact that IRAK and MyD88 have death domains.

The premiere tool of reverse genetics is gene targeting, and the limitations of gene targeting are imposed by two factors. First, extraneous phenotypic changes (foremost lethality) may obfuscate the phenomenon that is sought (in the present instance, TLR signals). Second, in the absence of an hypothetical framework or outright "clue," it is not easy to know what to target. Forward genetic methods (Fig. 2) can overcome both of these limitations, although they have distinct limitations of their own. Random mutagenesis creates alleles that are viable and discrete in their phenotypic effects, and the approach is an unbiased one: it will ultimately result in the discovery of all genes required to support a given biological phenomenon, provided that it is pursued with relentlessness and vigor.

As recently reported *(146)*, novel mutations induced by *N*-ethyl-*N*-nitrosourea are capable of blocking LPS signaling, at least in large part. Because screens have not yet approached saturation of the genome, it is anticipated that many new genes encoding proteins required for LPS signaling may yet be found. These may potentially include novel components of the LPS receptor and signaling proteins that contribute to the activation of numerous proteins activated by LPS. The same sort of screens may disclose proteins that contribute to adjuvant effects wrought by TNF and other molecules. As such, it might ultimately be possible to separate some of the "toxic" effects of these inducers from the beneficial effect of adjuvanticity. Forward genetic methods have disclosed two new adapter proteins, TRIF and TRAM. TRIF was originally designated as Lps2, so named because a mutation at this locus closely mimicked the classic LPS mutation. TRIF is required for all TLR3 signals and about half of TLR4 signals, including the adjuvant effect of LPS.

## CONCLUSIONS AND FUTURE DIRECTIONS

From the foregoing discussion, it should be evident that the unity of the receptors that sense microbes and those that contribute to adjuvant effect was entirely predictable, and in fact, was a basic tenet in the microbial pathogenesis field for many decades. The problem of finding these receptors—in the event, the Toll-like receptors—was solved by concerted inquiry into the LPS receptor, long a "holy grail" in microbial pathogenesis circles because LPS so faithfully mimicked the effects of an authentic infection. However, the identification of the TLRs is only a starting point. It has become abundantly clear that these proteins serve as essential "gateways" to cell activation, but signal by way of a complex network of intracellular molecules, and not all of these have been identified. As all signaling pathways ramify, it may be possible to contemplate blocking the LPS signal entirely or partially, as suits the circumstance. The same applies to all signals of microbial origin. One might therefore envision a situation in which adjuvants no longer provoke the untoward responses that they do at present. However, it might be pointed there is no assurance that such an outcome can be achieved. The history of attempts to split the "good" effects of infection from the "bad" effects is a long one. It began in the time of William Coley *(147–151)*, who noted the tumorolytic properties of bacterial products, and attempts to dissociate the toxicity of an infection from this beneficial side effect. The purification of TNF, the endogenous mediator of Coley's toxins, did not alleviate the problem of toxicity. Time will tell whether an analogous distinction between the desired and the undesirable can be achieved at the level of the TLRs or beyond.

## REFERENCES

1. Westphal O, Westphal U, Sommer T. The history of pyrogen research. In: Schlessinger D, ed. Microbiology-1977. Washingtion, DC: American Society of Microbiology, 1977, pp. 221–238.
2. Rietschel ET, Westphal O. Endotoxin: historical perspectives. In: Brade H, Opal SM, Vogel SN, Morrison DC, eds. Endotoxin in Health and Disease. Basel: Marcel Dekker, Inc., 1999, pp. 1–30.
3. Von Bergmann E. Schwefelsaures Sepsin. Centralbl Med Wissensch 1868;32: 497–498.
4. Von Bergmann E. Zur Lehre von der putriden Intoxikation. Dtsch Z Chir 1872; 1:373–398.
5. Parnas J. Peter Ludwig Panum: great Danish pathologist and discoverer of endotoxin. Dan Med Bull 1976;23:143–146.
6. Pfeiffer R. Untersuchungen über das Choleragift. Z Hygiene 1892;11:393–412.
7. Shear MJ, Andervont HB. Chemical treatment of tumors. III. Separation of hemorrhage-producing fraction of B. coli filtrate. Proc Soc Exp Biol Med 1936;34: 323–325.
8. Hartwell JL, Shear MJ, Adams JR Jr. Chemical treatment of tumors. VII. Nature of the hemorrhage-producing fraction from Serratia marcescens (Bacillus prodigiosus) culture filtrate. J Natl Canc Inst 1943;4:107–122.
9. Kasai N. Chemical studies on the lipid component of endotoxin, with special emphasis on its relation to biological activities. Ann NY Acad Sci 1966;133:486–507.
10. Luderitz O, Galanos C, Lehmann V, et al. Lipid A: chemical structure and biological activity. J Infect Dis 1973;128:29.
11. Osborn MJ, Rick PD, Lehmann V, Rupprecht E, Singh M. Structure and biogenesis of the cell envelope of gram-negative bacteria. Ann NY Acad Sci 1974; 235: 52–65.

12. Osborn MJ. Studies on gram-negative cell wall .1. Evidence for role of 2-keto-deoxyoctonate in lipopolysaccharide of Salmonella Typhimurium. Proc Natl Acad Sci USA 1963;50:499.
13. Nikaido H. Galactose-sensitive mutants of *Salmonella* I. Metabolism of galactose. Biochim Biophys Acta 1960;48:460–469.
14. Nikaido H, Naide Y, Makela PH. Biosynthesis of O-antigenic polysaccharides in Salmonella. Ann NY Acad Sci 1966;133:299–314.
15. Nikaido H. Studies on the biosynthesis of cell wall polysaccharide in mutant strains of Salmonella, II. Proc Natl Acad Sci USA 1962;48:1542–1548.
16. Finkelstein RA. Observations on mode of action of endotoxin in chick embryos. Proc Soc Exp Biol Med 1964;115:702–707.
17. Beeson PB. Development of tolerance to typhoid bacterial pyrogen and its abolition by reticulo-endothelial blockade. Proc Soc Exp Biol Med 1947;61:248–250.
18. Beeson RB. Tolerance of bacterial pyrogens. II. Role of the reticulo-endothelial system. J Exp Med 1947;86:39–44.
19. Heppner G, Weiss DW. High susceptibility of strain A mice to endotoxin and endotoxin-red blood cell mixtures. J Bacteriol 1965;90:696–703.
20. Coutinho A, Forni L, Melchers F, Watanabe T. Genetic defect in responsiveness to the B cell mitogen lipopolysaccharide. Eur J Immunol 1977;7:325–328.
21. Watson J, Riblet R. Genetic control of responses to bacterial lipopolysaccharides in mice. I. Evidence for a single gene that influences mitogenic and immuno-genic respones to lipopolysaccharides. J Exp Med 1974;140:1147–1161.
22. Coutinho A, Meo T. Genetic basis for unresponsiveness to lipopolysaccharide in C57BL/10Cr mice. Immunogenetics 1978;7:17–24.
23. Moore RN, Goodrum KJ, Berry LJ. Mediation of an endotoxic effect by macro-phages. J Reticuloendothel Soc 1976;19:187–197.
24. Michalek SM, Moore RN, McGhee JR, Rosenstreich DL, Mergenhagen SE. The primary role of lymphoreticular cells in the mediation of host responses to bacterial endotoxin. J Infec Dis 1980;141:55–63.
25. Beutler B, Mahoney J, Le Trang N, Pekala P, Cerami A. Purification of cachectin, a lipoprotein lipase-suppressing hormone secreted by endotoxin-induced RAW 264.7 cells. J Exp Med 1985;161:984–995.
26. Beutler B, Greenwald D, Hulmes JD, et al. Identity of tumour necrosis factor and the macrophage-secreted factor cachectin. Nature 1985;316:552–554.
27. Beutler B, Milsark IW, Cerami A. Passive immunization against cachectin/tumor necrosis factor (TNF) protects mice from the lethal effect of endotoxin. Science 1985;229:869–871.
28. Pfeffer K, Matsuyama T, Kündig TM, et al. Mice deficient for the 55 kd tumor necrosis factor receptor are resistant to endotoxic shock, yet succumb to L. mono-cytogenes infection. Cell 1993;73:457–467.
29. Car BD, Eng VM, Schnyder B, et al. Interferon gamma receptor deficient mice are resistant to endotoxic shock. J Exp Med 1994;179:1437–1444.
30. Carswell EA, Old LJ, Kassel RL, Green S, Fiore N, Williamson B. An endotoxin-induced serum factor that causes necrosis of tumors. Proc Natl Acad Sci USA 1975; 72:3666–3670.
31. Helson L, Green S, Carswell E, Old LJ. Effect of tumour necrosis factor on cultured human melanoma cells. Nature 1975;258:731–732.

32. Shakhov AN, Collart MA, Vassalli P, Nedospasov SA, Jongeneel CV. kappaB-type enhancers are involved in lipopolysaccharide-mediated transcriptional activation of the tumor necrosis factor $\alpha$ gene in primary macrophages. J Exp Med 1990;171:35–47.
33. Han J, Thompson P, Beutler B. Dexamethasone and pentoxifylline inhibit endotoxin-induced cachectin/TNF synthesis at separate points in the signalling pathway. J Exp Med 1990;172:391–394.
34. O'Brien AD, Rosenstreich DL, Scher I, Campbell GH, MacDermott RP, Formal SB. Genetic control of susceptibility to Salmonella typhimurium in mice: role of the LPS gene. J Immunol 1980;124:20–24.
35. Rosenstreich DL, Weinblatt AC, O'Brien AD. Genetic control of resistance to infection in mice. CRC Crit Rev Immunol 1982;3:263–330.
36. Hagberg L, Hull R, Hull S, McGhee JR, Michalek SM, Svanborg Eden C. Difference in susceptibility to gram-negative urinary tract infection between C3H/HeJ and C3H/HeN mice. Infect Immun 1984;46:839–844.
37. Macela A, Stulik J, Hernychova L, Kroca M, Krocova Z, Kovarova H. The immune response against *Francisella tularensis* live vaccine strain in Lps[n] and Lps[d] mice. FEMS Immunol Med Microbiol 1996;13:235–238.
38. Tobias PS, Soldau K, Ulevitch RJ. Isolation of a lipopolysaccharide-binding acute phase reactant from rabbit serum. J Exp Med 1986;164:777–793.
39. Tobias PS, Soldau K, Ulevitch RJ. Identification of a lipid A binding site in the acute phase reactant lipopolycaccharide binding protein. J Biol Chem 1989;264:10867–10871.
40. Schumann RR, Leong SR, Flaggs GW, et al. Structure and function of lipopolysaccharide binding protein. Science 1990;249:1429–1431.
41. Wright SD, Ramos RA, Tobias PS, Ulevitch RJ, Mathison JC. CD14, a receptor for complexes of lipopolysaccharide LPS and LPS binding protein. Science 1990;249:1431–1433.
42. Watson J, Riblet R, Taylor BA. The response of recombinant inbred strains of mice to bacterial lipopolysaccharides. J Immunol 1977;118:2088–2093.
43. Watson J, Kelly K, Largen M, Taylor BA. The genetic mapping of a defective LPS response gene in C3H/HeJ mice. J Immunol 1978;120:422–424.
44. Weinstein SL, Gold MR, DeFranco AL. Bacterial lipopolysaccharide stimulates protein tyrosine phosphorylation in macrophages. Proc Natl Acad Sci USA 1991;88:4148–4152.
45. Dearden-Badet MT, Revillard JP. Requirement for tyrosine phosphorylation in lipopolysaccharide-induced murine B-cell proliferation. Immunol 1993;80:658–660.
46. Dong Z, Qi X, Xie K, Fidler IJ. Protein tyrosine kinase inhibitors decrease induction of nitric oxide synthase activity in lipopolysaccharide-responsive and lipopolysaccharide-nonresponsive murine macrophages. J Immunol 1993;151:2717–2724.
47. Geng Y, Zhang B, Lotz M. Protein tyrosine kinase activation is required for lipopolysaccharide induction of cytokines in human blood monocytes. J Immunol 1993;151:6692–7000.
48. Han J, Lee J-D, Tobias PS, Ulevitch RJ. Endotoxin induces rapid protein tyrosine phosphorylation in 70Z/3 cells expressing CD14. J Biol Chem 1993;268:25009–25014.

49. Han J, Lee JD, Bibbs L, Ulevitch RJ. A MAP kinase targeted by endotoxin and hyperosmolarity in mammalian cells. Science 1994;265:808–811.
50. Reimann T, Büscher D, Hipskind RA, Krautwald S, Lohmann-Matthes M-L, Baccarini M. Lipopolysaccharide induces activation of the Raf-1/MAP kinase pathway: a putative role for Raf-1 in the induction of the IL-1β and the TNF-α genes. J Immunol 1994;153:5740–5749.
51. Geppert TD, Whitehurst CE, Thompson P, Beutler B. LPS signals activation of TNF biosynthesis through the RAS/RAF-1/MEK/MAPK pathway. Mol Med 1994; 1:93–103.
52. Poltorak A, Smirnova I, He XL, et al. Genetic and physical mapping of the *Lps* locus-identification of the toll-4 receptor as a candidate gene in the critical region. Blood Cells Molecules & Diseases 1998;24:340–355.
53. Poltorak A, He X, Smirnova I, et al. Defective LPS signaling in C3H/HeJ and C57BL/10ScCr mice: mutations in *Tlr4* gene. Science 1998;282:2085–2088.
54. Poltorak A, Smirnova I, Clisch R, Beutler B. Limits of a deletion spanning *Tlr4* in C57BL/10ScCr mice. J Endotoxin Res 2000;6:51–56.
55. Yang R-B, Mark MR, Gray A, et al. Toll-like receptor-2 mediates lipopolysaccharide-induced cellular signalling. Nature 1998;395:284–288.
56. Kirschning CJ, Wesche H, Merrill AT, Rothe M. Human toll-like receptor 2 confers responsiveness to bacterial lipopolysaccharide. J Exp Med 1998;188:2091–2097.
57. Takeuchi O, Hoshino K, Kawai T, et al. Differential roles of TLR2 and TLR4 in recognition of Gram-negative and Gram-positive bacterial cell wall components. Immunity 1999;11:443–451.
58. Poltorak A, Ricciardi-Castagnoli P, Citterio A, Beutler B. Physical contact between LPS and Tlr4 revealed by genetic complementation. Proc Natl Acad Sci USA 2000; 97:2163–2167.
59. Lien E, Means TK, Heine H, et al. Toll-like receptor 4 imparts ligand-specific recognition of bacterial lipopolysaccharide. J Clin Invest 2000;105:497–504.
60. da Silva CJ, Soldau K, Christen U, Tobias PS, Ulevitch RJ. Lipopolysaccharide is in close proximity to each of the proteins in its membrane receptor complex: transfer from CD14 to TLR4 and MD-2. J Biol Chem 2001;276:21129–21135.
61. Shimazu R, Akashi S, Ogata H, et al. MD-2, a molecule that confers lipopolysaccharide responsiveness on Toll-like receptor. J Exper Med 1999;189:1777–1782.
62. Akashi S, Nagai Y, Ogata H, et al. Human MD-2 confers on mouse Toll-like receptor 4 species-specific lipopolysaccharide recognition. Int Immunol 2001;13:1595–1599.
63. Nomura N, Miyajima N, Sazuka T, et al. Prediction of the coding sequences of unidentified human genes. I. The coding sequences of 40 new genes KIAA0001-KIAA0040 deduced by analysis of randomly sampled cDNA clones from human immature myeloid cell line KG-1. DNA Res 1994;1:27–35.
64. Taguchi T, Mitcham JL, Dower SK, Sims JE, Testa JR. Chromosomal localization of TIL, a gene encoding a protein related to the Drosophila transmembrane receptor Toll, to human chromosome 4p14. Genom 1996;32:486–488.
65. Medzhitov R, Preston-Hurlburt P, Janeway CA, Jr. A human homologue of the Drosophila Toll protein signals activation of adaptive immunity. Nature 1997;388: 394–397.

66. Rock FL, Hardiman G, Timans JC, Kastelein RA, Bazan JF. A family of human receptors structurally related to Drosophila Toll. Proc Natl Acad Sci USA 1998; 95:588–593.
67. Takeuchi O, Kawai T, Sanjo H, et al. TLR6: a novel member of an expanding Toll-like receptor family. Gene 1999;231:59–65.
68. Du X, Poltorak A, Wei Y, Beutler B. Three novel mammalian toll-like receptors: gene structure, expression, and evolution. Eur Cytokine Netw 2000;11:362–371.
69. Chuang TH, Ulevitch RJ. Cloning and characterization of a sub-family of human toll-like receptors: hTLR7, hTLR8 and hTLR9. Eur Cytokine Netw 2000;11:372–378.
70. Chuang T, Ulevitch RJ. Identification of hTLR10: a novel human Toll-like receptor preferentially expressed in immune cells. Biochim Biophys Acta 2001;1518: 157–161.
71. Underhill DM, Ozinsky A, Hajjar AM, et al. The Toll-like receptor 2 is recruited to macrophage phagosomes and discriminates between pathogens. Nature 1999; 401:811–815.
72. Hayashi F, Smith KD, Ozinsky A, et al. The innate immune response to bacterial flagellin is mediated by Toll- like receptor 5. Nature 2001;410:1099–1103.
73. Hemmi H, Takeuchi O, Kawai T, et al. A Toll-like receptor recognizes bacterial DNA. Nature 2000;408:740–745.
74. Alexopoulou L, Holt AC, Medzhitov R, Flavell RA. Recognition of double-stranded RNA and activation of NF-kappaB by Toll-like receptor 3. Nature 2001; 413:732–738.
75. Takeuchi O, Sato S, Horiuchi T, et al. Cutting edge: role of Toll-like receptor 1 in mediating immune response to microbial lipoproteins. J Immunol 2002;169: 10–14.
76. Takeuchi O, Kawai T, Muhlradt PF, et al. Discrimination of bacterial lipoproteins by Toll-like receptor 6. Int Immunol 2001;13:933–940.
77. Hemmi H, Kaisho T, Takeuchi O, et al. Small anti-viral compounds activate immune cells via the TLR7 MyD88-dependent signaling pathway. Nat Immunol 2002;3:196–200.
78. Tauszig S, Jouanguy E, Hoffmann JA, Imler JL. Toll-related receptors and the control of antimicrobial peptide expression in Drosophila. Proc Natl Acad Sci USA 2000;97:10520–10525.
79. Belvin MP, Anderson KV. A conserved signaling pathway: the Drosophila toll-dorsal pathway. Annu Rev Cell Dev Biol 1996;12:393–416.
80. Gay NJ, Keith FJ. Drosophila Toll and IL-1 receptor. Nature 1991;351:355–356.
81. Lemaitre B, Nicolas E, Michaut L, Reichhart JM, Hoffmann JA. The dorsoventral regulatory gene cassette spatzle/Toll/cactus controls the potent antifungal response in Drosophila adults. Cell 1996;86:973–983.
82. Sun SC, Lindstrom I, Lee JY, Faye I. Structure and expression of the attacin genes in Hyalophora cecropia. Eur J Biochem 1991;196:247–254.
83. Reichhart JM, Meister M, Dimarcq JL, et al. Insect immunity: developmental and inducible activity of the Drosophila diptericin promoter. EMBO J 1992;11: 1469–1477.

84. Rutschmann S, Jung AC, Hetru C, Reichhart JM, Hoffmann JA, Ferrandon D. The Rel protein DIF mediates the antifungal but not the antibacterial host defense in Drosophila. Immunity 2000;12:569–580.
85. Rutschmann S, Kilinc A, Ferrandon D. Cutting edge: the toll pathway is required for resistance to gram-positive bacterial infections in Drosophila. J Immunol 2002; 168:1542–1546.
86. Hoshino K, Takeuchi O, Kawai T, et al. Cutting edge: Toll-like receptor 4 (TLR4)-deficient mice are hyporesponsive to lipopolysaccharide: Evidence for TLR4 as the Lps gene product. J Immunol 1999;162:3749–3752.
87. Lewis PA, Loomis D. The formation of anti-sheep hemolytic amboceptor in the normal and tuberculous guinea pig. J Exp Med 1924;40:503.
88. Lewis PA, Loomis D. II. Anaphylaxis in the guinea pig as affected by the inheritance. J Exp Med 1925;41:327–335.
89. Dienes L, Schoenheit EW. The reproduction of tuberculin hypersensitiveness in guinea pigs with various protein substances. Am Rev Tub 1929;20:92–105.
90. Hanks JH. The mechanism of tuberculin hypersensitiveness. J Immunol 1935;28: 107–121.
91. Freund J. Hemorrhages in tuberculous guinea pigs at the site of injection or irritants following intravascular injections of injurious substances (Shwartzman phenomenon). J Exp Med 1934;60:669–685.
92. Freund J, Casals J, Hosmer E. Sensitization and antibody formation after injection of tubercle bacilli and paraffin oil. SEBM 1937;37:509–513.
93. Casals J, Freund J. Sensitization and antibody formation in monkeys injected with tubercle bacilli in paraffin oil. JIM 1939;36:399–404.
94. Freund J, Casals-Ariet J, Genghof D. The synergistic effect of paraffin-oil combined with heat-killed tubercle bacilli. JIM 1940;37:67–79.
95. Freund J, Gottschalk R. Standardization of tuberculin with the aid of guinea pigs sensitized by killed tuberculosis bacilli in liquid petroleum. Arch Pathol 1942;34: 73–74.
96. Saenz A. Acriossement de l'etat allergique et titragede la sensibilite tuberculinique conferes au cobaye par l'innoculation sous-cutane des bacilles tuberculex morts enrobes dans l'huile de vaseline. CR 1935;120:1050–1053.
97. Saenz A. Retard de dispersion des germes de surinfection chez les cobayes pares avec des bacilles tuberculex morts enrobes dans l'huile de vaseline. CR 1937;124: 1161–1164.
98. Saenz A. Vaccination du cobaye contre la tuberculose avec des bacilles morts enrobes dans l'huile de vaseline. CR 1937;125:495–498.
99. Freund J, McDermott K. Sensitization to horse serum by means of adjuvants. SEBM 1942;49:548–553.
100. Rasmussen N. Freund's adjuvant and the realization of questions in postwar immunology. Hist Stud Phys Biol Sci 1993;23:337–366.
101. Pieroni RE, Levine L. Adjuvant principle of pertussis vaccine in the mouse. Nature 1966;211:1419–1420.
102. Uchitel IY, Khasman EL. Mechanism of adjuvant action of nonspecific stimulators of antibody formation. Fed Proc Transl Suppl 1965;24:500–506.

103. Grinstein S, Kierszenbaum F, Ferraresi RW. The adjuvant action of Escherichia coli lipopolysaccharide and of its lipid fraction on antibody production. Rev Immunol Ther Antimicrob 1966;30:141–149.
104. Neter E. Endotoxins and the immune response. Curr Top Microbiol Immunol 1969; 47:82–124.
105. Berger FM. The effect of endotoxin on resistance to infection and disease. Adv Pharmacol 1967;5:19–46.
106. Skidmore BJ, Chiller JM, Weigle WO. Immunologic properties of bacterial lipopolysaccharide LPS. IV. Cellular basis of the unresponsiveness of C3H/HeJ mouse spleen cells to LPS-induced mitogenesis. J Immunol 1977;118:274–281.
107. Skidmore BJ, Chiller JM, Weigle WO, Riblet R, Watson J. Immunologic properties of bacterial lipopolysaccharide LPS. III. Genetic linkage between the in vitro mitogenic and in vivo adjuvant properties of LPS. J Exp Med 1976;143:143–150.
108. Skidmore BJ, Morrison DC, Chiller JM, Weigle WO. Immunologic properties of bacterial lipopolysaccharide LPS. II. The unresponsiveness of C3H/HeJ mouse spleen cells to LPS-induced mitogenesis is dependent on the method used to extract LPS. J Exp Med 1975;142:1488–1508.
109. Skidmore BJ, Chiller JM, Morrison DC, Weigle WO. Immunologic properties of bacterial lipopolysaccharide (LPS): correlation between the mitogenic, adjuvant, and immunogenic activities. J Immunol 1975;114:770–775.
110. Weigle WO, Skidmore BJ. Mechanism of activation and tolerance induction in b lymphocytes. Transplant Rev 1975;23:250–257.
111. Chiller JM, Skidmore BJ, Morrison DC, Weigle WO. Relationship of the structure of bacterial lipopolysaccharides to its function in mitogenesis and adjuvanticity. Proc Natl Acad Sci USA 1973;70:2129–2133.
112. Ribi E, Cantrell JL, Takayama K, Qureshi N, Peterson J, Ribi HO. Lipid A and immunotherapy. Rev Infect Dis 1984;6:567–572.
113. Chase JJ, Kubey W, Dulek MH, Holmes CJ, Salit MG, Pearson FC, III et al. Effect of monophosphoryl lipid A on host resistance to bacterial infection. Infect Immun 1986;53:711–712.
114. Masihi KN, Lange W, Brehmer W, Ribi E. Immunobiological activities of nontoxic lipid A: enhancement of nonspecific resistance in combination with trehalose dimycolate against viral infection and adjuvant effects. Int J Immunopharmacol 1986;8:339–345.
115. Tomai MA, Solem LE, Johnson AG, Ribi E. The adjuvant properties of a nontoxic monophosphoryl lipid A in hyporesponsive and aging mice. J Biol Response Mod 1987;6:99–107.
116. Baker PJ, Hiernaux JR, Fauntleroy MB, Stashak PW, Prescott B, Cantrell JL, et al. Ability of monophosphoryl lipid A to augment the antibody response of young mice. Infect Immun 1988;56:3064–3066.
117. Schenck JR, Hargie MP, Brown MS, Ebert DS, Yoo AL, McIntire FC. The enhancement of antibody formation by Escherichia coli lipopolysaccharide and detoxified derivatives. J Immunol 1969;102:1411–1422.
118. Youmans GP, Youmans AS. Allergenicity of mycobacterial ribosomal and ribonucleic acid preparations in mice and guinea pigs. J Bacteriol 1969;97:134–139.
119. Youmans AS, Youmans GP. Factors affecting immunogenic activity of mycobacterial ribosomal and ribonucleic acid preparations. J Bacteriol 1969;99:42–50.

120. Casavant CH, Youmans GP. The induction of delayed hypersensitivity in guinea pigs to poly U and poly A:U. J Immunol 1975;114:1506–1509.
121. Casavant CH, Youmans GP. The adjuvant activity of mycobacterial RNA preparations and synthetic polynucleotides for induction of delayed hypersensitivity to purified protein derivative in guinea pigs. J Immunol 1975;114:1014–1022.
122. Bultmann B, Finger H, Heymer B, Schachenmayr W, Hof H, Haferkamp O. Adjuvancy of streptococcal nucleic acids. Z Immunitatsforsch Exp Klin Immunol 1975;148:425–430.
123. Saito R, Tanaka A, Sugiyama K, Azuma I, Yamamura Y. Adjuvant effect of cord factor, a mycobacterial lipid. Infect Immun 1976;13:776–781.
124. Ribi E, Milner KC, Granger DL, et al. Immunotherapy with nonviable microbial components. Ann NY Acad Sci 1976;277:228–238.
125. Schmidtke JR, Johnson AG. Regulation of the immune system by synthetic polynucleotides. I. Characteristics of adjuvant action on antibody synthesis. J Immunol 1971;106:1191–1200.
126. Nauciel C, Fleck J, Martin JP, Mock M, Nguyen-Huy H. Adjuvant activity of bacterial peptidoglycans on the production of delayed hypersensitivity and on antibody response. Eur J Immunol 1974;4:352–356.
127. Migliore-Samour D, Bouchaudon J, Floc'h F, et al. A short lipopeptide, representative of a new family of immunological adjuvants devoid of sugar. Life Sci 1980;26:883–888.
128. Werner GH, Maral R, Floch F, Migliore-Samour D, Jolles P. Adjuvant and immuno-stimulating activities of water-soluble substances extracted from Mycobacterium tuberculosis var. hominis. Biomedicine 1975;22:440–452.
129. Jolles P, Migliore-Samour D, Maral R, Floc'h F, Werner GH. Low molecular weight water-soluble peptidoglycans as adjuvants and immunostimulants. Z Immunitatsforsch Exp Klin Immunol 1975;149:331–340.
130. Collins T, Lapierre LA, Fiers W, Strominger JL, Pober JS. Recombinant human tumor necrosis factor increases mRNA levels and surface expression of HLA-A,B antigens in vascular endothelial cells and dermal fibroblasts in vitro. Proc Natl Acad Sci USA 1986;83:446–450.
131. Chang RJ, Lee SH. Effects of interferon-gamma and tumor necrosis factor-alpha on the expression of an Ia antigen on a murine macrophage cell line. J Immunol 1986;137:2853–2856.
132. Hathcock KS, Laszlo G, Pucillo C, Linsley P, Hodes RJ. Comparative analysis of B7-1 and B7-2 costimulatory ligands: expression and function. J Exp Med 1994;180:631–640.
133. Southern SO, Swain SL, Dutton RW. Induction of the H-2 D antigen during B cell activation. J Immunol 1989;142:336–342.
134. Rehli M, Poltorak A, Schwarzfischer L, Krause SW, Andreesen R, Beutler B. PU.1 and interferon consensus sequence binding protein ICSBP regulate the myeloid expression of the human Toll-like receptor 4 gene. J Biol Chem 2000;275:9773–9781.
135. Fukui A, Inoue N, Matsumoto M, et al. Molecular cloning and functional characterization of chicken toll-like receptors: a single chicken toll covers multiple molecular patterns. J Biol Chem 2001;276:47143–47144.

136. Kanthack AA. Acute leucocytosis produced by bacterial products. The British Med J 1892;1301–1303.
137. Suzuki N, Suzuki S, Duncan GS, et al. Severe impairment of interleukin-1 and Toll-like receptor signalling in mice lacking IRAK-4. Nature 2002;416:750–756.
138. Fitzgerald KA, Palsson-McDermott EM, Bowie AG, et al. Mal MyD88-adapter-like is required for Toll-like receptor-4 signal transduction. Nature 2001;413: 78–83.
139. Horng T, Barton GM, Medzhitov R. TIRAP: an adapter molecule in the Toll signaling pathway. Nat Immunol 2001;2:835–841.
140. Toshchakov V, Jones BW, Perera PY, et al. TLR4, but not TLR2, mediates IFN-beta-induced STAT1alpha/beta-dependent gene expression in macrophages. Nat Immunol 2002;3:392–398.
141. Doyle S, Vaidya S, O'Connell R, et al. IRF3 Mediates a TLR3/TLR4-Specific Antiviral Gene Program. Immunity 2002;17:251.
142. Gottar M, Gobert V, Michel T, et al. The Drosophila immune response against Gram-negative bacteria is mediated by a peptidoglycan recognition protein. Nature 2002;416:640–644.
143. Van Dullemen HM, Van Deventer SJH, Hommes DW, et al. Treatment of Crohn's disease with anti-tumor necrosis factor chimeric monoclonal antibody (cA2). Gastroenterology 1995;109:129–135.
144. Elliott MJ, Maini RN, Feldmann M, et al. Treatment of rheumatoid arthritis with chimeric monoclonal antibodies to tumor necrosis factor a. Arthritis Rheumatol 1993;36:1681–1690.
145. Adachi O, Kawai T, Takeda K, et al. Targeted disruption of the MyD88 gene results in loss of IL-1- and IL-18-mediated function. Immunity 1998;9:143–150.
146. Brieger L, Fraenkel C. I. Untersuchungen uber Bakteriengifte. Berliner Klinische Wochenschrift 1890;11:241–271.
147. Coley WB. The treatment of malignant tumors by repeated inoculations of erysipelas; with a report of ten original cases. Am J Med Sci 1893;105:487–511.
148. Coley WB. Treatment of inoperable malignant tumors with toxins of erysipelas and the Bacillus prodigiosus. Trans Am Surg Assoc 1894;12:183–212.
149. Coley WB. Further observations upon the treatment of malignant tumors with the mixed toxins of erysipelas and Bacillus prodigiosus with a report of 160 cases. Bull Johns Hopkins Hosp 1896; 65:157–162.
150. Coley WB. The therapeutic value of the mixed toxins of the streptococcus of erysipelas in the treatment of inoperable malignant tumors, with a report of 100 cases. Am J Med Sci 1896;112:251–281.
151. Coley WB. Late results of the treatment of inoperable sarcoma by the mixed toxins of erysipelas and Bacillus prodigiosus. Am J Med Sci 1906;131:375–430.

# 2
# Dendritic Cells

## Targets for Immune Modulation by Microbes and Immunologists

### Bali Pulendran, Anshu Agrawal, Stephanie Dillon, and Sudhanshu Agrawal

## INTRODUCTION

Since the original description of Th1 and Th2 T cells by Mosman and Coffman some 15 years ago (1), there has been a profusion of knowledge about the cytokines that influence the type of Th response. Thus, interleukin 4 (IL)-4 is known to induce IL-4 production in T cells; conversely IL-12 and interferon (IFN)γ are known to induce IFNγ production by T cells. However, the original sources of these cytokines in vivo, and the mechanisms that initiate one or another response, are less clear. Recent developments from several labs point to a potential role for dendritic cells (DCs) in orchestrating this decision. Here, we present our current view of DC development in vivo and then review the literature that suggest that distinct DC subsets may direct Th responses differently. These ideas are discussed in the context that the Th polarizing potentials of DC subsets are not fixed, but are rather plastic. Given their pivotal roles in immunity, DCs represent prime targets for immune modulation by both microbes, and immunologists. Some examples of immune modulation by microbes, and prospects for clinical utility are briefly considered.

## THE DC SYSTEM

Since its observation more than 25 years ago as an accessory cell of the immune system (2), the dendritic cell (DC) has assumed center stage as the key initiator of adaptive immunity. DCs are scattered throughout the body, including the various portals of microbe entry, in which they reside in an immature form. Immature DCs are "immunological sensors" alert for potentially dangerous microbes and are capable of decoding and integrating such signals, and then

From: *Vaccine Adjuvants: Immunological and Clinical Principles*
Edited by: C. J. Hackett and D. A. Harn, Jr. © Humana Press Inc., Totowa, NJ

ferrying this information to the T-cell areas of secondary lymphoid organs, in which naïve T cells are. Here, in a mature form they present this information to T lymphocytes, thus initiating an immune response. DCs can also tune the immune response, by modulating either the amplitude, or the type of the response (2–5). We now know that there are several different types of DCs (2–5). Recent evidence suggests that different subpopulations of DCs are capable of inducing distinct types of responses (6–8). However, the function of DCs also appears to be modulated by microbes and the environment (9–11).

## DC SUBSETS

Like lymphocytes, DCs consist of multiple subsets that differ in phenotype, function, and microenvironmental localization (1–5). It is not known whether this heterogeneity reflects distinct lineages or DCs at different stages of maturation, or both.

Mouse DCs that are characterized as "mature" express high levels of the integrin-$\alpha$ CD11c and class II major histocompatibility complex, and the costimulatory molecules CD80 and CD86. In the secondary lymphoid organs of mice, at least four subsets of "mature" DCs have been described: CD8$\alpha^+$ DCs, CD8$\alpha^-$ CD4$^+$ DCs, CD8$\alpha^-$ CD4$^-$ DCs, and Langerhans cell-derived DCs (LCDCs) (1–5). CD8$\alpha^+$ DCs are located in the thymic cortex and T-cell areas of secondary lymphoid organs, although CD8$\alpha^-$ DCs occur in the marginal zones of the spleens, subcapsular sinuses of the lymph nodes, and the subepithelial dome of Peyer's patch (1–5). LCs, which are the precursors of LCDCs are found in the epithelial layers of the skin and mucosa and contain unique structures called Birbeck granules, the development of which is dependent on expression of Langerin (12). As LCs migrate to the T-cell areas of lymph nodes they mature into LCDCs.

More recently, a precursor DC subset with a plasmacytoid morphology, the ability to secrete large amounts of interferon-$\alpha$ in culture, and that can generate mature DCs in culture has been described (13–15). This plasmacytoid precursor DC (pDC) subset is similar to its human counterparts (discussed below), and secrete copious amounts of interferon-$\alpha$ when stimulated with CpG DNA or certain viruses.

Early studies suggested that the CD8$\alpha^+$ DCs can develop from progenitor cell populations, which also yield T, B, and NK cells (16), although whether the same progenitor cell yields DCs and lymphoid cells is not known. However recent evidence suggests that CD8$\alpha^+$ DCs can also develop from a myeloid precursor (4), suggesting that lymphoid and myeloid precursors may have some plasticity in their developmental potentials. More recently, a common precursor population yielding CD8$^+$ and CD8$^-$ murine DCs, but devoid of myeloid or lymphoid differentiation potential has been characterized (17). Given this confusion, the developmental origins of DC subsets is at present a subject of intense debate.

In human skin two subsets of immature DCs are found in distinct microenvironments; LCs in the epidermis and interstitial DCs in the dermis *(2–5)*. These two subsets also appear in culture of hematopoietic progenitor cells, driven by granulocyte-macrophage colony-stimulating factor (GM-CSF) plus tumor necrosis factor-$\alpha$. In the blood, two subsets of DCs are identified, the CD11c$^+$ subset, which differentiates into mature CD11c$^+$ DCs in response to inflammatory stimuli, and the CD11c$^-$ subset, which differentiates into pDCs in response to IL-3 *(18)*. pDCs appear to be the principal source of type-1 interferons in response to viruses *(19,20)*. Cytokines such as Flt3-Ligand, GM-CSF, and granulocyte colony-stimulating factor, induce the development of these DC subsets in vivo *(21–26)*.

## DCs AND IMMUNOLOGICAL TOLERANCE

### Central Tolerance

The idea that certain DC subsets could induce self-tolerance was experimentally addressed by showing that splenic DCs, if introduced into fetal thymic organ culture, could induce negative selection *(27)*. However, subsequent studies have shown that other antigen-presenting cells such as thymic cortical epithelial cells can also induce thymic negative selection *(27)*. This suggests that the developmental stage of the thymocyte is crucial for negative selection, although it does not exclude some unique tolerogenic feature that thymic DCs may have. Indeed the transfer of thymic DCs has been shown to induce tolerance to myelin basic protein and limit experimental allergic encephalomyelitis *(28)*, and the role of thymic DCs in negative selection in vivo, has been confirmed by the targeted expression of class II myosin heavy chain molecules on CD11c$^+$ DCs *(29)*.

### Peripheral Tolerance

The question of whether certain DC subsets can induce self-tolerance in the periphery (or at least downmodulate an ongoing T-cell response) has received much attention recently, and two broad scenarios have been envisioned. One concept is that all DCs have a the capacity to induce either immunity or tolerance, depending on the maturation or activation state of the DCs *(30)*. It was originally proposed that immature DCs *(31,32)*, or those exposed to cytokines such as IL-10, transforming growth factor -$\beta$, or prostaglandin E2 (PGE2), which maintain DCs in an immature state and can induce tolerance *(33–37)*. More recent evidence suggests that tolerance is induced by DCs that are mature but not activated, although immunity is induced by DCs that are fully activated *(38)*.

The second concept is that there is a specialized DC subset dedicated for peripheral tolerance induction. In mice, there is evidence that the CD8$\alpha^+$ DC subset in mice can limit the proliferation of both CD4$^+$ and CD8$^+$ T cells in vitro *(39,40)*. Thus it has been suggested that the CD8$\alpha^+$ DCs play a role in inducing self-tolerance in the periphery *(41)*. Consistent with this notion, one study suggests that in DBA/2 mice, CD8$\alpha^+$ DCs are weaker than the CD8$\alpha^-$ DCs at eliciting DTH responses against a poorly immunogenic tumor peptide *(42)*. In these studies, the CD8$\alpha^-$ DCs were found to inhibit the function of CD8$\alpha^-$ DCs. The relevance of these observations to peripheral tolerance induction in vivo remains to be determined. However, recent studies suggest that steady state targeting of DC antigen receptors with low doses of antigen leads to deletion of corresponding T cells, and unresponsiveness to antigenic challenge with strong adjuvants *(43)*. There is also new evidence that DCs can contribute to the expansion of T cells that regulate or suppress other immune T cells *(44,45)*.

## DCs AND THE CONTROL OF ADAPTIVE IMMUNITY

### DC Subsets

There is evidence that distinct DC subsets can induce different Th responses. In mice, freshly isolated CD8$\alpha^+$ and CD8$\alpha^-$ DCs from spleens *(6–8)* or Peyer's patch *(46)* induce Th1 and Th2 responses, respectively. CD8$\alpha^+$ DCs can be induced to secrete IL-12 *(7,26,47,48)*, which is essential for their Th1 induction *(7)*. IL-10 appears to be important for optimal Th2 induction by CD8$\alpha^-$ DCs *(49)*. Consistent with this differential skewing, cytokines which differentially expand these DC subsets in vivo promote different responses. Thus, GM-CSF, which preferentially expands CD8$\alpha^-$ DCs in mice, elicits Th2 responses, although Flt3-L, which expands both DC subsets, elicits both Th1 and Th2 responses *(6)*. In humans, monocyte-derived CD11c$^+$ DCs and CD11c$^-$ pDCs can induce Th1 and Th2/Th0 responses in vitro, respectively *(8,26)*. However, the extent of polarization by these cells may differ according to their method of isolation and maturation *(20)* or the ratio of dendritic cells to T cells *(50)*. As with mice, IL-12 secretion by CD11c$^+$ DCs seem essential for their Th1 induction *(8)*, but the factors that induce Th2 responses are unknown.

### Microbes

The nature of the microbe also plays an important role in tuning the response, by modulating DC function. For example, viruses stimulate IFN$\alpha$ from the plasmacytoid CD11c$^-$ precursors *(19,20)* and induce their differentiation into DCs that induce IFN$\gamma$- and IL-10-producing T cells *(51)*; however IL-3 induces CD11c$^-$ precursors to differentiate into Th2-inducing DCs *(19,51)*. Different forms of the fungus *Candida albicans* instruct an immature, murine DC cell line to induce either Th1 or Th2 responses *(52)*. As stated above, the immune system can discriminate between different microbes through receptors, such as Toll-like receptors (TLRs). This is reminiscent of the situation in *Drosophila*, in which bacterial and fungal infections signal through distinct TLRs to elicit different classes of antimicrobial peptides *(53–55)*. In mammals too, it is now clear that different microbial stimuli induce qualitatively distinct immune responses. For example, *Escherichia coli* lipopolysaccharide (LPS) induces a Th1 response, but LPS from the oral bacterium *Porphyromonas gingivalis*, which signals through TLR2 *(56)* skews toward a Th2 response *(57)*. Consistent with this, *E. coli* LPS, but not *P. gingivalis* LPS induces IL-12 in the splenic CD8$\alpha^+$ DCs *(57)*. Similar results have been obtained with the synthetic TLR 2 ligand, Pam-3-cys *(58–60)*. Thus, Pam-3-cys, *E. coli* LPS, flagellin, and schistosome egg antigens (SEA) activate human DCs to secrete different cytokine profiles. *E. coli* LPS and flagellin induce IL-12(p70), but Pam-3-cys and SEA do not do so, but can induce the Th2-inducing or regulatory cytokine, IL-10. Although *E. coli* LPS and flagellin induce Th1 responses, Pam-3-cys and SEA favor a Th2 bias *(58)*. In the mouse system, almost identical results are evident; Pam-3-cys induces very little IL-12 (p70) in splenic CD8$\alpha^+$ DCs compared to *E. coli* LPS *(59)*. Consistent with their differential cytokine induction in DCs, Pam-3-cys and *E. coli* LPS induced Th2- and Th1-biased responses, respectively *(58–60)*. These studies are supported by several other reports, which suggest that signaling via TLR2 may result in Th2 or T-regulatory responses *(61–64)*.

## The Microenvironment

Cytokines secreted by activated T cells in the lymph node or in the periphery can also modulate DC function. Thus Th1-inducing DCs, when exposed to IL-10, transforming growth factor-$\beta$, induce Th2-like responses *(33–37)*. Conversely, IFN$\gamma$ can instruct DCs to acquire some Th1-inducing capacity *(11)*. These results are consistent with observations that DCs in distinct microenvironments induce different Th responses. For example, Peyer's patch or respiratory tract DCs prime Th2 responses, although total spleen DCs prime Th1/Th0 responses *(43,65)*.

If one DC subset is capable of generating any type of response, depending on the microbial stimuli, then why evolve so many different subsets with different functions? One solution would be to have functionally different DC subsets capable of recognizing different microbial stimuli, because they express distinct, but overlapping repertoires of TLRs (Fig. 1). Indeed, consistent with this model recent studies suggest that in humans *(66,67)* and in mice (Pulendran, et al., unpublished data) different DC subsets express distinct but overlapping repertoire of TLRs. Thus, at the site of an infection, microbial stimuli 1 and 2 may preferentially activate immature DC1s and DC2s, which express quite different TLRs, and which have some genetic propensity to generate Th1 and Th2 responses respectively (Fig. 1). However, the DCs would have some plasticity in that stimulus 1 may prompt DC2s toward a Th1-inducing mode, and stimu-

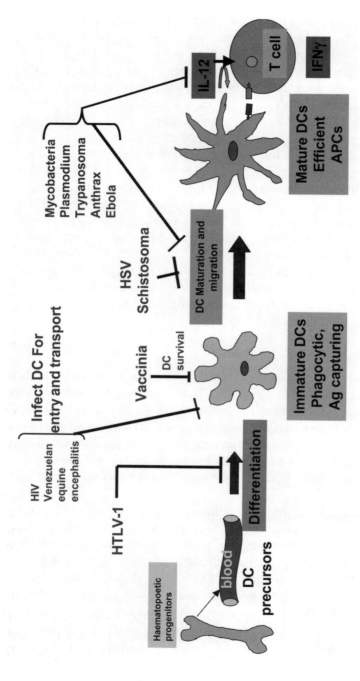

**Fig. 1.** The microbe's box of tricks. Pathogens have evolved several strategies to modulate various aspects of dendritic cell (DC) biology. For example, human immunodeficiency virus and Venezuelan equine encephalitis virus target DCs in the periphery and hitch a ride to the draining lymph nodes; vaccinia virus kills DCs (although the consequences of this for adaptive immunity is debatable); herpes simplex virus, schistosomes, mycobacteria, plasmodium parasites, anthrax, and ebola interfere with DC maturation and migration.

lus 2 may prompt DC1s toward a Th2-inducing mode (Fig. 1). A further level of regulation may occur in the draining lymph node, during the early stages of the response. Th1 and Th2 cytokines made by T cells could suppress DC2s and DC1s respectively, to amplify the response. Thus IL-10 and IFNγ suppress the function of DC1s and DC2s, respectively. However later in the response, Th2 cytokines may enhance the Th1-induction by DCs *(9)*, to prevent a runaway Th2 response. In this model therefore, the immune response is a multiparametric function of the microbe, microbe-recognition receptors, the genetic hardwiring of the DCs, and the environment and cytokines.

## TURNING DOWN THE VOLUME

DCs may also play crucial roles in downregulating the immune responses. For instance, DCs may express molecules that inhibit T-cell expansion. B7 molecules on DCs engage CTLA-4 on activated T cells and inhibit their proliferation, and B7-H1 molecules on antigen-presenting cells engage inducible costimulator receptor on activated T cells and induce IL-10, which dampens T-cell activation *(68)*. In principle, these molecules may be upregulated on the same DCs that initially primed the T cells, or may be constitutively expressed on a specialized subset of DCs dedicated for switching off T cells *(39,40,42)*. Thus these regulatory DCs may capture and present antigens from stimulatory DCs to terminate an ongoing T-cell response. Indeed, as stated above, DCs that capture apoptotic cells do not stimulate T cells efficiently and presentation of antigens from apoptotic cells may result in immunological tolerance *(30,32, 62)*. A discrete population of DCs in the rat Peyer's patch have been shown to transport apoptotic cells from the intestinal epithelium to the lymph nodes, suggesting a possible mechanism through which oral tolerance may occur *(69)*.

## THE MICROBE'S BOX OF TRICKS

Cells that play such crucial roles in the immune response must also be the prime targets of many a conspirator wishing to manipulate the immune system. This appears to be the case with many pathogens, and at least a few immunologists. Pathogens have evolved a remarkably wide array of strategies to subvert DC function, (and adaptive immunity), in almost every conceivable way.

### Trick 1: Impairment of DC Recruitment, Maturation, and Survival

One mechanism of subversion is impairment of DC maturation or survival, as observed with erythrocytes infected with the malaria parasite *Plasmodium falciparum (70)*, or with human T cell leukemia virus 1 (HTLV-1), or with *Trypanoma cruzi (71)*, or with herpes simplex virus *(72)*, or measles virus *(73–75)*, or canarypox or vaccinia viruses, which eventually kill DCs *(76,77)*. Furthermore, poxviruses and herpesviruses encode secreted homologues of chemokine receptors that act as chemokine antagonists to prevent the recruitment of additional DCs to infection sites *(78,79)*, and *Schistosoma mansoni* suppresses Langerhans cell migration from the epidermis via a parasite-derived homologue of PGD2 *(80)*. Our recent work suggests that *Bacillus anthracis* lethal toxin inhibits mitrogen-activated protein kinase signaling in DCs to impair DC function and adaptive immunity *(81)*, and that infection of DCs with Ebola or Lassa viruses results in an inhibition of DC maturation and function *(82)*.

### Trick 2: Highjacking DCs

Pathogens may also highjack DCs to control to immune system. Thus human immunodeficiency virus (HIV)-1 gp-120 uses the "Trojan Horse" strategy by binding to DC-specific adhesion molecule-3-grabbing nonintegrin, a lectin expressed on DCs, facilitating transport of the virus to the lymph nodes, in which it infects CD4$^+$ T cells *(83)*. Interaction of HIV-infected DCs with memory or activated T cells favors HIV replication. Furthermore, Venezuelan equine encephalitis virus targets LCs, which serve as replication sites and transport the virus into the draining lymph node *(84)*.

### Trick 3: Messing With T-Cell Activation

Microbes have devised several ways to impair T-cell activation. As mentioned above, several microbes can inhibit DC maturation, thus preventing efficient T-cell priming. This effect may be because of inhibition of factors contributing to T-cell proliferation and differentiation. Another mechanism of impeding T-cell immunity is via the apoptosis of T cells by virally infected DCs. For instance, measles virus and human cytomegalovirus render DCs cytotoxic through the upregulation of both FasL/CD95L and tumor necrosis factor-related apoptosis-inducing ligand on DCs *(85,86)*. The virus sensitizes the activated T cells, which are otherwise resistant to these molecules. The bacterium *Bordetella pertussis*, which is the causative agent of whooping cough, has crafted a strategy to generate antigen-specific T regulatory cells (Tr cells) to suppress protective Th1 responses *(87)*. During acute infection with *B. pertussis*, Tr cells specific for *B. pertussis* filamentous hemagglutinin (FHA) and pertactin, which are generated at the mucosal surfaces, secrete IL-10 but neither IL-4 nor IFN-, and suppress the Th1 responses against *B. pertussis*, and unrelated pathogens. The generation of Tr cells is mediated by FHA, which inhibits DC IL-12 secretion but promotes their secretion of IL-10.

## THE IMMUNOLOGIST'S QUEST

The microbes offer us valuable lessons in our quest for immune modulation in the clinic. The growing list of strategies used by microbes offer us many insights into the untapped potential that lie within these cells. Already, much progress has been made in eliciting tumor immunity in humans using adoptive therapy of DCs loaded with tumor antigens *(88)*. The ultimate challenge is to design vaccines that induce optimally effective immunities in different clinical settings by modulating DC function in vivo. Microbes have taken evolutionary time scales to learn the art of immune modulation. Immunologists of the 21st century will surely take a much shorter time to master this art!

## ACKNOWLEDGMENTS

Supported by grants from the National Institutes of Health.

## REFERENCES

1. Mosmann TR, Coffman RL. TH1 and TH2 cells: different patterns of lymphokine secretion lead to different functional properties. Annu Rev Immunol 1989;7: 145–173.
2. Steinman RM, Cohn ZA. Identification of a novel cell type in peripheral lymphoid organs of mice. I. Morphology, quantitation, tissue distribution. J Exp Med 1973; 137:1142–1162.
3. Banchereau J, Steinman RM. Dendritic cells and the control of immunity. Nature 1998;392:245–252.
4. Shortman K, Liu Y-J. Mouse and human dendritic cell subtypes. Nature Rev Immunol 2002;2:151–161.
5. Pulendran B, Maraskovsky E, Banchereau J, Maliszewski C. Modulating the immune response with dendritic cells and their growth factors. Trends Immunol 2001; 22:41–47.
6. Pulendran B, Smith JL, Caspary G, et al. Distinct dendritic cell subsets differentially regulate the class of immune response in vivo. Proc Natl Acad Sci USA 1999; 96:1036–1041.
7. Maldonado-Lopez R, De Smedt T, Michel P, et al. CD8alpha+ and CD8alpha– subclasses of dendritic cells direct the development of distinct T helper cells in vivo. J Exp Med 1999;189:587–592.
8. Rissoan MC, Soumelis V, Kadowaki N, et al. Reciprocal control of T helper cell and dendritic cell differentiation [see comments]. Science 1999;283:1183–1186.
9. Pulendran B, Palucka K, Banchereau J. Sensing pathogens and tuning immune responses. Science 2001;293:253–256.
10. Lanzavecchia A, Sallusto F. Regulation of T-cell immunity by dendritic cells. Cell 2001;106:263–266.
11. Kalinski P, Hikens CM, Wierenga EA, Kapsenberg ML. T-cell priming by type-1 and type-2 polarized dendritic cells: the concept of a third signal. Immunol Today 1999;20:561–567.
12. Valladeau J, Ravel O, Dezulter-Dambuyant C, et al. Langerin, a novel C-type lectin specific to Langerhans cells, is an endocytic receptor that induces the formation of Birbeck granules. Immunity 2000;12:71–81.
13. Asselin-Paturel C, Boonstra A, Dalod M, et al. Mouse type I IFN-producing cells are immature APCs with plasmacytoid morphology. Nature Immunol 2001;2: 1144–1150.

14. Nakano H, Yanagita M, Gunn MD. CD11c+ B220+ Gr-1+ cells in mouse lymph nodes and spleen display characteristics of plasmacytoid dendritic cells. J Exp Med 2001;194:1171–1178.
15. Bjorck P. Isolation and characterization of plasmacytoid dendritic cells from Flt3-Ligand and granulocyte-macrophage colony stimulating factor treated mice. Blood 2001;98:3520–3526.
16. Ardavin C, Wu L, Li CL, Shortman K. Thymic dendritic cells and T cells develop simultaneously in the thymus from a common precursor population. Nature 1993; 362:761–763.
17. del Hoyo GM, Martin P, Vargas HH, Ruiz S, Arias CF, Ardavin C. Characterization of a common precursor population for dendritic cells. Nature 2002;415:1043–1047.
18. Grouard G, Rissoan MC, Filgueira L, Durand I, Banchereau J, Liu YJ. The enigmatic plasmacytoid T-cells develop into dendritic cells with interleukin-3 (IL)-3 and CD40-ligand. J Exp Med 1996;184:1101–1111.
19. Siegal FP, Kadowaki N, Shodell M, et al. The nature of the principle type 1 interferon-producing cells in human blood. Science 1999;284:1835–1837.
20. Cella M, Jarrossay D, Facchett F, et al. Plasmacytoid monocytes migrate to inflamed lymph nodes and produce large amounts of type-1 interferon. Nat Med 1999;5:919–923.
21. Maraskovsky E, Brasel K, Teepe M, et al. Dramatic increase in the numbers of functionally mature dendritic cells in Flt3 ligand-treated mice: multiple dendritic cell subpopulations identified. J Exp Med 1996;184:1953–1962.
22. Pulendran B, Lingappa J, Kennedy MK, et al. Developmental pathways of dendritic cells in vivo: distinct function, phenotype, and localization of dendritic cell subsets in FLT3 ligand-treated mice. J Immunol 1997;159:2222–2231.
23. Shurin MR, Pandharipande PP, Zorina TD, et al. FLT3 ligand induces the generation of functionally active dendritic cells in mice. Cell Immunol 1997;179:174–184.
24. Pulendran B, Smith JL, Jenkins M, Schoenborn M, Maroskovsky E, Maliszeski CR. Prevention of peripheral tolerance by a dendritic cell growth factor: flt3 ligand as an adjuvant. J Exp Med 1998;188:2075–2082.
25. Maraskovsky E, Daro E, Roux E, et al. In vivo generation of human dendritic cell subsets by Flt3-Ligand. Blood 2000;96:878–884.
26. Pulendran B, Banchereau J, Burkeholder S, et al. Flt3-ligand and granulocyte colony-stimulating factor mobilize distinct human dendritic cell subsets in vivo. J Immunol 2000;165:566–572.
27. Sprent J, Webb SR. Intrathymic and extrathymic clonal deletion of T cells. Curr Opin Immunol 1995;7:196–205.
28. Khoury SJ, Wu ZY, Zhang HP, et al. Suppression of experimental autoimmune encephalomyelitis by oral administration of myelin basic protein. III. Synergistic effect of lipopolysaccharide. Cell Immunol 1990;131:302–310.
29. Brocker T, Riedinger M, Karjalainen K. Targeted expression of major histocompatibility complex (MHC) class II molecules demonstrates that dendritic cells can induce negative but not positive selection of thymocytes in vivo. J Exp Med 1997; 185:541–550.

30. Steinman RM, Nussenzweig MC. Avoiding horror autotoxicus: the importance of dendritic cells in peripheral T cell tolerance. Proc Natl Acad Sci USA 2002;99: 351–358.
31. Dhodapkar M, Steinman RM, Krasovsky J, Munz C, Bhardwaj N. Antigen-specific inhibition of effector T cell function in humans after injection of immature dendritic cells. J Exp Med 2001;193:233–238.
32. Steinman RM, Turley S, Mellman I, Inaba K. The induction of tolerance by dendritic cells that have captured apoptotic cells. J Exp Med 2000;191:411–416.
33. Caux C, Massacrier C, Vandervliet B, Barthelemy C, Liu YJ, Banchereau J. Interleukin 10 inhibits T cell alloreaction induced by human dendritic cells. Int Immunol 1994;6:1177–1785.
34. Kalinski P, Schuitemaker JH, Hilkens CM, Kapsenberg ML. Prostaglandin E2 induces the final maturation of IL-12-deficient CD1a+CD83+ dendritic cells: the levels of IL-12 are determined during the final dendritic cell maturation and are resistant to further modulation. J Immunol 1998;161:2804–2809.
35. Steinbrink K, Wolfl M, Jonuleit H, Knop J, Enk AH. Induction of tolerance by IL-10-treated dendritic cells. J Immunol 1997;159:4772–4780.
36. Liu L, Rich BE, Inobe J, Chen W, Weiner HL. A potential pathway of Th2 development during primary immune response. IL-10 pretreated dendritic cells can prime naive CD4+ T cells to secrete IL-4. Adv Exp Med Biol 1997;417:375–381.
37. Takeuchi M, Kosiewicz MM, Alard P, Streilein JW. On the mechanisms by which transforming growth factor-beta 2 alters antigen-presenting abilities of macrophages on T cell activation. Eur J Immunol 1997;27:1648–1656.
38. Albert ML, Jegatheesan M, Darnell RB. Dendritic cell maturation is required for cross-tolerization of CD8+ T cells. Nature Immunol 2001;11:1010–1017.
39. Suss G, Shortman K. A subclass of dendritic cells kills CD4 T cells via Fas/Fas-ligand-induced apoptosis. J Exp Med 1996;183:1789–1796.
40. Kronin V, Winkel K, Suss G, et al. A subclass of dendritic cells regulates the response of naive CD8 T cells by limiting their IL-2 production. J Immunol 1996; 157:3819–3827.
41. Smith AL, de St Groth BF. Antigen-pulsed CD8alpha+ dendritic cells generate an immune response after subcutaneous injection without homing to the draining lymph node. J Exp Med 1999;189:593–598.
42. Grohmann U, Bianchi R, Belladonna ML, et al. IL-12 acts selectively on CD8 alpha– dendritic cells to enhance presentation of a tumor peptide in vivo. J Immunol 1999;163:3100–3105.
43. Steinman RM, Hawiger D, Nussenzweig MC. Tolerogenic dendritic cells. Annu Rev Immunol 2003:21:685–711.
44. Heath WR, Carbone FR. 2001. Cross-presentation, dendritic cells, tolerance and immunity. Annu Rev Immunol 2001;19:47–64.
45. Walker LSK, Abbas AK. The enemy within: keeping self-reactive T cells at bay in the periphery. Nat Rev Immunol 2002;2:11–19.
46. Iwasaki A, Kelsall BL. Freshly isolated Peyer's patch, but not spleen, dendritic cells produce interleukin 10 and induce the differentiation of T helper type 2 cells. J Exp Med 1999;190:229–239.

47. Sousa CR, Hieny S, Scharton-Kersten T, et al. In vivo microbial stimulation induces rapid CD40 ligand-independent production of interleukin 12 by dendritic cells and their redistribution to T cell areas. J Exp Med 1997;186:1819–1829.
48. Ohteki T, Fukao T, Suzue K, et al. Interleukin 12-dependent interferon gamma production by CD8 alpha+ lymphoid dendritic cells. J Exp Med 1999;189:1981–1986.
49. Maldanado-Lopez R, Maliszewski C, Urbain J, Moser M. Cytokines regulate the capacity of CD8alpha(+) and CD8alpha(−) dendritic cells to prime Th1/Th2 cells in vitro. J Immunol 2001;167:4345–4350.
50. Tanaka H, Demeure CE, Rubio M, Delespresse G, Sarfati M. Human monocyte-derived dendritic cells induce naive T cell differentiation into T helper cell type 2 (Th2) or Th1/Th2 effectors. Role of stimulator/responder ratio. J Exp Med 2000; 192:405–412.
51. Kadowaki N, Antonenko S, Lau JY, Liu YJ. Natural interferon-alpha/beta producing cells link innate and adaptive immunity. J Exp Med 2000;192:219–226.
52. d'Ostiani CF, Del Sero G, Bacci A, et al. Dendritic cells discriminate between yeasts and hyphae of the fungus Candida albicans. Implications for initiation of T helper immunity in vitro and in vivo. J Exp Med 2000;191:1661–1674.
53. Tzou P, De Gregorio E, Lemaitre B. How Drosophila combats microbial infection: a model to study innate immunity and host-pathogen interactions. Curr Opin Microbiol 2002;5:102–110.
54. Janeway CA Jr, Mezhitov R. Innate immune recognition. Annu Rev Immunol 2002; 20 :197–216.
55. Hoffman JA, Kafatos FC, Janeway CA Jr, Ezekowiz RAB. Phylogenetic perspectives in immunity. Science 1999;284:1313–1318.
56. Hirschfeld M, Weis JJ, Toshchakov V, et al. Signaling by toll-like receptor 2 and 4 agonists results in differential gene expression in murine macrophages. Infect Immun 2001;69:1477–1482.
57. Pulendran B, Kumar P, Cutler CW, Mohamadzadeh M, Van Dyke T, Banchereau J. Lipopolysaccharides from distinct pathogens induce different classes of immune responses in vivo. J Immunol 2001;167:5067–5076.
58. Agrawal S, Agrawal A, Doughty B, et al. Cutting edge: different Toll-like receptor agonists instruct dendritic cells to induce distinct Th responses via differential modulation of extracellular signal-regulated kinase-mitogen-activated protein kinase and c-Fos. J Immunol 2003;171:4984–4989.
59. Dillon S, Agrawal A, Van Dyke T, et al. A Toll-like receptor 2 ligand stimulates Th2 responses in vivo, via induction of extracellular signal-regulated kinase mitogen-activated protein kinase and c-Fos in dendritic cells. J Immunol 2004;172: 4733–4743.
60. Redecke V, Hacker H, Datta SK, et al. Cutting edge: activation of Toll-like receptor 2 induces a Th2 immune response and promotes experimental asthma. J Immunol 2004;172:2739–2743.
61. Re F, Strominger JL. Toll-like receptor 2 (TLR2) and TLR4 differentially activate human dendritic cells. J Biol Chem 2001;276:37692–37699.
62. Netea MG, Sutmuller R, Hermann C, et al. Toll-like receptor 2 suppresses immunity against Candida albicans through induction of IL-10 and regulatory T cells. J Immunol 2004;172:3712–3718.

63. Sing A, Rost D, Tvardovskaia N, et al. Yersinia V-antigen exploits toll-like receptor 2 and CD14 for interleukin 10-mediated immunosuppression. Exp Med 2002; 196:1017–1024.
64. van der Kleij D, Latz E, Brouwers JF, et al. A novel host-parasite lipid cross-talk. Schistosomal lysophosphatidylserine activates toll-like receptor 2 and affects immune polarization. J Biol Chem 2002;277:48122–48129.
65. Stumbles PA, Thomas JA, Pimm CL. Resting respiratory tract dendritic cells preferentially stimulate T helper cell type 2 (Th2) responses and require obligatory cytokine signals for induction of Th1 immunity. J Exp Med 1998;188:2019–2031.
66. Kadowaki B, Ho S, Antonenko S, et al. Subsets of human dendritic cell precursors express different Toll-like receptors and respond to different microbial antigens. J Exp Med 2001;194:863–869.
67. Jarrossay D, Napolitani G, Colonna M, Sallusto F, Lanzavecchia A. Specialization and complementarity in microbial molecule recognition by human myeloid and plasmacytoid dendritic cells. Eur J Immunol 2001;31:3388–3393.
68. Linsey PS. T cell activation: you can't get good help. Nature Immunol 2001;2: 139,140.
69. Huang FP, Platt N, Wykes M, et al. A discrete subpopulation of dendritic cells transports apoptotic intestinal epithelial cells to T cell areas of mesenteric lymph nodes. J Exp Med 2000;191:435–444.
70. Urban BC, Kaneko O, Dvorak JA. Plasmodium falciparum-infected erythrocytes modulate the maturation of dendritic cells. Nature 1999;400:73–77.
71. Van Overtvelt L, Vanderkeyde W, Verhasselt V, et al. *Trypanosoma cruzi* infects human dendritic cells and prevents their maturation: inhibition of cytokines, HLA-DR, and costimulatory molecules. Infect Immun 1999;67:4033–4040.
72. Salio M, Cella M, Suter M, Lanzavecchia A. Inhibition of dendritic cell maturation by herpes simplex virus. Eur J Immunol 1999;29:3245–3253.
73. Grosjean I, Caux C, Bella C, et al. Measles virus infects human dendritic cells and blocks their allostimulatory properties for CD4+ T cells. J Exp Med 1997;186: 801–812.
74. Fugier-Vivier I, Servet-Delprat C, Rivailler P, Rissoan NC, Liu YJ, Rabourdin-Combe C. Measles virus suppresses cell-mediated immunity by interfering with the survival and functions of dendritic and T cells. J Exp Med 1997;186:813–823.
75. Servet-Delprat C, Bausinger H, Manie S, et al. Measles virus induces abnormal differentiation of CD40 ligand-activated human dendritic cells. J Immunol 2000;164:1753–1760.
76. Norbury CC, Malide D, Gibbs JS, Bennink JR, Yewdell JK. Visualizing priming of virus-specific CD8+ T cells by infected dendritic cells in vivo. Nat Immunol 2002;3:265–271.
77. Engelmayer J, Larsson M, Subklewe M, et al. Vaccinia virus inhibits the maturation of human dendritic cells: a novel mechanism of immune evasion. J Immunol 1999;163:6762–6768.
78. Tortorella D, Gewurz BE, Furman MH, Schust DJ, Ploegh HL. Viral subversion of the immune system. Ann Rev Immunol 2000;18:861–926.
79. McFadden G, Murphy PM. (2000). Host-related immunodmodulators encoded by poxviruses and herpesviruses. Curr Opin Microbiol 2000;3:371–378.

80. Angeli V, Faveeuw C, Roye C, et al. Role of the parasite-derived prostaglandin D2 in the inhibition of epidermal Langerhans cell migration during schistosomiasis infection. J Exp Med 2001;193:1135–1147.
81. Agrawal A, Lingappa J, Leppla SH, et al. Impairment of dendritic cells and adaptive immunity by anthrax lethal toxin. Nature 2003;424:329–334.
82. Mahanty S, Hutchinson K, Agarwal S, McRae M, Rollin PE, Pulendran B. Cutting edge: impairment of dendritic cells and adaptive immunity by Ebola and Lassa viruses. J Immunol 2003;170:2797–2801.
83. Geijtenbeek TB, Kwon DS, Torensma R, et al. DC-SIGN, a dendritic cell specific-HIV-1-binding protein that enhances trans-infection of T cells. Cell 2000; 151:673–684.
84. MacDonald GH, Johnston RE. Role of dendritic cell targeting in Venezuelan equine encephalitis virus pathogenesis. J Virol 2000;74:914–922.
85. Vidalain PO, Azocar O, Lamouille B, Astier A, Rabourdin-Combe C, Servet-Delprat C. Measles virus induces functional TRAIL production by human dendritic cells. J Virol 2000;74:556–559.
86. Servert-Delprat C, Vidalain PO, Azocar O, Le Deist F, Fischer A, Rabourdin-Combe C. Consequences of Fas-mediated human dendritic cell apoptosis induced by measles virus. J Virol 2000;74:4387–4393.
87. McGurik P, McCann C, Mills KH. Pathogen-specific T regulatory 1 cells induced in the respiratory tract by a bacterial molecule that stimulates interleukin-10 production by dendritic cells: a novel strategy for evasion of protective T helper type 1 responses by Bordetella pertussis. J Exp Med 2002;195:221–231.
88. Dhodapkar MV, Steinman RM, Sapp M, et al. Rapid generation of broad T-cell immunity in humans after a single injection of mature dendritic cells. J Clin Invest 1999;104:173–180.

# 3

# Achieving Transcriptional Specificity in NF-κB-Dependent Inflammatory Gene Expression

Gioacchino Natoli

## INTRODUCTION

One of the most daunting problems in research on transcriptional regulation is to understand how specificity is achieved, that is, how a relatively small number of signal transduction pathways and transcription factors can activate transcription from different sets of genes in response to different stimuli.

When applied to transcriptional regulation of inflammatory genes, the same problem could be reformulated the following way: how different microbial stimuli and inflammatory cytokines—which trigger very similar receptors and activate largely overlapping or identical signal transduction pathways and transcription factors—can induce transcriptional outputs that are plastically adapted to each stimulus. It is rather obvious that achieving transcriptional specificity is a particularly relevant task in the context of the antimicrobial response; rapid and successful elimination of any pathogen requires that the antimicrobial apparatus does its best to adapt the response to each type of pathogen.

A central component of the inflammatory response is the NF-κB family of transcription factors, which is almost invariably activated in response to any type of inflammatory stimulus and is required for transcription of an impressive number of inflammatory genes *(1–3)*. After a brief overview of the NF-κB system, I will discuss recent studies, carried out in our and other laboratories, aiming at explaining how different sets of NF-κB-dependent genes are induced in response to different inflammatory stimuli.

## THE NF-κB/REL FAMILY OF TRANSCRIPTION FACTORS

In mammalian cells, NF-κB exists as a collection of homo- and heterodimers composed of five distinct proteins bearing a conserved domain required for dimerization, nuclear localization and interaction with the IκBs, the Rel homology domain: RelA/p65, cRel, RelB, NF-κB1/p50 (and its precursor p105), NF-κB2/

From: *Vaccine Adjuvants: Immunological and Clinical Principles*
Edited by: C. J. Hackett and D. A. Harn, Jr. © Humana Press Inc., Totowa, NJ

p52 (and its precursor p100) *(4–6)*. Although almost all combinations are virtually possible (and at least 12 different dimers have been identified in living cells), the most abundant and extensively characterized species is the p65-p50 heterodimer, and very often the term NF-κB is used to describe this species.

With a few exceptions NF-κB dimers are found in the cytoplasm of unstimulated cells as inactive complexes bound to inhibitory proteins, the IκBs (IκBα, IκBβ and IκBε) and the two precursors p100 and p105 *(7)*. The inhibitors contain carboxy-terminal ankyrin repeats that mediate binding to the Rel homology domain of NF-κB dimers and prevent their nuclear accumulation. Conversely, the amino-terminal region mediates stimulus-induced degradation of the IκBs, a process required for NF-κB activation in response to the great majority of stimuli.

The key steps leading to signal-induced degradation of the IκBs have been clarified in the recent years *(5,8)*. First, the amino-terminal serines undergoing rapid phosphorylation in response to stimulation have been identified and shown to be essential for subsequent IκB degradation *(9,10)*. Second, a multi-component IκB-kinase complex (IKK) has been identified *(11)*, its components have been cloned *(12–18)*, and its general role as a bridge between membrane receptors and NF-κB activation has been formally demonstrated *(19–21)*. Third, amino-terminal IκB phosphorylation has been demonstrated to generate a novel docking site for ubiquitin ligases responsible for poli-ubiquitylation of IκBs, which is the final event targeting the IκBs for proteasomal degradation *(22)*. The whole process is usually complete in just a few minutes.

## NF-κB REGULATION IN THE NUCLEUS AND CHROMATIN ORGANIZATION AND ACCESSIBILITY OF NF-κB SITES

In a simple-minded view, IκB degradation is followed by a rapid entry of NF-κB dimers in the nucleus, in which they bind degenerated 9-11nt recognition sites contained in the promoters and enhancers of several inducible genes *(23)*. NF-κB recruitment is only a minute part of a very complex process involving protein–protein and protein–DNA interactions ultimately leading to the assembly of multiprotein complexes (made of both sequence-specific and general transcription factors) and to transcriptional activation.

What until recently has been given little attention is the fact that, like any other DNA-binding protein, also NF-κB has to deal with the fact that DNA is not naked (as in in vitro DNA-binding assays) but complexed to histones and non-histone proteins to form the chromatin *(24)*. Organization of DNA into chromatin has a major consequence: that accessibility to the underlying genome is limited by histone–DNA interactions and by the higher order folding of chromatin. Thus, a canonical high affinity NF-κB binding site (as it can be defined on the basis of in vitro DNA-binding assays) may be not accessible in vivo and thus it may not support NF-κB recruitment. In order to understand the impact of chromatin organization on NF-κB-dependent gene expression, we have started analyzing NF-κB recruitment to endogenous target genes in intact cells using the Chromatin Immunoprecipitation (ChIP) assay *(25)*. In the ChIP assay, cells are mildly fixed in formaldehyde, which promotes the formation of covalent protein–DNA crosslinks, thus preserving relevant protein–DNA interactions and preventing postlysis movements of DNA-binding proteins or nucleosomes. After lysis, nuclear extracts are sonicated to shear the chromatin into fragments of an average size between 500 and 1500 bp and aliquots of the extracts are immunoprecipitated with the desired antibody. After stringent washing the protein–DNA complexes are extracted, crosslinks are reverted by heating, and immunoprecipitated DNA is analyzed by polymerase chain reaction with promoter-specific primers. It is expected that promoters and enhancers bound by the immunoprecipitated protein will be enriched in the immunoprecipitates obtained with a specific but not with a control antibody. Therefore, this assay provides a very simple and extremely relevant piece of information: *whether a protein is bound to a specific chromatin region, in a specific moment and in intact cells.* By applying the ChIP assay to the study of NF-κB physiology, we have found that in macrophages—in which NF-κB is rapidly activated by lipopolysaccharide (LPS) stimulation—recruitment of p65/RelA to target genes occurs in two temporally distinct phases *(26)*: some genes (e.g., IκBα) recruit NF-κB immediately after its nuclear entry (i.e., starting at about 10 minutes after stimulation), although recruitment to other genes (e.g., interleukin [IL]-6) occurs with much slower kinetics. This kinetic complexity in NF-κB recruitment correlates very well with gene-specific profiles of NF-κB-dependent transcriptional induction, thus providing the molecular basis for such phenomenon. The simplest explanation for the existence of a gene-specific timing of NF-κB recruitment is the existence of reversible physical barriers that prevent exposure of NF-κB sites: the time required for such reversion dictates the kinetic of NF-κB recruitment. Indeed, genes recruiting NF-κB with fast kinetics are able to recruit transfected NF-κB subunits in the absence of any stimulation, thus indicating that the NF-κB site is available for binding; conversely, genes recruiting NF-κB with slow kinetics do not recruit transfected NF-κB proteins unless stimulated with LPS. We called the genes of the first group "constitutively and immediately accessible" (CIA) and the genes of the second group "genes with regulated and late accessibility" (RLA). The properties of these two groups of NF-κB targets are shown in Fig. 1. CIA genes have exposed NF-κB sites and therefore recruit NF-κB immediately after its nuclear entry, and with a similar efficiency no matter what is the stimulus used to induce its activation. Very often, these promoters tend to have high constitutive levels of histone acetylation. Conversely, NF-κB sites in RLA genes are not accessible unless the promoter is properly modified

# TWO CLASSES OF
# NF-κB-DEPENDENT GENES

## CONSTITUTIVELY AND IMMEDIATELY ACCESSIBLE

- exposed and accessible NF-κB site
- recruitment of transfected NF-κB proteins in the absence of stimulus
- immediate NF-κB recruitment

## GENES WITH REGULATED AND LATE ACCESSIBILITY

- NF-κB site not accessible before stimulation
- do not recruit transfected NF-κB proteins
- variable time gap between nuclear entry and recruitment
- promoter modifications preceding recruitment (transcription factor recruitment/acetylation)
- increased accessibility with proper prestimulation

**Fig. 1.** A classification of NF-κB target genes based on accessibility of the DNA-binding site. Kinetic analysis of p65 recruitment to target genes in lipopolysaccharide-stimulated macrophages and dendritic cells indicate the existence of two distinct groups of NF-κB targets, which differ in the accessibility of target site.

in response to stimulation. Because transcription of these genes is NF-κB-dependent, they will not be transcribed unless changes in accessibility take place before NF-κB extrusion from the nucleus. Very often these promoters have low basal levels of histone acetylation; acetylation is dramatically increased by LPS stimulation and in several cases this modification clearly precedes NF-κB recruitment. Moreover, we have found that at some RLA genes, prestimulation with agonists (such as interferon-γ) that do not activate transcription on their own, can induce promoter remodeling and increase accessibility to NF-κB (thus partially explaining their ability to synergize with LPS and inflammatory cytokines). Our interpretation of these results is that, considering the increase in acetylation as evidence of ongoing remodeling events, chromatin structure at these promoters has to be modified to make the NF-κB site accessible. Additional evidence in support of this model comes from studies previously carried out in Steven Smale's lab: in the interleukin 12 (IL-12) p40 subunit promoter, a strategically positioned nucleosome covers the cRel-binding site *(27,28)*. This nucleosome is rapidly remodeled after activation in a cRel-independent manner. Although this has not been directly proven, the final outcome of this remodeling event may well be to increase the accessibility of the cRel binding site.

The most important aspect of this model is that not all NF-κB activators are necessarily able to provide the signals enhancing the accessibility of the NF-κB sites contained in RLA genes. Consequently, RLA genes are transcribed in response to only specific NF-κB inducers. Keeping a subset of NF-κB-dependent promoters in a NF-κB-inaccessible state that can be quickly reversed if a proper stimulus is delivered, represents a very simple and effective strategy that significantly contributes to shape different patterns of NF-κB-dependent transcription in response to different NF-κB activators.

Another important issue to consider is that the accessibility state of a NF-κB site in a specific gene appears to be differentially regulated in different cell types thus fulfilling the specific needs of individual tissues. For instance in fibroblasts gene-specific differences in the kinetics of NF-κB recruitment are much less obvious than in macrophages.

## THE NF-κB/P38 MITOGEN-ACTIVATED PROTEIN KINASE CONNECTION

Stimulation of receptors for microbial products and inflammatory cytokines also leads to the activation of the mitogen-activated protein kinase (MAPK) pathways. p38 (which is actually a family of four proteins) *(29)* appears to be the MAPK most obviously required for the induction of the inflammatory response. Indeed, one of the groups that originally identified p38, purified it as the receptor of a novel class of experimental anti-inflammatory drugs *(30)*.

Because the p38 MAPK pathway is activated simultaneously to NF-κB in response to inflammatory agonists, we thought it interesting to test if it may contribute to regulate NF-κB recruitment to chromatin. Indeed, apart from phosphorylating and activating target transcription factors (whose actual list is probably far from complete) *(29)*, p38 mediates the induction of a specific histone modification, namely histone H3 phosphorylation at Ser10, in response to inflammatory agonists *(31)*. H3-Ser10 phosphorylation has been demonstrated to promote transcriptional activation in yeast *(32)*, although evidence in mammalian cells is mostly correlative *(31)*. In human monocyte-derived dendritic cells this histone modification occurs only in response to stimulation and is entirely p38-dependent (because p38 does not phosphorylate H3-Ser10, it probably acts through a downstream kinase such as MSK-1). Moreover, H3-Ser10 phosphorylation is highly regional and not widespread, as it can be detected only at some genes but not at others. A striking correlation we noticed is that all the genes in which this modification was detected required p38 for transcriptional activation. Even more strikingly, p38 was required for NF-κB recruitment to the genes undergoing H3-Ser10 phosphorylation, thus indicating that p38 is part of the regulatory circuitry controlling NF-κB access to chromatin (Fig. 2). In this context, the different extent (intensity and duration) to which inflammatory

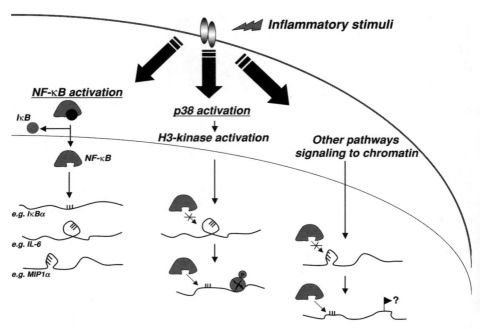

**Fig. 2.** Modulation of NF-κB access to chromatin by p38 and other signaling pathways. Three model promoters are shown: IκBα, whose NF-κB site (represented by three lines) is constitutively accessible to NFκB; interleukin (IL)-6 and macrophage inflammatory protein (MIP)-1α, whose site is buried in chromatin and not accessible to NF-κB. p38 activation is required to make the NF-κB site in the IL-6 gene accessible, possibly by triggering H3-Ser10 phosphorylation and subsequent chromatin remodeling. Conversely, the MIP-1a gene is switched into an open conformation in a p38-independent manner.

stimuli activate the p38 MAPK may determine differences in NF-κB recruitment to specific targets and ultimately lead to differences in gene expression patterns.

A recent study has also confirmed that p38 is required for transcriptional activation of a subset of NF-κB-dependent genes, including genes required for survival of activated macrophages *(33)*.

Overall, these results indicate that one major function of p38 is to regulate activation of selected NF-κB-dependent genes; because the genes coregulated by NF-κB and p38 are numerous, it is possible and likely that different mechanisms are implicated in this synergistic response. First of all p38 can regulate recruitment of NF-κB to chromatin, as we have shown for IL-8 and MCP-1 in dendritic cells. In this case, p38 may directly signal chromatin modifications ultimately leading to increased accessibility of high affinity NF-κB binding sites;

alternatively p38 may directly or indirectly phosphorylate transcription factors that increase NF-κB binding to low-affinity sites. Second, p38 may activate transcription factors cooperating with NF-κB in transcriptional activation but not required for NF-κB binding. In this case, we should expect that inhibition of p38 with selective chemical inhibitors does not affect recruitment of NF-κB to target genes but impairs transcriptional induction.

It is clear that because the identification of protein-kinase targets is still an extremely complex and experimentally inefficient task, it will take time before the list of transcription factors targeted by p38 is significantly expanded and the mechanisms of the synergism between p38 and NF-κB are thoroughly understood.

## NOT ONLY CHROMATIN:
## OTHER SOURCES OF SPECIFICITY IN THE NF-κB SYSTEM

A careful analysis of the anatomy of the NF-κB system *(4,5,34)* allows unveiling several other sources of specificity. The most obvious one is the presence of several dimers. Each dimer has a different DNA-binding surface and as a consequence it may show some preference toward one or more of the several possible NF-κB sites *(35)*. Thus, we can imagine that the reason why the system is composed of so many dimers is that this allows expanding the number of target genes (more dimers = more target sites). However, the real situation is far more complicated. Indeed, in vitro most NF-κB dimers are able to bind in a highly redundant fashion and with comparable affinities to several canonical and noncanonical NF-κB sites *(23)*. The reason for this behavior is the remarkable flexibility of the DNA-binding domain of NF-κB proteins *(35)*, which allows them to adapt their own conformation to different DNA-binding sites. For this reason, it is still impossible to predict (based on the DNA sequence) whether a NF-κB-dependent gene is regulated in a redundant or dimer-specific fashion. However, analysis of knockout mice and cells lacking individual NF-κB proteins has demonstrated some specificity of NF-κB proteins in the induction of some target genes (although others are regulated in an apparently redundant fashion). For instance, IL-12 p40 synthesis in macrophages is specifically dependent on cRel *(36)*; conversely, p65 is required for the synthesis of IL-6, macrophage inflammatory protein 2 (MIP-2) and inducible nitric oxide synthase in fibroblasts *(37)*. Thus the system is organized to provide both redundancy and specificity.

In this regard, it should be also considered that each dimer has a different affinity toward the IκBs and therefore release of different dimers may be differentially regulated *(7)*. For instance, RelB-p52 dimers are largely insensitive to IκB-mediated inhibition: they are sequestered in the cytoplasm mainly through association with p100, and are released in response to a NIK/IKKα pathway that is different from the one regulating release of most other dimers *(38,39)*. It follows that both the representation of different dimers in a specific cell type and the ability of each stimulus to activate the signaling pathways regulating release of different dimers affect transcriptional specificity in the NF-κB system.

A relevant and to date poorly appreciated source of specificity is the degeneracy in the sequence of the NF-κB site *(23)*. Variations in NF-κB site sequence have two main effects: first, as discussed above, they may promote a preferential recruitment of one or selected dimers. Second, the NF-κB site has an allosteric effect on the bound dimer, that is, it affects its conformation *(40)*. This means that the same dimer adopts different conformations when bound to different sites. Because a transcriptionally active promoter looks pretty much like a Chinese puzzle in which all pieces have to perfectly fit, it follows that differences in the conformation of the bound NF-κB dimer may have dramatic effects on transcriptional activation.

## CONCLUSIONS

More than 15 years after the discovery of NF-κB, and despite the tremendous effort put by many laboratories in understanding its physiology, several questions remain to be answered. Overall, we know far less about the mechanisms regulating NF-κB response in the nucleus than about mechanisms connecting NF-κB to signal transduction pathways. Chemical inhibitors of the IκB kinases have been already developed and are likely to exert dramatic anti-inflammatory effects. However, it is highly unlikely that indiscriminate inhibition of NF-κB will represent in the future a clinically relevant approach, as it will lead to severe immunosuppression and to several other dangerous side effects (such as massive apoptosis in cells/organs requiring NF-κB for expression of essential antiapoptotic genes). Ideally, drugs should be designed inhibiting induction of only selected subsets of NF-κB targets. To this aim, a prerequisite is to define molecular determinants regulating activation of specific genes by individual NF-κB dimers and to understand the rules explaining specificity and redundancy in the NF-κB system.

## ACKNOWLEDGMENTS

The work described in this manuscript was partially supported by the Swiss National Foundation.

## REFERENCES

1. Hatada EN, Krappmann D, Scheidereit C. NF-kappaB and the innate immune response. Curr Opin Immunol 2000;12:52–58.
2. Baldwin AS, Jr. The NF-kappa B and I kappa B proteins: new discoveries and insights. Annu Rev Immunol 1996;14:649–683.

3. Ghosh S, May MJ, Kopp EB. NF-kappa B and Rel proteins: evolutionarily conserved mediators of immune responses. Annu Rev Immunol 1998;16:225–260.
4. Verma IM, Stevenson JK, Schwarz EM, Van Antwerp D, Miyamoto S. Rel/NF-kappa B/I kappa B family: intimate tales of association and dissociation. Genes Dev 1995;9:2723–2735.
5. Rothwarf DM, Karin M. The NF-kappa B activation pathway: a paradigm in information transfer from membrane to nucleus. Sci STKE 1999;1999:RE1.
6. May MJ, Ghosh S. Rel/NF-kappa B and I kappa B proteins: an overview. Semin Cancer Biol 1997;8:63–73.
7. Whiteside ST, Israel A. I kappa B proteins: structure, function and regulation. Semin Cancer Biol 1997;8:75–82.
8. Karin M, Ben-Neriah Y. Phosphorylation meets ubiquitination: the control of NF-[kappa]B activity. Annu Rev Immunol 2000;18:621–663.
9. Brown K, Gerstberger S, Carlson L, Franzoso G, Siebenlist U. Control of I kappa B-alpha proteolysis by site-specific, signal-induced phosphorylation. Science 1995; 267:1485–1488.
10. DiDonato J, Mercurio F, Rosette C, et al. Mapping of the inducible IkappaB phosphorylation sites that signal its ubiquitination and degradation. Mol Cell Biol 1996;16:1295–1304.
11. Chen ZJ, Parent L, Maniatis T. Site-specific phosphorylation of IkappaBalpha by a novel ubiquitination-dependent protein kinase activity. Cell 1996;84:853–862.
12. DiDonato JA, Hayakawa M, Rothwarf DM, Zandi E, Karin M. A cytokine-responsive IkappaB kinase that activates the transcription factor NF-kappaB. Nature 1997; 388:548–554.
13. Regnier CH, Song HY, Gao X, Goeddel DV, Cao Z, Rothe M. Identification and characterization of an IkappaB kinase. Cell 1997;90:373–383.
14. Mercurio F, Zhu H, Murray BW, et al. IKK-1 and IKK-2: cytokine-activated IkappaB kinases essential for NF-kappaB activation. Science 1997;278:860–866.
15. Woronicz JD, Gao X, Cao Z, Rothe M, Goeddel DV. IkappaB kinase-beta: NF-kappaB activation and complex formation with IkappaB kinase-alpha and NIK. Science 1997;278:866–869.
16. Yamaoka S, Courtois G, Bessia C, et al. Complementation cloning of NEMO, a component of the IkappaB kinase complex essential for NF-kappaB activation. Cell 1998;93:1231–1240.
17. Rothwarf DM, Zandi E, Natoli G, Karin M. IKK-gamma is an essential regulatory subunit of the IkappaB kinase complex. Nature 1998;395:297–300.
18. Mercurio F, Murray BW, Shevchenko A, et al. IkappaB kinase (IKK)-associated protein 1, a common component of the heterogeneous IKK complex. Mol Cell Biol 1999;19:1526–1538.
19. Li ZW, Chu W, Hu Y, et al. The IKKbeta subunit of IkappaB kinase (IKK) is essential for nuclear factor kappaB activation and prevention of apoptosis. J Exp Med 1999;189:1839–1845.
20. Li Q, Van Antwerp D, Mercurio F, Lee KF, Verma IM. Severe liver degeneration in mice lacking the IkappaB kinase 2 gene. Science 1999;284:321–325.
21. Makris C, Godfrey VL, Krahn-Senftleben G, et al. Female mice heterozygous for IKK gamma/NEMO deficiencies develop a dermatopathy similar to the human X-linked disorder incontinentia pigmenti. Mol Cell 2000;5:969–979.

22. Yaron A, Hatzubai A, Davis M, et al. Identification of the receptor component of the IkappaBalpha-ubiquitin ligase. Nature 1998;396:590–594.
23. Grilli M, Chiu JJ, Lenardo MJ. NF-kappa B and Rel: participants in a multiform transcriptional regulatory system. Int Rev Cytol 1993;143:1–62.
24. Kornberg RD, Lorch Y. Twenty-five years of the nucleosome, fundamental particle of the eukaryote chromosome. Cell 1999;98:285–294.
25. Hecht A, Strahl-Bolsinger S, Grunstein M. Mapping DNA interaction sites of chromosomal proteins. Crosslinking studies in yeast. Methods Mol Biol 1999;119: 469–479.
26. Saccani S, Pantano S, Natoli G. Two waves of nuclear factor kappaB recruitment to target promoters. J Exp Med 2001;193:1351–1359.
27. Weinmann AS, Plevy SE, Smale ST. Rapid and selective remodeling of a positioned nucleosome during the induction of IL-12 p40 transcription. Immunity 1999; 11:665–675.
28. Weinmann AS, Mitchell DM, Sanjabi S, et al. Nucleosome remodeling at the IL-12 p40 promoter is a TLR-dependent, Rel-independent event. Nat Immunol 2001; 2:51–57.
29. Kyriakis JM, Avruch J. Mammalian mitogen-activated protein kinase signal transduction pathways activated by stress and inflammation. Physiol Rev 2001;81:807–869.
30. Lee JC, Laydon JT, McDonnell PC, et al. A protein kinase involved in the regulation of inflammatory cytokine biosynthesis. Nature 1994;372:739–746.
31. Saccani S, Pantano S, Natoli G. p38-Dependent marking of inflammatory genes for increased NF-kappa B recruitment. Nat Immunol 2002;3:69–75.
32. Lo WS, Duggan L, Tolga NC, et al. Snf1—a histone kinase that works in concert with the histone acetyltransferase Gcn5 to regulate transcription. Science 2001; 293:1142–1146.
33. Jin Mo Park FRG, Zhi-Wei Li, Karin M. Macrophage apoptosis by anthrax lethal factor through p38 MAP kinase inhibition. Science 2002;297:2048–2051.
34. Siebenlist U, Franzoso G, Brown K. Structure, regulation and function of NF-kappa B. Annu Rev Cell Biol 1994;10:405–455.
35. Huxford T, Malek S, Ghosh G. Structure and mechanism in NF-kappa B/I kappa B signaling. Cold Spring Harb Symp Quant Biol 1999;64:533–540.
36. Sanjabi S, Hoffmann A, Liou HC, Baltimore D, Smale ST. Selective requirement for c-Rel during IL-12 P40 gene induction in macrophages. Proc Natl Acad Sci USA 2000;97:12705–12710.
37. Ouaaz F, Li M, Beg AA. A critical role for the RelA subunit of nuclear factor kappaB in regulation of multiple immune-response genes and in Fas-induced cell death. J Exp Med 1999;189:999–1004.
38. Solan NJ, Miyoshi H, Carmona EM, Bren GD, Paya CV. RelB cellular regulation and transcriptional activity are regulated by p100. J Biol Chem 2002;277:1405–1418.
39. Senftleben U, Cao Y, Xiao G, et al. Activation by IKKalpha of a second, evolutionary conserved, NF-kappa B signaling pathway. Science 2001;293:1495–1499.
40. Chen-Park FE, Huang DB, Noro B, Thanos D, Ghosh G. The kappa B DNA sequence from the HIV-LTR functions as an allosteric regulator of HIV transcription. J Biol Chem 2002;22:22.

# 4

# Adjuvants and the Initiation of T-Cell Responses

## Matthew F. Mescher,
## Julie M. Curtsinger, and Marc Jenkins

## INTRODUCTION

Despite extensive study and use of adjuvants that promote initiation of T-cell responses, we are only now beginning to understand the mechanistic basis for the adjuvant effect. This rapidly increasing understanding is a result of several factors including advances in our fundamental understanding of the requirements of T-cell activation, a developing appreciation of the importance of innate immunity in T-cell activation, and realization that dendritic cells (DCs) play the central role as antigen-presenting cells (APCs) to activate T cells. Furthermore, previous studies of adjuvants were largely empirical although new approaches are allowing much more detailed and quantitative studies of the in vivo activation of antigen (Ag)-specific T cells. Impetus for studying the mechanisms by which adjuvants influence T-cell responses is provided by their tremendous importance in developing vaccination strategies to prevent and treat diseases. In addition to the classical adjuvant formulations, most of which include bacterial cell wall components, numerous other substances with adjuvant effects have been described and the list continues to grow. The ability to activate DCs and induce production of inflammatory cytokines is emerging as a critical feature shared by most if not all adjuvants, and recent studies are beginning to suggest ways in which these cytokines contribute to T-cell proliferation and differentiation. This chapter examines the requirements for effective activation of T-cell responses and discusses how adjuvants and their effects on DCs can or might contribute at each stage.

## VISUALIZING THE EFFECTS OF ADJUVANT ON IN VIVO T-CELL RESPONSES

The development of methods that allow direct visualization of Ag-specific T-cell responses in vivo has allowed major advances to be made in our understanding

From: *Vaccine Adjuvants: Immunological and Clinical Principles*
Edited by: C. J. Hackett and D. A. Harn, Jr. © Humana Press Inc., Totowa, NJ

of the effects of adjuvants on these responses. Until recently, the earliest events in Ag-specific T-cell activation could not be directly examined in vivo; the frequency of naïve T cells specific for a given Ag is very low in a normal animal and there was no means to identify the small number of Ag-specific T cells before activation. Thus, responses initiated by in vivo challenge with Ag could only be indirectly assessed by isolating lymphocytes from various sites and measuring functional responses. In most cases this required in vitro restimulation, thereby limiting the analysis to only the cells that could be restimulated in this way.

The development of mice expressing a transgenic T-cell antigen receptor (TCR) of known Ag specificity overcame some of these limitations. In these mice, all of the T cells are specific for the Ag and almost all express the appropriate coreceptor, CD4 for class II-restricted TCRs and CD8 for class I-restricted TCRs. However, a normal immune response cannot be studied in these animals because of the complete skewing to a single Ag specificity and T-cell subset. This limitation was removed when it was found that small numbers of T cells from TCR transgenic mice could be adoptively transferred into normal mice and their responses tracked by identifying the cells using either a clonotypic mAb specific for the transgenic TCR or using a recipient mouse congenic for a surface marker such as Thy 1 or CD45 *(1,2)*. When the T cells are transferred by intravenous (iv) injection in appropriate numbers they equilibrate in the recipient's immune system within 6 hours *(3)* and constitute 0.1 to 0.5% of the T cells in the lymph nodes (LN) and spleen. Thus, they are present in sufficient numbers to allow enumeration and characterization by flow cytometry, but are a small enough population that the immune system remains relatively normal. The TCR transgenic T cells survive and retain a naïve phenotype for at least 60 days following transfer, and when the animal is challenged with Ag their response can be followed by isolating cells from various sites during the course of the response and determining the number and activation status of the Ag-specific T cells by flow cytometry (Fig. 1).

An alternative means of visualizing Ag-specific T cells directly ex vivo or in situ employs major histocompatibility complex (MHC) protein–peptide complexes to detect the specific cells *(4–6)*. TCRs interact with peptide-MHC complexes with relatively low affinity, too low for monomeric binding to be retained for a sufficient time to allow detection by flow cytometry. When dimers or multimers are used the increased avidity of binding to the cell stabilizes the interaction sufficiently to allow analysis by flow cytometry or histochemistry. However, the low frequency of naïve T cells specific for most Ags is below the limit of detection by these means. Thus, MHC protein–peptide complexes are very effective for studying T-cell responses once initial clonal expansion has occurred, but in most cases they cannot be used to study the earliest events in the activation process.

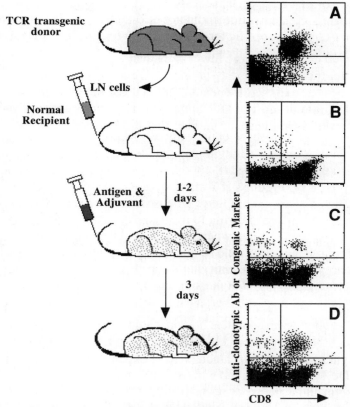

**Fig. 1.** Visualizing an antigen-specific T-cell response in vivo. Adoptive transfer of a small number of lymph node (LN) T cells from a TCR transgenic mouse (A) to a normal recipient (B) results in a population of antigen-specific T cells in the spleen and lymph nodes that can be detected by flow cytometry using either an anticlonotypic Ab specific for the TCR or a congenic marker, along with an anti-CD4 or anti-CD8 mAb (C). On challenge with antigen and adjuvant the specific T cells undergo clonal expansion (D), and can be characterized by gating on the population and staining with mAbs specific for activation markers.

Using the adoptive transfer approach, Jenkins and coworkers were able for the first time to directly assess the effects of adjuvants on T-cell responses. The adjuvant effect, termed immunology's "dirty little secret" by Janeway *(7)*, was finally brought into the light. Beginning with the seminal work of Dresser *(8,9)*, it was found that challenge with soluble Ag resulted in tolerance induction although injection of the same Ag along with a bacterial cell wall adjuvant caused a productive response. Tracking adoptively transferred CD4 T cells revealed that soluble Ag activated the T cells in the LN and spleen and caused substantial clonal expansion at these sites that peaked on day 3 *(1,10)*. Within a few days, however, the number of Ag-specific cells declined precipitously so that by day 10 to 15 there were fewer cells than were present before challenge. Furthermore, these cells were hyporesponsive after re-exposure to Ag. Thus, activation occurred in the absence of adjuvant but the outcome was tolerance because of failure of most of the cells to survive, and because of induction of nonresponsiveness in the small number that did survive.

Challenge with the same peptide Ag along with lipopolysaccharide (LPS) as an adjuvant resulted in a comparable initial clonal expansion of the Ag-specific T cells, peaking at day 3 at levels only about twofold higher than in the absence of adjuvant. However, following the peak of clonal expansion the decline in numbers of Ag-specific cells was much less when adjuvant was used, and an expanded population persisted for a prolonged time. Furthermore, the remaining cells responded rapidly on rechallenge with the Ag. Thus, adjuvant converted a tolerizing response to one that yielded an expanded, responsive memory population.

Similar results have been obtained in experiments examining responses of adoptively transferred CD8 T cell, although in this case the presence of adjuvant appears to have a greater effect on the initial clonal expansion *(11)*. Thus, challenge with peptide Ag in complete Freund's adjuvant resulted in extensive clonal expansion of the Ag-specific cells in the draining LN, although challenge with peptide Ag alone resulted in much weaker expansion. As in the case of CD4 T cells, CD8 T cells challenged with peptide alone persisted in only low numbers long term and were hyporesponsive *(11,12)*, whereas cells challenged with peptide and adjuvant persisted long term as an expanded, responsive memory population *(11)*.

When adoptively transferred mice are challenged with Ag and adjuvant by iv injection, clonal expansion of the Ag-specific T cells occurs in all LN and in the spleen. By contrast, subcutaneous injection of Ag in Freund's adjuvant results in clonal expansion predominantly in the draining LN, and activated Ag-specific T cells only appear in significant numbers in the spleen and distant nodes after day 3 as the cells begin to migrate out of the draining LN following the initial expansion *(2,10,11)*. The mineral oil emulsion of Freund's adjuvant likely causes the Ag to remain sequestered in the region of the injection, thereby limiting the amount of Ag that reaches distant LN or spleen. When Ag is injected subcutaneously along with an adjuvant that does not include mineral oil, for example LPS or cytokines, expansion is somewhat favored in draining LN, but also occurs in distant LN and spleen. An antigen depot effect of complete Freund's adjuvant (CFA) was long considered to be a possible mechanism by which this adjuvant enhanced T-cell responses, by providing for prolonged presence of the Ag at a localized site *(13)*. In fact, this does not appear to be a major factor in the adjuvant effect *(10,14)* and, if anything, may somewhat limit responses by preventing the Ag from reaching distant sites and activating additional T cells at those locations. Thus, a depot effect does not appear to play a major role in the ability of adjuvant to support development of effective T-cell responses. Instead, the effects of adjuvants appear to result from their ability to activate DC so that they can effectively deliver the signals needed to stimulate T cells to undergo a productive response. The following sections discuss the nature of these required signals, and the ways in which adjuvants stimulate DC to provide them.

## THE REQUIREMENTS
## FOR CLONAL EXPANSION OF NAÏVE T CELLS

Lafferty and Cunningham *(15)* first proposed that lymphocyte activation requires two signals, with signal 1 being provided by the Ag-specific receptor and signal 2 by a second receptor–ligand interaction, and a wealth of data has accumulated in support of this model *(16–20)*. More recent evidence has suggested that a third signal is also required, at least for CD8 T cells, and that the presence or absence of "signal 3" determines whether effective activation or tolerance induction occurs in response to Ag and costimulation *(11,21–24)*.

### Signal 1: TCR Interaction With Ag

To become activated, naïve T cells must recognize peptide Ag bound to class I or class II MHC protein on an APC. This is not sufficient for full activation, however, and can instead lead to the induction of anergy *(20)*, a nonresponsive state characterized by an inability of the T cells to produce interleukin (IL)-2 on restimulation. For full activation to occur, the T cell must receive a second signal via a costimulatory receptor. Although there are reports of costimulation-independent activation of T cells using anti-TCR mAb or high densities of class I/peptide Ag complexes, naïve T cells appear to require both signal 1 and signal 2 to respond to normal physiological levels of Ag in most circumstances. Whether or not naïve T cells encounter sufficient Ag in lymphoid organs to receive an effective signal 1 can be influenced by adjuvants (*see* Signal 1: Mitigation of DC to Lymph Nodes and Processing and Presentation of Ag1).

### Signal 2: Costimulation

Experimental support for a two-signal model for T-cell activation was first provided by the observation that chemically fixed APC could not fully activate T cells despite displaying Ag on the cell surface *(25)*. Subsequent work demonstrated that binding of the CD28 receptor on the T cell to its ligands, B7-1 or B7-2, on the APC could provide the second signal necessary to activate the cells *(16,18)*, and a wealth of data has accumulated to support the importance of this interaction. More recently, several additional receptor-ligand systems have been shown to have costimulatory activity for T cells including leucocyte function-associated antigen (LFA)-1/intercellular adhesion molecule (ICAM) and several members of the tumor necrosis factor (TNF)-superfamily *(26)*. LFA-1 is expressed on naïve T cells, and may have some role in providing costimulation to initiate responses, particularly for CD8 T cells *(27)*. The other costimulatory receptors are expressed predominantly on activated T cells and this, together with the tissue distribution of the ligands, suggests that they may have roles in the T-cell response subsequent to the initial activation of naïve cells, perhaps in sustaining and extending responses *(28)*. CD28 binding to B7 ligands appears be the major provider of signal 2 to naïve T cells to initiate responses *(29)*.

### Signal 3: Cytokines

Although two signals are necessary to activate naïve T cells, they may not be sufficient, at least for CD8 T cells. This was first suggested in experiments using artificial APC made by immobilizing class I/peptide Ag and B7-1 ligand on cell-size microspheres and examining their ability to stimulate highly purified T cells from TCR transgenic mice. Memory CD8 T cells responded well to the microspheres by proliferating and developing effector functions, but naïve cells did not respond despite expressing the same TCR *(22)*. This suggested that some additional signal was required for the naïve cells to respond. There have been numerous reports of cytokines augmenting cytotoxic T-lymphocyte (CTL) responses, but in most cases it was not determined whether the effect of the cytokine was directly on the CD8 T cell or the APC, to either increase Ag or costimulatory ligand levels or induce production of another cytokine. When a panel of cytokines was examined for effects in the artificial APC system it was found that addition of IL-12 resulted in vigorous proliferation and development of effector functions by the naïve CD8 T cells *(22)*. The response of the naïve cells depended on all three signals, Ag, costimulation, and IL-12. A number of other cytokines including IL-1, IL-2, IL-4, IL-6, IL-7, and IL-15 did not support the response. The ability of IL-12 to augment CTL responses has been known for some time *(30)*, but its ability to provide a requisite third signal to naïve cells had not previously been appreciated.

Using the adoptive transfer approach, IL-12 was also found to provide a critical third signal to support in vivo activation of CD8 T cells. IL-12 was as effective as CFA in supporting peptide Ag-specific clonal expansion, development of effector function and establishment of a long-lived, responsive memory population *(11,24)*. The response to Ag and IL-12 was dependent on costimulation because it could be largely prevented by blocking CD28/B7 interactions, that is, signal 2 was still required. Furthermore, IL-12 was acting by providing a third signal directly to the T cells, because it was effective when the adoptive transfer recipient was IL-12R deficient, and thus the only cells in the mouse that expressed an IL-12R were the transferred CD8 T cells *(24)*. Thus, like the conventional adjuvants CFA and LPS, the presence or absence of IL-12 determined whether peptide Ag resulted in full activation or tolerance induction. IL-12 has also been shown to be an effective adjuvant for supporting the expansion of Ag-specific CD8 T cells in melanoma patients immunized with tumor antigen peptides *(31)*.

When TCR transgenic CD8 T cells were adoptively transferred into IL-12 deficient mice, peptide and CFA was still able to stimulate a vigorous response indicating that IL-12 was not the only thing that could provide the third signal for activation *(11)*. Recent studies have demonstrated that interferon (IFN)$\alpha$ can also act as a third signal to stimulate responses. Like IL-12, IFN$\alpha$ supports proliferation and development of effector function in vitro, and acts as a potent adjuvant in vivo *(32)*. Additionally, immunization with peptide and either IL-12 or IFN$\alpha$ results in protective immunity in a B16 melanoma lung metastases model (Popescu and Mescher, manuscript in preparation). Whether there are additional cytokines and/or surface ligands on APC that can also provide the third signal to CD8 T cells remains to be determined.

There is some data to suggest that CD4 T cells may also require a third signal for productive activation, and that IL-1 may provide this signal. Stimulation of naïve CD4 T cells with Ag and B7 on microspheres is substantially increased when IL-1, but not IL-12, is added to the cultures *(22)*. Furthermore, IL-1 was as effective as LPS in enhancing the clonal expansion and persistence of adoptively transferred CD4 T cells in response to peptide or protein Ag *(10)*. TNF-$\alpha$ had similar effects in vivo, possibly as a result of its ability to induce IL-1 production *(33)*. By contrast, although IL-12 could skew the response toward a TH1 response it did not enhance clonal expansion or persistence of the CD4 T cells *(10)*. It remains to be determined whether these adjuvant effects of IL-1 and/or TNF-$\alpha$ result from direct delivery of a third signal to the CD4 T cells in vivo.

These findings suggest that at least one critical function of adjuvants in stimulating CD8 T-cell responses, and possibly CD4 T-cell responses, is induction of the third signal required to support clonal expansion, development of effector function and survival of a responsive memory population (Fig. 2). Interestingly, the data available thus far suggests that the relevant cytokines are different for the different T-cell subsets, with IL-1 but not IL-12 being effective for CD4 T cells and IL-12 but not IL-1 being effective for CD8 T cells. Many of the commonly used adjuvants do, in fact, stimulate production of these "third signal" cytokines by DC.

Several events must occur in order for naïve T cells to undergo maximal clonal expansion after in vivo exposure to Ag. Ag first has to be delivered to the secondary lymphoid organs in which the T cells reside, and be processed and presented on class I or class II MHC proteins so that it can be recognized by the

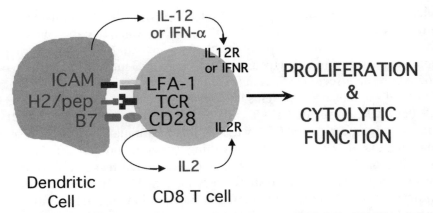

**Fig. 2.** Three signals are required for activation of naïve CD8 T cells. Signals 1 and 2 are provided by the TCR and costimulatory receptors including CD28 and leucocyte function-associated antigen-1. Signal 3 can be provided by IL-12 or IFNα. Stimulation of DC with adjuvants increases the surface expression of B7 costimulatory ligands and upregulates production of signal 3 cytokines.

TCR to deliver signal 1. The cell presenting the Ag must also express ligands for a costimulatory receptor, probably B7 ligands for the CD28 receptor in most cases, to deliver signal 2 to the T cell. Then, at least in the case of CD8 T cells, an appropriate cytokine may need to be present to deliver signal 3 to allow full activation and avoid tolerance induction. It has become clear over the past several years that DC are the cells primarily responsible for presenting Ag to T cells, and can satisfy all of these requirements for activating a response. They have efficient machinery for taking up extracellular Ag, processing it and loading the peptides onto class I and II MHC proteins, they can deliver Ag to T cells by migrating from peripheral sites of Ag deposition to secondary lymphoid organs, they express ligands for costimulatory receptors on T cells, and they can produce an array of inflammatory cytokines, some of which can provide the third signal to the T cell (Fig. 2). However, the ability of a DC to transport Ag to the T cells and optimally deliver each of the necessary signals requires that it first be activated and undergo a maturation process. Many, if not all, conventional adjuvants activate this maturation process by binding to receptors expressed on the surface of the DC.

## ACTIVATION OF DENDRITIC CELLS: TOLL-LIKE RECEPTORS AND ADJUVANTS

Toll-like receptors (TLRs) are expressed on macrophages and DCs in which they recognize conserved molecular patterns on products of microbial metabolism, termed pathogen-associated molecular patterns. They are structurally related to the Toll family of proteins found in *Drosophila*, which play important roles in antimicrobial defense *(34)*. The first evidence for a functional role in immunity for mammalian Toll-like proteins was provided in 1997 by Janeway and coworkers *(35)* for human TLR4. A wealth of data characterizing the structure and function of the mammalian TLR family has subsequently accumulated *(36)*. There are at least 10 members of the family (TLR1 through TLR10) and numerous ligands for these receptors have been identified. Almost all of the ligands are conserved microbial products. The different TLR are specific for different ligands, but most if not all of them can recognize multiple ligands. Included in the array of molecules identified as TLR ligands are most of the conventional adjuvants such as lipids and glycolipids, including LPS, lipoteichoic acid, polynucleotides, including bacterial deoxyribonucleic acid (DNA) and double-stranded ribonucleic acid (RNA) (produced on viral infection), lipoproteins, and yeast zymosan.

Signaling through TLRs activates the NF-κB pathway and results in induction of a variety of genes that function in host defense. These include effector molecules of innate immunity such as antimicrobial peptides and nitric oxide synthase, and molecules with roles in adaptive responses, including chemokines, MHC proteins, costimulatory molecules, and inflammatory cytokines. Signaling pathways activated by TLR include both shared pathways, activated by all of the receptors, and pathways specific to a given TLR. Thus, TLR engagement by most adjuvants will result in some common activation events, although adjuvants may differ with respect to other activation events depending on which TLR is involved *(36–38)*. Adding to this complexity is the fact that there are several different subsets of DC *(39,40)* and they can express different sets of TLRs, so adjuvants may have differing effects depending on the DC subset that expresses the TLR for a given adjuvant. Furthermore, the same TLR can induce different cytokines depending on the DC subset that it is expressed on; for example, TLR7 ligation results in IFNα production by plasmacytoid DCs, but IL-12 production by myeloid DCs *(41)*. Thus, although engagement of TLR by different adjuvants results in many common events associated with DC maturation, the full spectrum of changes that occur may differ from one adjuvant to another in ways that influence T-cell activation and differentiation.

## THE EFFECTS OF DC ACTIVATION
## ON STIMULATION OF NAÏVE T CELLS

### Signal 1: Migration of DC to Lymph Nodes
### and Processing and Presentation of Ag

DC are located in the T-cell areas of the secondary lymphoid organs in most nonlymphoid tissues. The DC in the secondary lymphoid organs consist of several subpopulations that can be separated broadly into subsets that arrived recently from the blood or nonlymphoid tissues *(42–44)*. For example, LNs contain blood-derived DC that entered via blood vessels and Langerhans cells that migrated from the skin via afferent lymphatic vessels. The rate of DC migration from nonlymphoid organs is thought to be relatively low under normal uninflamed conditions. However, in the presence of inflammation, most DC in the inflamed tissue migrate to the lymph nodes because of changes in expression of chemokine receptors, and undergo functional changes known collectively as DC maturation *(45,46)*. In the absence of inflammation, immature tissue DC, for example Langerhans cells of the skin are efficient at uptake of particulate and fluid phase Ag. When immature DC are stimulated in vitro by TLR ligands or by inflammatory cytokines, produced in response to adjuvants, further Ag uptake is inhibited, and the already internalized Ag is processed to produce peptide-class II MHC complexes that are then shuttled to the surface *(47)*. Inflammation also reduces the turnover of peptide-class II MHC complexes on the surface of DCs *(48)* and induces components of the MHC I peptide processing machinery *(49)*. Thus, inflammation caused by adjuvants would lead to much greater antigen presentation because many immature DCs would migrate from the tissue of antigen deposition into the lymphoid organs in which naïve T cells reside, and in the process mature to display more stable surface and abundant peptide–MHC complexes.

### Signal 2: Costimulation

In addition to increasing expression of MHC protein-peptide complexes in response to maturation agents like adjuvants, DC also upregulate expression of adhesion molecules and costimulatory ligands including LFA-3 (CD58), ICAM-1 (CD54), B7-1 (CD80), and B7-2 (CD86). Splenic DC express relatively low levels of B7-1 and B7-2, and both increase within 6 h of injection of LPS, with B7-2 expression increasing five- to sixfold and B7-1 somewhat less *(50)*. The increased expression of CD28 ligands could enhance the ability of DC to provide signal 2 to T cells. Support for this comes from the observation that the ability of LPS to enhance IL-2 production and proliferation by antigen-stimulated CD4 T cells requires that these T cells express CD28 *(51)*. However, this experiment does not rule out the possibility that basal CD28 signaling is necessary for the T cells to respond to some other signal stimulated by the adjuvant, for example, a cytokine. This in fact is the case for CD8 T cells. When IL-12R deficient mice received Ag-specific CD8 T cells by adoptive transfer and were then challenged with peptide Ag and IL-12 the T cells responded vigorously *(24)*. The response depended on CD28 signaling, because it was largely blocked by administration of CTLA4-Ig, which binds to CD80 and CD86 and prevents their interaction with CD28. Costimulation was presumably provided by the basal levels of B7 ligands expressed on the recipient APC, because these cells lacked IL-12R and would not be stimulated to upregulate the ligands.

CD28-dependent costimulation induces IL-2 production by naïve T cells, thus providing an important growth factor to support proliferation, at least in vitro. The importance of IL-2 as a growth factor in the initial proliferation of naïve T cells in vivo is less clear, however. CD4 T cells that lack IL-2 or IL-2R undergo essentially normal in vivo clonal expansion in response to a TCR stimulus *(52–54)*. Furthermore, LPS enhances Ag-dependent clonal expansion of naïve CD4 T cells in vivo in the absence of IL-2, although the response remains dependent on CD28 *(50)*. Similarly, early expansion of virus-specific CD8 T cells in secondary lymphoid tissues was shown to be IL-2 independent, although IL-2 did play a role in supporting continued clonal expansion in nonlymphoid tissue later in the response *(55)*. Thus, although costimulation is critical for initiating responses of naïve T cells, it appears likely that this is largely mediated by pathways that do not involve IL-2 as an autocrine growth factor.

## Cytokine Production: Multiple Roles

DC are capable of secreting a wide array of cytokines including IL-1, IL-2, IL-6, IL-7, IL-12, IL-15, IL-18, and type I IFNs. Which cytokines a DC produces is a function of its lineage and the way in which the cell is activated; engagement of different TLR and other surface receptors results in production of different cytokines in many instances. These cytokines have profound influences on the adaptive T-cell response by providing a third signal for the initial activation of the T cells and by directing the differentiation of the responding cells. It appears likely that the relative efficacies of different adjuvants for inducing protective or therapeutic T-cell responses to a given Ag or microorganism will be greatly influenced by the cytokines induced by each adjuvant.

## The Third Signal for Initiating the Response of Naïve T Cells

In order for naïve CD8 T cells to be activated to undergo clonal expansion and develop effector function they must receive signals 1 and 2, but also require a third signal that can be provided by IL-12 or IFNα *(22,24,32)*. Recent studies suggest that one subset of DC is ideally suited to provide all three signals to activate CD8 T cells. Three subclasses of murine DC can be distinguished based on their surface expression of CD8α and CD4; CD4–8+, CD4+8–, and CD4–8– *(56,57)*. The CD8– DC subsets most effectively activate class II restricted CD4 T cells, whereas CD8+ DC are more efficient for cross-presentation of Ag to CD8 T cells *(58)*. This is, in part, a result of this subset being the most efficient in shuttling Ag into the class I pathway *(59)*. Additionally, however, CD8+ DC produce high levels of IL-12 and IFNα on stimulation through TLR or CD40, although CD8– DC produce little of either cytokine *(60,61)*. Thus, DC of this subset appear to be ideally suited for activating CD8 T cells because of their ability to optimally provide all three signals required to initiate responses.

Either IL-12 or IFNα can provide the third signal in vivo that is needed to support maximal CD8 T-cell clonal expansion, development of effector functions and establishment of a long-lived memory population *(11,24,32)*. Furthermore, either supports development of protective or therapeutic CD8-mediated antitumor immunity when administered along with peptide Ag *(62)*. Whether there are differences in the responses at the levels of effector or memory cells, for example with respect to trafficking and tissue distribution, remains to be determined. Additionally, further studies are needed to determine if activation of CD4 T cells depends on a third signal delivered directly to the T cells, and whether activated DC can provide this signal.

## T-Cell Survival and Memory

To mount an effector response and develop a responsive memory population, T cells not only have to undergo clonal expansion, they also have to survive in sufficient numbers to be effective. Recent evidence suggests that cytokines produced by DC in response to adjuvants also influence this aspect of T-cell responses. Antiapoptotic proteins of the Bcl-2 family, including Bcl-2 and Bcl-$X_L$, are induced on TCR and CD28 ligation and help promote survival. However, Marrack and coworkers showed that this was not sufficient and that adjuvant could contribute to long-term survival in a manner that did not depend on effects on members of the Bcl-2 family *(62,63)*. More recently, using gene array analysis, the same group showed that adjuvants promote in vivo survival of T cells by inducing expression of Bcl-3, a member of the IκB gene family, and suggested that this might be mediated by inflammatory cytokines induced by the adjuvant *(64)*. This appears to be the case, as recent experiments have demonstrated that in vitro stimulation of naïve CD8 T cells with Ag and B7-1 does not upregulate Bcl-3, but it is upregulated when IL-12 is present and there is a concomitant increase in survival *(65)*. This suggests that signal 3 not only helps to initiate CD8 T-cell responses, but that it programs the cells for more effective survival. It was also found that IL-1, a putative third signal for CD4 T cells *(10,22)*, stimulates upregulation of Bcl-3 in these cells *(65)*. Consistent with the apparent requirement for distinct third signals for CD4 and CD8 T cells, IL-12 did not upregulate Bcl-3 in CD4 T cells and IL-1 did not upregulate Bcl-3 in CD8 T cells.

IL-15, another cytokine produced by DC in response to adjuvants such as LPS and double-stranded RNA *(66)*, is required to support the continuing survival of memory CD8 T cells by driving a low level of proliferative self-renewal of these cells *(67–69)*. Schluns et al. *(70)* have recently shown that IL-15 can act early in a virus-specific CD8 response to extend the primary proliferative phase of the response and yield a large memory pool. Over the first 5 to 6 days after infection with vesicular stomatitis virus, virus-specific CD8 cells underwent similar clonal expansion in normal and IL-15 deficient mice. Beyond that time, however, the number of Ag-specific CD8 cells continued to expand in normal mice but declined in IL-15 deficient mice, and the IL-15 deficient mice developed a smaller memory pool. Thus, adjuvant-induced production of IL-15 by DC may make a significant contribution to the size of the effector and memory populations that develop following initial activation of the T cells.

As in the case of CD8 T cells, immune memory for the CD4 T-cell subset is dependent on the survival of antigen-specific cells at the end of the primary response *(71,72)*. Such surviving memory CD4 T cells are located in secondary lymphoid and nonlymphoid organs. Initial exposure to antigen during the primary response must occur in the presence of an adjuvant for maximal numbers of memory CD4 T cells to survive in the secondary lymphoid organs, and for these cells to retain the capacity to produce IL-2 abundantly and rapidly *(1,10, 73)*. Additionally, an adjuvant must be present at the time of initial exposure to antigen for antigen-specific CD4 T cells to survive as memory cells in nonlymphoid organs *(74)*. The memory CD4 T cells that are present in nonlymphoid tissues after immunization with antigen plus adjuvant produce more IFNγ after in vivo re-challenge with antigen, than the cells present in the lymph nodes. The generation of memory CD4 T cells with IFNγ production potential in nonlymphoid organs probably depends on initial antigen recognition in the presence of an adjuvant because acquisition of IFNγ production potential by CD4 T cells is related to exposure to IL-12 *(75)* and multiple cell divisions *(76)*, both of which occur maximally in the presence of adjuvant-related inflammation.

*Shaping the T-Cell Response*

In addition to providing a third signal to initiate T-cell responses, cytokines produced in response to adjuvants also have roles in shaping the resulting T-cell responses by influencing the effector functions that the cells develop and the migration patterns of the effector cells. As one example, IL-12 cannot provide a third signal to support the initial activation of CD4 T cells, but once they have become activated IL-12 directs their development down the TH1 pathway *(10)*. Thus, the same cytokine that can provide the third signal to initiate CD8 responses also directs CD4 T-cell development to helper cells that can support the CD8 response. Inflammatory cytokines can also regulate the expression on T cells of a variety of receptors that mediate adhesion and migration. Thus, the spectrum of cytokines produced in response to a particular adjuvant interacting with specific TLRs will determine not only whether a T-cell response occurs, but will also determine the nature of the T-cell responses and the trafficking and locations of the resulting effector cells.

## BYPASSING THE USE OF CONVENTIONAL ADJUVANTS

Conventional adjuvants, bacterial and viral products, rapidly induce an innate response to both deal immediately with microorganisms by a variety of effector mechanisms, and to support induction of adaptive T-cell responses. Although this is beneficial when the challenge is with live infectious agents, it may be preferable to avoid some of the inflammatory sequelae when the goal is to induce T-cell immunity using defined protein or peptide antigens. In fact, these unwanted effects preclude the use of some of the most potent adjuvants for human immunizations.

One approach to bypassing conventional adjuvants is the use of isolated DC that have been activated and loaded with antigen in vitro, and then administered. This is receiving considerable attention as a means of activating T cells for tumor immunotherapy, and some promising results are being obtained *(77)*. Although potentially useful for therapeutic immunization for serious diseases, the time and labor intensity of this individualized approach will preclude its use for protective immunization on any large scale.

A second approach for bypassing conventional adjuvants is use of Ab or reagents that bind receptors on DC and directly activates them to mature and effectively present antigen. In this regard, anti-CD40 mAb have received the greatest attention *(78)*. Ligating CD40 on DCs stimulates their maturation, and upregulates expression of costimulatory ligands *(79)* and production of cytokines including IL-12 *(80)*. As a result, in vivo administration of anti-CD40 along with antigen can induce strong T-cell responses.

Finally, use of peptide antigens and the appropriate cytokine(s) may make it possible to bypass the need for DC activation altogether. Systemic administration of peptide likely results in presentation of the antigen on APC by binding directly to MHC proteins on the cell surface, avoiding the need to activate intracellular antigen-processing pathways. Because this will include APC resident in the spleen and lymph nodes, migration of the Ag-bearing DC to these sites is not necessary. Finally, if the appropriate cytokine is administered along with peptide to provide the third signal, potent T-cell activation will ensue. This has been demonstrated in murine adoptive transfer systems using IL-1 and peptide to induce CD4 T-cell responses *(10)* and IL-12 and peptide to induce potent CD8 cytolytic responses *(11,24)*. Similarly, administration of peptide and IL-12 to melanoma patients was shown to increase antigen-specific CD8 T-cell responses, using tetramers to detect the expanded T-cell population *(31)*. It remains to be determined whether such strategies provide protective or therapeutic immunity. It may be the case that additional cytokines will be needed to skew responses in the appropriate way, or modify the migration properties of the cells, depending on the organism or disease that the response is directed against.

## CONCLUSION

The importance of adjuvants for eliciting T-cell responses has been appreciated for many years, but the reasons for this have only recently begun to be understood. Now, however, immunology's "dirty little secret" *(7)* has been revealed as a complex interplay between the innate and adaptive responses, and a detailed understanding of the molecular and cellular basis of the adjuvant effect is rapidly developing. The major developments contributing to this growing understanding have been the realization that DC play the central role as APCs, the discovery that DCs use TLR to recognize components of adjuvants to lead to their activation, and the ability to visualize and quantitatively assess T-cell responses in vivo. The findings are already suggesting novel approaches for protective and therapeutic immunization, and hold great promise for rational design of vaccine strategies in the future.

## REFERENCES

1. Kearney E, Pape K, Loh D, Jenkins M. Visualization of peptide-specific T cell immunity and peripheral tolerance induction in vivo. Immunity 1994;1:327–339.
2. Pape K, Kearney E, Khoruts A, et al. Use of adoptive transfer of T-cell antigen-receptor-transgenic T cell for the study of T-cell activation in vivo. Immunol Rev 1997;156:67–78.
3. Rogers WO, Weaver CT, Kraus LA, Li J, Li L, Bucy RP. Visualization of antigen-specific T cell activation and cytokine expression in vivo. J Immunol 1997;158: 649-657.
4. Altman JD, Moss PAH, Goulder PJR, et al. Phenotypic analysis of antigen-specific T lymphocytes. Science 1996;274:94–96.
5. Kozono H, White J, Clements J, Marrack P, Kappler J. Production of soluble MHC class II proteins with covalently bound single peptides. Nature 1994;369:151–154.
6. O'Herrin SM, Lebowitz MS, Bieler JG, et al. Analysis of the expression of peptide-major histocompatibility complexes using high affinity soluble divalent T cell receptors. J Exp Med 1997;186:1333–1345.
7. Janeway CA Jr. Approaching the asymptote? Evolution and revolution in immunology. Cold Spring Harb Symp Quant Biol 1989;54:1–13.
8. Dresser DW. Effectiveness of lipid and lipidophilic substances as adjuvants. Nature 1961;191:1169–1171.
9. Dresser DW. Specific inhibition of antibody production. II. Paralysis induced in adult mice by small quantities of protein antigen. Immunology 1962;5:378–388.
10. Pape KA, Khoruts A, Mondino A, Jenkins MK. Inflammatory cytokines enhance the in vivo clonal expansion and differentiation of antigen-activated CD4+ T cells. J Immunol 1997;159:591–598.
11. Schmidt CS, Mescher MF. Adjuvant effect of IL-12: conversion of peptide antigen administration from tolerizing to immunizing for CD8$^+$ T cells in vivo. J Immunol 1999;163:2561–2567.

64                                                                      *Mescher et al.*

12. Kyburz D, Aichele P, Speiser D, Hengartner H, Zinkernagel R, Pircher H. T cell immunity after a viral infection versus T cell tolerance induced by soluble viral peptides. Eur J Immunol 1993;23:1956–1962.
13. Jennings R, Simms JR, Heath AW. Adjuvants and delivery systems for viral vaccines—mechanisms and potential. Dev Biol Stand 1998;92:19–28.
14. van der Heijden PJ, Bokhout BA, Bianchi AT, Scholten JW, Stok W. Separate application of adjuvant and antigen: the effect of a water-in- oil emulsion on the splenic plaque-forming cell response to sheep red blood cells in mice. Immunobiology 1986;171:143–154.
15. Lafferty KJ, Cunningham AJ. A new analysis of allogeneic interactions. Aust J Exp Biol Med Sci 1975;53:27–42.
16. Allison JP. CD28-B7 interactions in T cell activation. Curr Opin Immunol 1994;6:414–419.
17. Janeway CA, Bottomly K. Signals and signs for lymphocyte responses. Cell 1994;76:275–285.
18. Jenkins MK, Johnson JG. Molecules involved in T-cell costimulation. Curr Opin Immunol 1993;5:361–367.
19. Lafferty KJ, Prowse SJ, Simeonovic CJ, Warren HS. Immunobiology of tissue transplantation: a return to the passenger leukocyte concept. Annu Rev Immunol 1983;1:143–173.
20. Mueller D, Jenkins M, Schwartz R. Clonal expansion vs functional clonal inactivation. Annu Rev Immunol 1989;7:445–480.
21. Albert ML, Jegathesan M, Darnell RB. Dendritic cell maturation is required for the cross-tolerization of CD8+ T cells. Nat Immunol 2001;2:1010–1017.
22. Curtsinger JM, Schmidt CS, Mondino A, et al. Inflammatory cytokines provide third signals for activation of naive CD4+ and CD8+ T cells. J Immunol 1999;162:3256–3262.
23. Hernandez J, Aung S, Marquardt K, Sherman LA. Uncoupling of proliferative potential and gain of effector function by CD8(+) T cells responding to self-antigens. J Exp Med 2002;196:323–333.
24. Schmidt CS, Mescher MF. Peptide Ag priming of naive, but not memory, CD8 T cells requires a third signal that can be provided by IL-2. J Immunol 2002;168:5521–5529.
25. Jenkins M, Schwartz R. Antigen presentation by chemically modified splenocytes induces antigen-specific T cell unresponsiveness in vitro and in vivo. J Exp Med 1987;165:302–319.
26. Watts TH, DeBenedette MA. T cell co-stimulatory molecules other than CD28. Curr Opin Immunol 1999;11:286–293.
27. Deeths MJ, Mescher MF. ICAM-1 and B7-1 provide similar but distinct costimulation for CD8+ T cells, while CD4+ T cells are poorly costimulated by ICAM-1. Eur J Immunol 1999;29:45–53.
28. Rogers PR, Song J, Gramaglia I, Killeen N, Croft M. OX40 promotes Bcl-xL and Bcl-2 expression and is essential for long-term survival of CD4 T cells. Immunity 2001;15:445–455.
29. Sharpe AH, Freeman GJ. The B7-CD28 superfamily. Nat Rev Immunol 2002;2:116–126.

30. Trinchieri G. Interleukin-12: A proinflammatory cytokine with immunoregulatory functions that bridge innate resistance and antigen-specific adaptive immunity. Ann Rev Immunol 1995;13:251–276.
31. Lee P, Wang F, Kuniyoshi J, et al. Effects of interleukin-12 on the immune response to a multipeptide vaccine for resected metastatic melanoma. J Clin Oncol 2001; 19:3836–3847.
32. Curtsinger JM, Valenzuela JO, Agarwal P, Lins D, Mescher MF. Cutting edge: type I interferons provide a third signal to CD8 T cells to stimulate clonal expansion and differentiation. J Immunol 2005;174:4465–4469.
33. Brouckaert P, Libert C, Everaerdt B, Takahashi N, Cauwels A, Fiers W. Tumor necrosis factor, its receptors and the connection with interleukin 1 and interleukin 6. Immunobiology 1993;187:317.
34. Lemaitre B, Nicolas E, Michaut L, Reichhart JM, Hoffmann JA. The dorsoventral regulatory gene cassette spatzle/Toll/cactus controls the potent antifungal response in Drosophila adults. Cell 1996;86:973–983.
35. Medzhitov R, Preston-Hurlburt P, Janeway CA Jr. A human homologue of the Drosophila Toll protein signals activation of adaptive immunity. Nature 1997;388: 394–397.
36. Medzhitov R. Toll-like receptors and innate immunity. Nature Rev Immunol 2001; 1:135–145.
37. Aderem A, Ulevitch RJ. Toll-like receptors in the induction of the innate immune response. Nature 2000;406:782–787.
38. Kaisho T, Akira S. Toll-like receptors as adjuvant receptors. Biochim Biophys Acta 2002;1589:1–13.
39. Liu YJ. Dendritic cell subsets and lineages, and their functions in innate and adaptive immunity. Cell 2001;106:259–262.
40. Shortman K, Liu YJ. Mouse and human dendritic cell subtypes. Nature Rev Immunol 2002;2:151–161.
41. Ito T, Amakawa R, Kaisho T, et al. Interferon-alpha and interleukin-12 are induced differentially by Toll-like receptor 7 ligands in human blood dendritic cell subsets. J Exp Med 2002;195:1507–1512.
42. Henri S, Vremec D, Kamath A, et al. The dendritic cell populations of mouse lymph nodes. J Immunol 2001;167:741–748.
43. Nakano H, Yanagita M, Gunn MD. CD11c(+)B220(+)Gr-1(+) cells in mouse lymph nodes and spleen display characteristics of plasmacytoid dendritic cells. J Exp Med 2001;194:1171–1178.
44. Ruedl C, Koebel P, Bachmann M, Hess M, Karjalainen K. Anatomical origin of dendritic cells determines their life span in peripheral lymph nodes. J Immunol 2000;165:4910–4916.
45. Banchereau J, Steinman RM. Dendritic cells and the control of immunity. Nature 1998;392:245–252.
46. Sallusto F, Lanzavecchia A. Understanding dendritic cell and T-lymphocyte traffic through the analysis of chemokine receptor expression. Immunol Rev 2000; 177:134–140.
47. Mellman I, Steinman RM. Dendritic cells: specialized and regulated antigen processing machines. Cell 2001;106:255–258.

48. Cella M, Engering A, Pinet V, Pieters J, Lanzavecchia A. Inflammatory stimuli induce accumulation of MHC class II complexes on dendritic cells. Nature 1997; 388:782–787.
49. Epperson DE, Arnold D, Spies T, Cresswell P, Pober JS, Johnson DR. Cytokines increase transporter in antigen processing-1 expression more rapidly than HLA class I expression in endothelial cells. J Immunol 1992;149:3297–3301.
50. De Smedt T, Pajak B, Muraille E, et al. Regulation of dendritic cell numbers and maturation by lipopolysaccharide in vivo. J Exp Med 1996;184:1413–1424.
51. Khoruts A, Mondino A, Pape KA, Reiner SL, Jenkins M. A natural immunological adjuvant enhances T cell clonal expansion through a CD28-dependent, IL-2-independent mechanism. J Exp Med 1998;187:225–236.
52. Kneitz B, Herrmann T, Yonehara S, Schimpl A. Normal clonal expansion but impaired Fas-mediated cell death and anergy induction in interleukin-2-deficient mice. Eur J Immunol 1995;25:2572–2577.
53. Leung DT, Morefield S, Willerford DM. Regulation of lymphoid homeostasis by IL-2 receptor signals in vivo. J Immunol 2000;164:3527–3534.
54. Lantz O, Grandjean I, Matzinger P, Di Santo JP. Gamma chain required for naive CD4+ T cell survival but not for antigen proliferation. Nat Immunol 2000;1: 54–58.
55. D'Souza WN, Schluns KS, Masopust D, Lefrancois L. Essential role for IL-2 in the regulation of antiviral extralymphoid CD8 T cell responses. J Immunol 2002; 168:5566–5572.
56. Kamath AT, Pooley J, O'Keeffe MA, et al. The development, maturation, and turnover rate of mouse spleen dendritic cell populations. J Immunol 2000;165: 6762–6770.
57. Vremec D, Pooley J, Hochrein H, Wu L, Shortman K. CD4 and CD8 expression by dendritic cell subtypes in mouse thymus and spleen. J Immunol 2000;164:2978–2986.
58. Pooley JL, Heath WR, Shortman K. Cutting edge: intravenous soluble antigen is presented to CD4 T cells by CD8– dendritic cells, but cross-presented to CD8 T cells by CD8+ dendritic cells. J Immunol 2001;166:5327–5330.
59. Heath WR, Carbone FR. Cross-presentation, dendritic cells, tolerance and immunity. Annu Rev Immunol 2001;19:47–64.
60. Maldonado-Lopez R, De Smedt T, Michel P, et al. CD8alpha+ and CD8alpha– subclasses of dendritic cells direct the development of distinct T helper cells in vivo. J Exp Med 1999;189:587–592.
61. Hochrein H, Shortman K, Vremec D, Scott B, Hertzog P, O'Keeffe M. Differential production of IL-12, IFN-alpha, and IFN-gamma by mouse dendritic cell subsets. J Immunol 2001;166:5448–5455.
62. Mitchell T, Kappler J, Marrack P. Bystander virus infection prolongs activated T cell survival. J Immunol 1999;162:4527–4535.
63. Vella AT, Mitchell T, Groth B, et al. CD28 engagement and proinflammatory cytokines contribute to T cell expansion and long-term survival in vivo. J Immunol 1997;158:4714–4720.
64. Mitchell TC, Hildeman D, Kedl RM, et al. Immunological adjuvantsd promote activated T cell survival via induction of Bcl-3. Nat Immunol 2001;2:397–402.

65. Valenzuela JO, Hammerbeck C, Mescher MF. Cutting edge: Bcl-3 upregulation by signal 3 cytokine (IL-12) prolongs survival of Ag-activated CD8 T cells. J Immunol 2005;174:600–604.
66. Mattei F, Schiavoni G, Belardelli F, Tough DF. IL-15 is expressed by dendritic cells in response to type I IFN, double-stranded RNA, or lipopolysaccharide and promotes dendritic cell activation. J Immunol 2001;167:1179–1187.
67. Ku CC, Murakami M, Sakamoto A, Kappler J, Marrack P. Control of homeostasis of CD8+ memory T cells by opposing cytokines. Science 2000;288:675–678.
68. Sprent J, Surh CD. Generation and maintenance of memory T cells. Curr Opin Immunol 2001;13:248–254.
69. Zhang X, Sun S, Hwang I, Tough DF, Sprent J. Potent and selective stimulation of memory-phenotype CD8+ T cells in vivo by IL-15. Immunity 1998;8:591–599.
70. Schluns KS, Williams K, Ma, A, Zheng XX, Lefrancois, L. Cutting edge: requirement for IL-15 in the generation of primary and memory antigen-specific CD8 T cells. J Immunol 2002;168:4827–4831.
71. Antia R, Pilyugin SS, Ahmed R. Models of immune memory: on the role of cross-reactive stimulation, competition, and homeostasis in maintaining immune memory. Proc Natl Acad Sci USA 1998;95:14926–14931.
72. Homann D, Teyton L, Oldstone MB. Differential regulation of antiviral T-cell immunity results in stable CD8+ but declining CD4+ T-cell memory. Nat Med 2001;7:913–919.
73. Pape KA, Merica R, Mondino A, Khoruts A, Jenkins MK. Direct evidence that functionally impaired CD4+ T cells persist in vivo following induction of peripheral tolerance. J Immunol 1998;160:4719–4729.
74. Reinhardt RL, Khoruts A, Merica R, Zell T, Jenkins MK. Visualizing the generation of memory CD4 T cells in the whole body. Nature 2001;410:101–105.
75. Murphy KM, Ouyang W, Farrar JD, et al. Signaling and transcription in T helper development. Annu Rev Immunol 2000;18:451–494.
76. Bird JJ, Brown DR, Mullen AC, et al. Helper T cell differentiation is controlled by the cell cycle. Immunity 1998;9:229–237.
77. Banchereau J, Schuler-Thurner B, Palucka AK, Schuler G. Dendritic cells as vectors for therapy. Cell 2001;106:271–274.
78. Grewal I, Flavell R. CD40 and CD154 in cell-mediated immunity. Ann Rev Immunol 1998;16:111–135.
79. Ranheim EA, Kipps TJ. Activated T cells induce expression of B7/BB1 on normal or leukemic B cells through a CD40-dependent signal. J Exp Med 1993;177:925–935.
80. Cella M, Scheidegger D, Palmer-Lehmann K, Lane P, Lanzavecchia A, Alber G. Ligation of CD40 on dendritic cells triggers production of high levels of interleukin-12 and enhances T cell stimulatory capacity: T-T help via APC activation. J Exp Med 1996;184:747–752.

# 5

# Mechanism for Recognition of CpG DNA

## Kiyoshi Takeda, Hiroaki Hemmi, and Shizuo Akira

### INTRODUCTION

Bacterial deoxyribonucleic acid (DNA) containing cytosine phosphate guanine (CpG) motifs, but not vertebrate DNA, activates innate immune cells. CpG motifs in vertebrate DNA are suppressed and usually methylated. In contrast, CpG motifs in bacterial DNA are observed at the expected frequency and unmethylated, which causes immune cell activation. CpG DNA activation of immune cells is reproducible in synthetic oligonucleotides containing CpG motifs. Treatment with CpG DNA induces a potent immune response dominated by Th1 cell-mediated cellular immunity, which prevents and cures several infectious and immune diseases in animal models. CpG DNA is therefore promising as a clinically useful agent for the treatment of several human diseases including cancer, allergy, and infectious diseases. The molecular mechanism of CpG DNA-induced cellular activation has been investigated intensively, and a signaling pathway is now being revealed. The critical components that recognize CpG DNA have recently been identified. In this chapter, we focus on the recent advances in the CpG DNA-induced activation of innate immune cells.

### CpG DNA IS A POTENT IMMUNOSTIMULANT

#### Discovery of Bacterial DNA As an Immunostimulant

The innate immune system recognizes specific patterns of microbial structures such as lipopolysaccharide (LPS) and lipoprotein. These structures have been called pattern-associated molecular patterns (PAMPs) (1–3). The features of PAMPs can be attributed to their ability to stimulate the innate immune cells and the commonly observed structures in several microbial organisms. The majority of PAMPs, including LPS and lipoprotein, are cell wall components of the pathogens. Bacterial DNA, although not a microbial cell wall component, has also been shown to possess the ability to activate innate immune cells (4–6). In the 1970s, treatment with *Mycobacterium bovis* or Bacillus Calmette and Guerin (BCG) was shown to be effective in causing the regression of cancer in several

From: *Vaccine Adjuvants: Immunological and Clinical Principles*
Edited by: C. J. Hackett and D. A. Harn, Jr. © Humana Press Inc., Totowa, NJ

experimental models and in humans. Tokunaga and colleagues tried to identify the responsible component in BCG, and found that the DNA fraction could induce regression of tumors in vivo and enhance natural killer (NK) cell activity in vitro *(7,8)*. Thus, they first demonstrated that bacterial DNA is a potent activator of innate immunity.

## Unmethylated CpG Motif Is Responsible for Immunostimulatory Activity of Bacterial DNA

Tokunaga and colleagues extended their work with synthetic oligodeoxynucleotides (ODNs), and further showed that the palindromic sequences, containing unmethylated CpG dinucleotides, are responsible for the immunostimulatory activity *(9,10)*. Independently of these studies, several investigators utilizing antisense ODNs became aware that antisense ODNs possessing nuclease-resistant phosphorothioate backbones activate immune cells. They tried to identify sequences in ODNs that activate the immune cells, and finally, Krieg and colleagues demonstrated that a simple sequence motif based on an unmethylated CpG dinucleotide (5'-Pu-Pu-CpG-Pyr-Pyr-3') accounts for the immunostimulatory activity of ODNs in the mouse *(11)*. Furthermore, like LPS, bacterial DNA containing unmethylated CpG dinucleotides was shown to induce lethal shock when co-administered with D-galactosamine in mice *(12,13)*. In this respect, bacterial DNA can be clarified as one of the PAMPs *(3)*.

The mammalian immune system is activated by bacterial DNA but not by vertebrate DNA This is because of structural differences. CpG motifs are observed at the expected frequency of 1:16 in bacterial genomic DNA. By contrast, the frequency of CpG motifs in vertebrate genomic DNA is below one-fourth of that predicted (CpG suppression) *(14)*. In addition to CpG, cytosines of CpG motifs in vertebrate genomic DNA are highly methylated (CpG methylation). Methylation at the C-5 position of the cytosine of the CpG motif is shown to eliminate immunostimulatory activity *(11)*. Thus, a distinct CpG frequency and methylation lead to the structural difference between bacterial and vertebrate DNA. The mammalian immune system appears to recognize these differences, and respond only to bacterial DNA.

## CpG DNA AS A VACCINE ADJUVANT

### DNA Vaccine

The development of vaccination has made a great contribution to protection for infectious diseases. Vaccination with a peptide antigen elicits antibody-mediated antigen-specific humoral immune responses, which are most effective for protection against viral and bacterial infection. However, peptide antigen is less effective against infectious diseases caused by intracellular organisms such as tuberculosis, malaria, and leishmaniasis. Cellular immunity characterized by a T helper 1(Th1)-biased immune response is required to combat these infectious organisms. In trials of vaccination against these organisms, we had difficulty in developing an effective vaccine using peptide antigens. The antigens can only be derived from live or live attenuated organisms, which is inconvenient for use worldwide both from a financial perspective and in terms of safety *(15)*. Intramuscular injection of bacteria-derived plasmid DNA including β-galactosidase (β-Gal) was demonstrated to induce strong expression of β-Gal in myocytes and monocytes at the injection sites in mice *(16)*. It has also been shown that administration of plasmid DNA-encoding human growth hormone elicits an antigen-specific immune response in mice *(17)*. Subsequently, injection of plasmid DNA encoding a bacterial or viral protein has been shown to be protective in several animal models of infection with enhancement of both humoral and Th1-biased cellular immunity *(18–23)*. From these findings, the plasmid DNA is now anticipated to be useful for prevention of several infectious diseases as a "vaccine DNA," and indeed is in the course of clinical trials *(15,24–26)*.

## CpG DNA As an Adjuvant for DNA Vaccine

The effect of the plasmid DNA as a potent DNA vaccine has now been attributed to the presence of CpG motifs present in the bacteria-derived plasmid backbone DNA. Induction of preferential Th1 response by CpG DNA treatment has been demonstrated in several animal models. CpG DNA administration provided increased interleukin (IL)-12 production and resistance to infection by intracellular pathogens such as *Listeria monocytogenes (27,28)*. CpG DNA induction of a strong Th1 response was also demonstrated in BALB/c mice infected with *Leishmania major*, which normally show a preferential Th2-type response *(29)*. In these mice, CpG DNA treatment augmented the production of IFNγ (increased Th1 response) and diminished the IL-4 production (decreased Th2 response). Important roles for CpG DNA as an adjuvant for vaccines have been demonstrated with reports that co-administration of CpG DNA and soluble peptide antigen induced Th1-skewed immune responses when compared with administration of peptide antigen alone *(30–33)*. The introduction of CpG motifs into the backbone of the plasmid DNA has been shown to improve the resultant antigen-specific humoral response and cellular immune response *(34–36)*. These studies indicate that CpG motifs in the plasmid DNA act as intrinsic adjuvants to enhance the protective immune response against pathogens *(33,37)*.

## CpG DNA-Induced Maturation of Dendritic Cells

The mechanism by which CpG DNA induces a strong Th1 response in several animal models is being clarified. Dendritic cells (DCs) are the main cells that link innate immunity (recognition of PAMPs and induction of inflammatory responses) with acquired immunity (antigen-specific immune responses;

e.g., Th1 responses). Several independent groups demonstrated that CpG DNA induced maturation of DCs such as production of IL-12, and expression of costimulatory molecules *(38–40)*. We therefore propose the following model: CpG DNA is recognized by and induces maturation of DCs, leading to production of IL-12. IL-12, in turn, induces the development of Th1 cells from naïve T cells to employ an effective immune response. Thus, DCs contribute to preferential Th1 responses in CpG DNA-treated animal models.

## CpG DNA-MEDIATED SIGNALING PATHWAY IN INNATE IMMUNE CELLS

### The Molecular Mechanism for Action of CpG DNA

Because of the promising effect of CpG DNA as an adjuvant for vaccines, much effort has been made to reveal the molecular mechanism behind the action of CpG DNA *(5,6,40)*. Notably, CpG DNA-mediated signaling pathways including cellular uptake of CpG DNA, translocation into endosome, and activation of signaling molecules leading to activation of transcription factors, have been clarified.

### Cellular Uptake of CpG DNA

Following binding to the cell surface receptor, CpG DNA is internalized into cells. Krieg and colleagues demonstrated that internalization of CpG DNA is an essential step in the activation of the immune cells using CpG DNA immobilized on Teflon fibers, or avidin-coated plates *(11)*. Tokunaga and colleagues demonstrated the activation of B cells by direct uptake of CpG DNA by lipofection, indicating that the binding of the CpG DNA to the cell surface receptor is not, but the internalization, is essential for cellular activation *(42)*. Additionally, recognition of CpG DNA by the cell surface receptor and uptake of CpG DNA appear to have no sequence specificity *(11,43)*. CpG DNA and non-CpG DNA were similarly taken up into the cells, and further, non-CpG DNA effectively competed with the uptake of CpG DNA *(44)*. Although Mac-1 (CD11b/CD18) was one of the candidates for the cell surface receptors for CpG DNA *(45)*, knockout mice lacking Mac-1 have been shown to have a normal capacity to internalize CpG DNA *(5)*. Therefore, the cell surface receptor for CpG DNA is still to be defined.

### Localization of CpG DNA in the Endosome

Following internalization, CpG DNA is rapidly localized to acidic vesicles of the endosomal–lysosomal compartment in mouse macrophages, which is similar to the endosomal localization of the antisense phosphorothioate ODN in the premyelocytic leukemic cell line HL60, *(44,46)*. Chloroqine inhibits the pH-dependent maturation of endosome by acting as a basic substance to neutralize acidification in the vesicle *(47)*. Bafilomycin A also prevents endosomal maturation by inhibiting acidification through the blocking of hydrogen-ion pumps *(48)*. These two compounds have been shown to block cellular activation in response to CpG DNA, but not to LPS or phorbol 12-myristate 13-acetate *(44,49–51)*. Treatment with these compounds does not affect the internalization or vesicular localization of CpG DNA *(44)*. These findings indicate that the CpG DNA-induced activation of immune cells requires endosomal maturation. There might be several explanations for the relation between the CpG DNA-induced cellular activation and the endosomal acidification. First, the endosomal acidification might enable the uptaken CpG DNA to dissociate from nonspecific cell surface receptors and bind to a specific receptor in the endosome. Second, the endosomal acidification might be essential for the release of the CpG DNA from the endosome to the cytoplasm in which a specific receptor exists. Alternatively, there might be an unknown mechanism for activation of a CpG DNA signaling pathway.

## CpG DNA-Induced Activation of Mitogen-Activated Protein Kinases

Several inflammatory stimuli, including PAMPs such as LPS, have been shown to activate mitogen-activated protein kinases (MAPKs). LPS has been shown to activate three types of MAPKs, that is, the p38 MAPK, the c-Jun NH2-terminal kinase (JNK), and the extracellular receptor kinases (ERKs). Like LPS, CpG DNA, when administered to macrophages, DCs, and B cells, has been shown to induce activation of p38 and JNK *(44,51)*. Treatment of macrophages with p38 inhibitor inhibited the CpG DNA-induced production of IL-12, and tumor necrosis factor-$\alpha$, indicating that p38 is indispensable for CpG DNA-induced cytokine production in macrophages *(44)*. Treatment of macrophages with bafilomycin A or chloroquine also abrogated CpG DNA-induced production of IL-12, and tumor necrosis factor-$\alpha$, and activation of p38 and JNK *(44,51)*. This indicates that endosomal maturation is essential for CpG DNA-induced activation of signal transduction pathways leading to inflammatory responses.

Activation of ERK is somewhat controversial. According to a report by Yi et al., CpG DNA did not seem to activate ERK in B cells and a macrophage cell line (J774) *(51)*. By contrast, ERK has been reported to be activated in response to CpG DNA in primary macrophages and the macrophage cell line RAW264.7 *(52)*. Even in this report, CpG DNA did not activate ERK in DCs *(52)*.

## CpG DNA-Induced Activation of Transcription Factors

As in the LPS signaling pathway, CpG DNA-induced activation of JNK leads to phosphorylation of the AP-1 family of transcription factors, and activation of p38 leads to activation of transcription factor ATF2 *(44,51)*.

In addition to these transcription factors, CpG DNA has been shown to activate NF-κB, a family of transcription factors responsible for several aspects of inflammatory and immune responses *(13,50,53)*. The subunits of NF-κB transcription factors activated by CpG DNA are mainly p50 and p65 components *(13)*. Acidification of endosome was shown to lead to the rapid generation of intracellular reactive oxygen species, followed by NF-κB activation *(50)*. Additionally, treatment with bafilomycin A or chloroquine inhibited activation of NF-κB transcription factors. These findings indicate that CpG DNA-induced activation of NF-κB also requires endosomal maturation *(44,51)*. Thus, the endosomal maturation is indispensable for activation of almost all of the CpG DNA-mediated signaling cascades.

## RECOGNITION OF MICROBIAL COMPONENTS BY INNATE IMMUNE CELLS

### Innate Immune Recognition of Pathogens in Drosophila

The immune response to invading microbial pathogens consists of innate and acquired immunity. Innate immune cells recognize PAMPs (such as LPS and lipoproteins) by the germline-encoded -nonclonal receptor. This receptor, which is called a pattern recognition receptor, is activated immediately after infection and controls expansion of microbial pathogens by induction of inflammatory response *(2,3)*. In contrast, acquired immunity exerts a highly sophisticated antigen-specific immune response against microbial pathogens in mammals. Therefore, mammalian innate immunity has long been considered to act only as a first line of host defense until the antigen-specific acquired immunity develops. However, *Drosophila* with no acquired immunity, show an effective host defense response against microbial invasion through synthesis of antimicrobial peptides *(54)*. The antimicrobial peptides have been shown to be induced through activation of the signaling pathways via two Toll receptors, Toll and 18-wheeler *(55,56)*. Toll is essential for induction of antifungal peptides, whereas 18-wheeler regulates induction of antibacterial peptides. Further, fruit flies mutated in Toll and 18-wheeler are susceptible to infection by fungi and bacteria, respectively. Thus, in *Drosophila*, at least two Toll family proteins discriminate between pathogens, and induce effective host defense responses *(54)*. The Toll family has now been expanded to include eight family members in *Drosophila (57)*. The function of these newly identified members remains to be defined.

### Identification of Toll-Like Receptors in Mammals

Medzhitov and Janeway made efforts to find a mammalian protein that is related to *Drosophila* Toll. This finally led to identification of a human homologue (now designated TLR4) *(58)*. Subsequently, several proteins related to the first identified human Toll have been identified, and are now called Toll-like receptors (TLRs). The TLR family now consists of at least 10 members (TLR1-TLR9 and one is deposited to DNA databases), and will expand *(59–62)*. The role of the TLR family, especially TLR2, and TLR4, in the recognition of pathogens is being rapidly established.

## Innate Immune Recognition by TLR2 and TLR4

Two independent groups analyzed the gene responsible for hypo-responsiveness to LPS in mice, and found mutations in the *Tlr4* gene *(63,64)*. In the C3H/HeJ mouse strain, a point mutation was found that resulted in an amino acid change from proline to histidine in the cytoplasmic region of TLR4. This single amino acid conversion has been shown to result in defective TLR4-mediated signaling *(65)*. Another LPS hypo-responsive strain, C57BL10/ScCr, was shown to be null mutated in the *Tlr4* gene *(63,64)*. Generation of mice genetically deficient in *Tlr4* by gene targeting also demonstrated that TLR4-deficient mice are hypo-responsive to LPS, confirming that TLR4 is an essential receptor for recognition of LPS *(65)*. Although initial studies with overexpression of TLR2, in human embryonic kidney 293 cells indicated that TLR2 confers LPS responsiveness *(66,67)*, subsequent studies in mice lacking TLR2 or chinese hamster ovary fibroblasts demonstrated that TLR2 is not involved in the recognition of LPS *(68,69)*. Repurification of LPS also demonstrated that TLR4, but not TLR2, is a receptor for LPS *(70,71)*. Further study indicated that TLR2 recognizes several cell wall components from a variety of microbial pathogens, including Gram-positive bacteria *(72–74)*, mycobacteria *(75–77)*, spirochetes *(78)*, and yeast *(79)*. Generation of TLR2-deficient mice revealed a pivotal role for TLR2 in the recognition of bacterial cell wall components, such as peptidoglycan from Gram-positive bacteria and lipoproteins in several kinds of microbial organisms *(68,80)*. As a result, TLR2-deficient mice were shown to be susceptible to infection by *Staphylococcus aureus (81)*.

Recently, a new feature of TLR-mediated recognition of microbial pathogens was reported. TLR1 and TLR6, both of which are highly homologous *(60)*, were shown to cooperate with TLR2, and discriminate between the patterns of pathogens *(82–84)*. Aderem and colleagues demonstrated that TLR6 combines with TLR2 to detect the specific pattern of peptidoglycan *(82)*. Functional interaction of TLR6 and TLR2 for discrimination between microbial lipopeptides was recently demonstrated in a study with TLR6-deficient mice *(85)*. In that report, TLR6-deficient macrophages were unresponsive to mycoplasma-derived dipalmitoyl lipopeptides, but responsive to dipalmitoyl lipopeptides derived from other bacteria; whereas TLR2-deficient macrophages were unresponsive to either type of lipopeptide. The study also indicates the existence of other TLRs that functionally associate with TLR2 for recognizing dipalmitoyl lipopeptides.

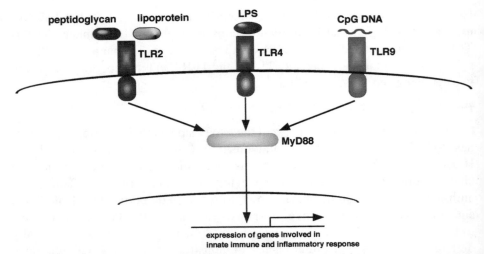

**Fig. 1.** Toll-like receptors (TLRs) in recognition of microbial components. Among 10 known mammalian TLR family members, TLR2, 4, and 9, have been implicated in recognition of bacterial components. TLR2 is responsible for recognition of peptidoglycan and lipoprotein, whereas TLR4 recognizes LPS. Recently TLR9 was shown to be a receptor for CpG DNA. Thus, the TLR family discriminates between the specific patterns of bacterial components.

Thus, the TLR family recognizes the PAMPs, and discriminates between their specific structures to activate innate immunity (Fig. 1) *(86,87)*.

## RECOGNITION OF CpG DNA BY INNATE IMMUNE CELLS

### *CpG DNA-Induced Cellular Activation Is TLR-Dependent*

The signaling pathway via the TLR family is highly homologous to that of the IL-1 receptor (IL-1R) family. The cytoplasmic portion of both TLR and IL-1R has a Toll/IL-1R homology domain, essential for signal transduction. Both TLR and IL-1R interact with an adaptor protein MyD88 in their Toll/IL-1R homology domains to transduce the signals to a downstream kinase, IL-1 receptor-associated kinase (IRAK) *(88–92)*. MyD88-deficient mice were shown to be unresponsive to the IL-1 family cytokines *(93)*. Additionally, MyD88-deficient mice showed no inflammatory responses to peptidoglycan and LPS, which are recognized by TLR2 and TLR4, respectively *(94,95)*. These results indicate that MyD88 is a critical adaptor in both IL-1R- and TLR- (at least, TLR2- and TLR4-) mediated signaling pathways.

The involvement of MyD88 in CpG DNA-induced cellular activation was also demonstrated *(96,97)*. In MyD88-deficient mice, CpG DNA-induced proliferation of B cells, cytokine production of macrophages, and maturation of DCs

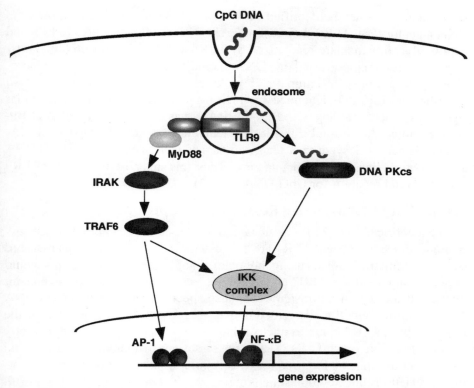

**Fig. 2.** Postulated signaling pathways induced by CpG DNA. CpG DNA binds to a nonspecific receptor on the cell surface, and is internalized into the cells. Internalization of CpG DNA induces maturation and acidification of endosome, the sequence-specific CpG DNA receptor (TLR9) exists. TLR9 may recognize CpG DNA there, and activate MyD88-dependent signaling pathways leading to activation of NF-κB. Additionally, acidification of endosome may allow CpG DNA to escape into the cytoplasm, in which another sequence-specific receptor (DNA-PKcs) exists. DNA-PKcs may recognize CpG DNA in the cytoplasm leading to activation of NF-κB.

were completely abolished. In contrast, CpG DNA-induced cellular activation was not impaired in TLR2- and TLR4-deficient mice, indicating that other members of the TLR family participate in the CpG DNA-mediated signaling pathway (Fig. 2).

## *TLR9 Is an Essential Receptor*
## *for CpG DNA-Induced Immune Response*

Subsequent to the indication of a role for the TLR family in CpG DNA recognition, experiments on gene deletion in mice led to elucidation of the CpG

DNA receptor. A newly identified TLR, TLR9, has been shown to be the CpG DNA receptor *(98)*. TLR9-deficient mice showed normal responses to LPS and peptidoglycan, which are recognized by TLR4 and TLR2, respectively. However, the cellular response to CpG DNA, including B-cell proliferation, macrophage production of inflammatory cytokines, and DC maturation, were all abolished in TLR9-deficient mice. CpG DNA-induced activation of intracellular signaling events, including NF-κB, JNK, IRAK, was also compromised in TLR9-deficient mice. Accordingly, TLR9-deficient mice were resistant to CpG DNA-induced lethal shock syndrome. Thus, cellular and in vivo responses to CpG DNA are not observed in TLR9-deficient mice. Thus, this study established that TLR9 is an essential receptor for CpG DNA (Fig. 2).

## Mechanism TLR9-Mediated Recognition of CpG DNA

The identification of TLR9 as an essential receptor for CpG DNA raised several questions. TLR2 and TLR4 are expressed on the cell surface as assessed by flowcytometric analysis using monoclonal antibodies *(99–102)*. This would indicate that ligands for TLR2 and TLR4 are recognized by receptors expressed on the cell surface. In contrast, the sequence-specific recognition of CpG DNA occurs within the cell as described above. At present, the localization of the CpG receptor, TLR9, remains unclear. However, structural features apparently indicate that, like other TLRs, TLR9, possesses a transmembrane portion and signal peptides that are required for extracellular transport of proteins, indicating that TLR9 is not a cytoplasmic protein *(98)*. It is intriguing whether TLR9, is expressed on endosomal membrane or extracellular membrane. Visualization of subcellular TLR9 localization will shed new light on the mechanism for recognition of CpG DNA by TLR9.

Another question is whether TLR9 directly binds to CpG DNA. Until now, no data has been published that indicates the direct binding of PAMPs with TLRs. This is probably because of the difficulty in manipulating PAMPs, such as LPS and lipopeptides. CpG DNA seems to be easier to manipulate than other PAMPs. Analysis of whether CpG DNA is recognized by TLR9 directly or indirectly will hopefully not only lead to elucidation of other mechanisms of CpG DNA recognition but also settle the question of whether bacterial components are the real ligands for TLRs (directly bind to TLRs) or not.

## DNA-PKcs As a Modulator for CpG DNA-Induced Immune Response

Independent of the identification of TLR9 as the CpG receptor DNA, another group has demonstrated the involvement of the catalytic subunit of DNA-dependent protein kinase (DNA-PKcs) in the CpG DNA-induced immune cell activation *(103)*. DNA-PKcs is a member of the phosphatidyl-inositol-3 kinase (PI-3K) family, localized in the nucleus and cytoplasm. In the nucleus, DNA-PKcs is activated in the process of repair of DNA double-stranded breaks caused by stress-induced damage from ionized radiation and by programmed DNA rearrangement (called VDJ recombination) during development of T and B cells *(104–106)*. However, the role of DNA-PKcs localized in the cytoplasm was unclear. Raz and colleagues demonstrated that macrophages from DNA-PKcs knockout mice did not produce inflammatory cytokines in response to CpG DNA. They further showed that CpG DNA-induced cellular activation in wild-type macrophages could be blocked by addition of wortmannin, an inhibitor of PI-3K, and that CpG DNA-induced activation of DNA-PKcs, in turn led to activation of NF-κB in vitro and in vivo. Thus, DNA-PKcs has been shown to be closely involved in the CpG DNA-induced immune responses.

## TLR9- and DNA-PKcs-Mediated Recognition of CpG DNA

Recent independent studies, identifying the involvement of TLR9 and DNA-PKcs in CpG DNA recognition, have made a great contribution to our understanding of the mechanism of CpG DNA-induced immune cell activation. When we consider that CpG DNA is a PAMP and that many PAMPs are recognized by TLR family members, the recognition of CpG DNA by TLR9 seems reasonable. This is emphasized by the finding that mice lacking MyD88, an essential adaptor molecule in the TLR-mediated signaling pathways, also showed no response to CpG DNA *(96,97)*. However, as described above, several questions remain to be answered before we can conclude that TLR9 is the real CpG DNA receptor.

Recognition of CpG DNA by DNA-PKcs seems rather unexpected and therefore exciting. But again, several points remain to be clarified before we can conclude that DNA-PKcs is the real CpG DNA receptor. It is well recognized that DNA-PKcs identifies DNA double-stranded breaks, but it is of interest how DNA-PKcs recognizes a specific sequence such as the CpG motifs. Secondly, a report that SCID mice lacking the catalytic activity of DNA-PK showed a normal response to CpG DNA seems contradictory to that of Raz and colleagues *(107)*. Finally, DNA-PKcs should recognize CpG DNA outside of the endosome, probably in the cytoplasm. If so, CpG DNA should escape from the endosome to the cytoplasm. Therefore, it is worth following the migration of CpG DNA from the surface via the endosome to the cytoplasm. Thus, there may exist an additional unveiled signaling event in the process of CpG DNA-induced cellular activation.

At present, a connection between TLR9 and DNA-PKcs in the recognition of CpG DNA can not easily be imagined. However, knockout of either molecule in mice disrupts the response to CpG DNA, indicating the critical involvement of both in the recognition of CpG DNA. Elucidation of the connection between TLR9 and DNA-PKcs is important if one is to fully understand the mechanism for recognition of CpG DNA.

## ACKNOWLEDGMENTS

We thank N. Tsuji for excellent secretarial assistance. This work was supported by grants from Special Coordination Funds of the Ministry of Education, Culture, Sports, Science and Technology; the Naito Foundation; and the Novartis Foundation for the Promotion of Science.

## REFERENCES

1. Janeway CA, Jr. Aproaching the asymptote? Evolution and revolution in immunology. Cold Spring Hab Symp Quant Biol 1989;54:1–13.
2. Medzhitov R, Janeway CA, Jr. Innate Immunity: the virtues of a nonclonal system of recognition. Cell 1997;91:295–298.
3. Medzhitov R, Janeway CA, Jr. Innate immunity: impact on the adaptive immune response. Curr Opin Immunol 1997;9:4–9.
4. Wagner H. Bacterial CpG DNA activates immune cells to signal infectious danger. Adv Immunol 1999;73:329–367.
5. Krieg AM, Hartmann GH, Yi A-K. Mechanism of action of CpG DNA. Curr Top Microbiol Immunol 2000;247:1–21.
6. Stacey KJ, Sester DP, Sweet MJ, Hume DA. Macrophage activation by immunostimulatory DNA. Curr Top Microbiol Immunol 2000;247:41–58.
7. Tokunaga T, Yamamoto H, Shimada S, et al. Antitumor activity of deoxyribonucleic acid fraction from mycobacterium bovis BCG. I. Isolation, physicochemical characterization, and antitumor activity. J Natl Cancer Inst 1984;72:955–962.
8. Yamamoto S, Kuramoto E, Shimada S, Tokunaga T. In vitro augmentation of natural killer cell activity and production of interferon-$\alpha/\beta$ and -$\gamma$ with deoxyribonucleic acid fraction from mycobacterium bovis BCG. Jpn J Cancer Res 1988; 79:866–873.
9. Kuramoto E, Yano O, Kimura Y, et al. Oligonucleotide sequences required for natural killer cell activation. Jpn J Cancer Res 1992;83:1128–1131.
10. Yamamoto S, Yamamoto T, Kataoka T, Kuramoto E, Yano O, Tokunaga T. Unique palindromic sequences in synthetic oligonucleotides are required to induce IFN and augment INF-mediated natural killer cells activity. J Immunol 1992;148:4072–4076.
11. Krieg AM, Yi A-K, Matson S, et al. CpG motifs in bacterial DNA trigger direct B cell activation. Nature 1995;374:546–549.
12. Sparwasser T, Miethke T, Lipford G, et al. Bacterial DNA causes septic shock. Nature 1997;386:336–337.
13. Sparwasser T, Miethke T, Lipford G, et al. Macrophages sense pathogens via DNA motifs: induction of tumor necrosis factor-$\alpha$-mediated shock. Eur J Immunol 1997;27:1671–1679.
14. Bird AP. Functions for DNA methylation in vertebrates. Cold Spring Harb Symp Quant Biol 1993;58:281–284.
15. Gurunathan S, Klinman D, Sedar RA. DNA vaccines: immunology, application and optimization. Annu Rev Immunol 2000;18:927–974.
16. Wolff JA, Malone RW, Williams P, et al. Direct gene transfer into mouse muscle in vivo. Science 1990;247:1465–1468.

17. Tang DC, de Vit M, Johnston SA. Genetic immunization is a simple method for eliciting an immune response. Nature 1992;356:152–154.

18. Ulmer JB, Donnelly JJ, Parker SE, et al. Heterologous protection against influenza by injection of DNA encoding a viral protein. Science 1993;259:1745–1749.

19. Sedegah M, Hedstrom R, Hobart P, Hoffman SL. Protection against malaria by immunization with plasmid DNA encoding circumsporozoite protein. Proc Natl Acad Sci USA 1994;91:9866–9870.

20. Boyer JD, Ugen KE, Wang B, et al. Protection of chimpanzees from high-dose heterologous HIV-1 challenge by DNA vaccination. Nat Med 1997;3:526–532.

21. Xu L, Sanchez A, Yang Z, et al. Immunization for Ebola virus infection. Nat Med 1998;4:37–42.

22. Lowrie DB, Silva CL, Colston MJ, Ragno S, Tascon RE. Protection against tuberculosis by a plasmid DNA vaccine. Vaccine 1997;15:834–838.

23. Gurunathan S, Sacks DL, Brown DR, et al. Vaccination with DNA encoding the immunodominant LACK parasite antigen confers protective immunity to mice infected with Leishmania major. J Exp Med 1997;186:1137–1147.

24. Wang R, Doolan DL, Le TP, et al. Induction of antigen specific cytotoxic T lymphocytes in humans by a malaria vaccine DNA. Science 1998;282:476–480.

25. Calarota S, Bratt G, Nordlund S, et al. Cellular cytotoxic response induced by DNA vaccination in HIV-I infected patients. Lancet 1998;351:1320–1325.

26. Gurunathan S, Wu C-Y, Freidag BL, Sedar RA. Vaccine DNA, a key for inducing long term cellular immunity. Curr Opin Immunol 2000;12:442–447.

27. Elkins KL, Rhinehart-Jones TR, Stibitz S, Conover JS, Klinman DM. Bacterial DNA containing CpG motifs stimulates lymphocyte-dependent protection of mice against lethal infection with intracellular bacteria. J Immunol 1999;162:2291–2298.

28. Krieg AM, Love-Homan L, Yi A-K, Harty JT. CpG DNA induces sustained IL-12, expression in vivo and resistance to Listeria monocytogenes challenge. J Immunol 1998;161:2428–2434.

29. Zimmermann S, Egeter O, Hausmann S, et al. CpG oligodeoxynucleotides trigger protective and curative Th1, responses in lethal murine leishmaniasis. J Immunol 1998;160:3627–3630.

30. Roman M, Martin-Orozco E, Goodman JS, et al. Immunostimulatory DNA sequences function as T helper-1-promoting adjuvants. Nat Med 1997;3:849–854.

31. Lipford GB, Bauer M, Blank C, Reiter R, Wagner H, Heeg, K. CpG-containing synthetic oligonucleotides promote B and cytotoxic T cell responses to protein antigen: a new class of vaccine adjuvants. Eur J Immunol 1997;27:2340–2344.

32. McCluskie MJ, Davis HL. CpG DNA is a potent enhancer of systemic and mucosal immune responses against hepatitis B surface antigen with intranasal administration to mice. J Immunol 1998;161:4463–4466.

33. Manders P, Thomas, R. Immunology of vaccines DNA, CpG motifs and antigen presentation. Inflamm Res 2000;49:199–205.

34. Sato Y, Roman M, Tighe H, et al. Immunostimulatory DNA sequences necessary for effective intradermal gene immunization. Science 1996;273:352–354.

35. Klinman DM, Yamshchikov G, Ishigatsubo Y. Contribution of CpG motifs to the immunogenicity of vaccines DNA. J Immunol 1997;158:3635–3642.

82

Takeda et al.

36. Klinman DM, Barnhart KM, Conover J. CpG motifs as immune adjuvants. Vaccine 1999;17:19–25.
37. Klinman DM, Verthelyi D, Takeshita F, Ishii KJ. Immune recognition of foreign DNA: a cure of bioterrorism? Immunity 1999;11:123–129.
38. Sparwasser T, Koch ES, Vabulas RM, et al. Bacterial DNA and immunostimulatory CpG oligonucleotides trigger maturation and activation of murine dendritic cells. Eur J Immunol 1998;28, 2045–2054.
39. Jakob T, Walker PS, Krieg AM, Udey MC, Vogel JC. Activation of cutaneous dendritic cells by CpG-containing oligodeoxynucleotides: a role for dendritic cells in the augmentation of Th1, responses by immunostimulatory DNA. J Immunol 1998;161:3042–3049.
40. Hartmann G, Weiner GJ, Krieg AM. CpDNA G, a potent signal for growth, activation, and maturation of human dendritic cells. Proc Natl Acad Sci USA 1999; 96: 9305–9310.
41. Hacker H. Signal transduction pathways activated by CpG-Curr DNA. Top Microbial Immunol 2000;247:77–921.
42. Yamamoto T, Yamamoto S, Kataoka T, Tokunaga T. Lipofection of synthetic oligodeoxyribonucleotide having a palindromic sequence of AACGTT to murine splenocytes enhances interferon production and natural killer activity. Microbiol Immunol 1994;38L831–836.
43. Kimua Y, Sonehara K, Kuramoto E, et al. Binding of oligoguanylate to scavenger receptors is required for oligonucleotides to augment NK cell activity and induce IFN. J Biochem 1994;116:991–994.
44. Hacker H, Mischak H, Miethke T, et al. CpG-DNA-specific activation of antigen-presenting cells requires stress kinase activity and is preceded by non-specific endocytosis and endosomal maturation. EMBO J 1998;17:6230–6240.
45. Benimetskaya L, Loike JD, Khaled Z, et al. Mac-1, (CD11b/CD18) is an oligodeoxynucleotide-binding protein. Nature Med 1997;3:414–420.
46. Tonkinson JL, Stein CA. Patterns of intracellular compartmentalization, trafficking and acidification of 5'-fluorescein labeled phophodiester and phosphorothioate oligodeoxynucleotides in HL60, cells. Nucleic Acids Res 1994;22:4268–4275.
47. Ohkuma S, Poole B. Cytoplasmic vacuolation of mouse peritoneal macrophages and the uptake into lysosomes of weakly basic substances. J Cell Biol 1981;90:656–664.
48. Yoshimori T, Yamamoto A, Moriyama Y, Futai M, Tashiro Y. Bafilomycin A1, a specific inhibitor of vacuolar-type H(+)-ATPase, inhibits acidification and protein degradation in lysosomes of cultured cells. J Biol Chem 1991;266:17707–17712.
49. MacFarlane DE, Manzel L. Antagonism of immunostimulatory CpG-oligodeoxynucleotides by quinacrine, chloroquine, and structurally related compounds. J Immunol 1998;160:1122–1131.
50. Yi A-K, Tuetken R, Redford T, Waldschmidt M, Kirsch J, Krieg AM. CpG motifs in bacterial DNA activates leukocytes through the pH-dependent generation of reactive oxygens species. J Immunol 1998;160:4755–4761.
51. Yi A-K, Krieg AM. Rapid induction of mitogen-activated protein kinases by immune stimulatory CpG DNA. J Immunol 1998;161:4493–4497.

52. Hacker H, Mischak H, Hacker G, et al. Cell type-specific activation of mitogen-activated protein kinases by CpG-DNA controls interleukin-12, release from antigen-presenting cells. EMBO J 1999;18:6973–3982.
53. Stacey KJ, Sweet M, Hume DA. Macrophages ingest and are activated by bacterial DNA. J Immunol 1996;157:2116–2122.
54. Hoffmann JA, Kafatos FC, Janeway CA Jr, Ezekowiz BRA. Phylogenetic perspectives in innate immunity. Science 1999;284:1313–1318.
55. Lemaitre B, Nicolas E, Michaut L, Reichhart, J-M, Hoffmann JA. The dorsoventral regulatory gene cassette spatzle/Toll/cactus controls the potent antifungal response in Drosophila adults. Cell 1996;86:973–983.
56. Williams MJ, Rodriguez A, Kimbrell DA, Eldon ED. The 18-wheeler mutation reveals complex antibacterial gene regulation in Drosophila host defense. EMBO J 1997;16:6120–6130.
57. Tauszig S, Jouanguy E, Hoffmann JA, Imler J-L. Toll-related receptors and the control of antimicrobial peptide expression in Drosophila. Proc Natl Acad Sci USA 2000;97:10520–10525.
58. Medzhitov R, Preston-Hurlburt P, Janeway CA Jr. A human homlogue of the Drosophila Toll protein signals activation of adaptive immunity. Nature 1997;388: 394–397.
59. Rock FL, Hardiman G, Timans JC, Kastelein RA, Bazan JF. A family of human receptors structurally related to Drosophila Toll. Proc Natl Acad Sci USA 1998; 95:588–593.
60. Takeuchi O, Kawai T, Sanjo H, et al. TLR6: a novel member of an expanding toll-like receptor family. Gene 1999;231:59–65.
61. Du X, Poltorak A, Wei Y, Beutler B. Three novel mammalian toll-like receptors: gene structure, expression, and evolution. Eur Cytokine Netw 2000;11:362–371.
62. Chuang, T-H, Ulevitch RJ. Cloning and characterization of a sub-family of human Toll-like receptors: hTLR7, hTLR8, and hTLR9. Eur Cytokine Netw 2000;11: 372–378.
63. Poltorak A, He X, Smirnova I, et al. Defective LPS signaling in C3H/HeJ and C57BL/10ScCr mice: mutation in Tlr4, gene. Science 1998;282:2085–2088.
64. Qureshi ST, Lariviere L, Leveque G, et al. Endotoxin-tolerant mice have mutations in Toll-like receptor 4 (Tlr4). J Exp Med 1999;189:615–625.
65. Hoshino K, Takeuchi O, Kawai T, et al. Cutting edge: Toll-like receptor 4 (TLR4)-deficient mice are hyporesponsive to lipopolysaccharide: evidence for TLR4, as the Lps hene product. J Immunol 1999;162:3749–3752.
66. Yang R-B, Mark MR, Gray A, et al. Toll-like receptor-2, mediates lipopolysaccharide-induced cellular signalling. Nature 1998;395:284–288.
67. Kirschning CJ, Wesche H, Ayres TM, Rothe M. Human Toll-like receptor 2, confers responsiveness to bacterial lipopolysaccharide. Exp J Med 1998;188:2091–2097.
68. Takeuchi O, Hoshino K, Kawai T, et al. Differential roles of TLR2, and TLR4, in recognition of Gram-negative and Gram-positive cell wall components. Immunity 1999;11:443–451.
69. Heine H, Kirschning CJ, Lien E, Monks BG, Rothe M, Golenbock DT. Cutting edge: Cell that carry a null mutation for Toll-like receptor 2, are capable for responding to endotoxin. J Immunol 1999;162:6971–6975.

70. Hirschfeld M, Ma Y, Weis JH, Vogel SN, Weis JJ. Cutting edge: repurification of lipopolysaccharide eliminates signaling through both human and murine Toll-like receptor 2. J Immunol 2000;165:618–622.
71. Tapping RI, Akashi S, Miyake K, Godowski PJ, Tobias RS. Toll-like receptor 4, bit not Toll-like receptor 2, is a signaling receptor for Escherichia and Salmonella lipopolysaccharides. J Immunol 2000;165:5780–5787.
72. Schwadner R, Dziarski R, Wesche H, Rothe M, Kirschning CJ. Peptidoglycan- and lipoteichoic acid-induced cell activation is mediated by Toll-like receptor 2. J Biol Chem 1999;274:17406–17409.
73. Aliprantis AO, Yang R-B, Mark MR, et al. Cell activation and apoptosis by bacterial lipoproteins through Toll-like receptor 2. Science 1999;285:736–739.
74. Yoshimura A, Lien E, Ingalls RR, Tuomanen E, Dziarski R, Golenbock, D. Cutting edge: recognition of Gram-positive bacterial cell wall components by the innate immune system occurs via Toll-like receptor 2. J Immunol 1999;165:1–5.
75. Brightbill HD, Libraty DH, Krutzik SR, et al. Host defense mechanisms triggered by microbial lipoproteins through Toll-like receptors. Science 1999;285:732–736.
76. Means TK, Wang S, Lien E, Yoshimura A, Golenbock DT, Fenton MJ. Human Toll-like receptors mediate cellular activation by Mycobacterium tuberculosis. J Immunol 1999;163:3920–3927.
77. Underhill DM, Ozinsky A, Smith KD, Aderem A. Toll-like receptor 2, mediates mycobacteria-induced proinflammatory signaling in macrophages. Proc Natl Acad Sci USA 1999;96:14459–14463.
78. Hirschfeld M, Kirschning CJ, Schwandner R, et al. Cutting edge: inflammatory signaling by Borrelia burgdorferi lipoproteins is mediated by Toll-like receptor 2. J Immunol 1999;163:2382–2386.
79. Underhill DM, Ozinsky A, Hajjar AM, et al. The Toll-like receptor 2, is recruited to macrophage phagosomes and discriminates between pathogens. Nature 1999; 401:811–815.
80. Takeuchi O, Kaufmann A, Grote K, et al. Cutting edge: preferentially the R-stero-isomer of the Mycoplasmal lipopeptide macrophage-activating lipopeptide-2, activates immune cells through a Toll-like receptor 2- and MyD88-dependent signaling pathway. J Immunol 2000;164:554–557.
81. Takeuchi O, Hoshino K, Akira S. Cutting edge: TLR2-deficient and MyD88-deficient mice are highly susceptible to Staphylococcus aureus infection. J Immunol 2000;165:5392–5396.
82. Ozinsky A, Underhill DM, Fontenot JD, et al. The repertoire for pattern recognition of pathogens by the innate immune system is defined by cooperation between Toll-like receptors. Proc Natl Acad Sci USA 2000;97:13766–13771.
83. Wyllie DH, Kiss-Toth E, Visintin A, et al. Evidence for an accessory protein function for Toll-like receptor 1, in anti-bacterial responses. J Immunol 2000;165:7125–7132.
84. Hajjar AM, O'Mahony DS, Ozinsky A, et al. Cutting edge: functional interactions between Toll-like receptor (TLR) 2, and TLR1, or TLR6, in response to phenol-soluble modulin. J Immunol 2001;166:15–19.
85. Takeuchi O, Kawai T, Muhlradt PF, et al. Discrimination of bacterial lipopeptides by Toll-like receptor 6. Int Immunol 2001;13:933–940.

86. Medzhitov R, Janeway CA Jr. Innate immunity. N Engl J Med 2000;343:338–344.
87. Aderem A, Ulevitch RJ. Toll-like receptors in the induction of the innate immune responses. Nature 2000;406:782–787.
88. Muzio M, Ni J, Feng P, Dixit VM. IRAK (Pelle) family member IRAK-2, and MyD88, as proximal mediators of IL-1, signaling. Science 1997;278,1612–1615.
89. Wesche H, Henzel WJ, Shillinglaw W, Li S, Cao Z. MyD88: an adaptor protein that recruits IRAK to the IL-1, receptor complex. Immunity 1997;7:837–847.
90. Muzio M, Natoli G, Saccani S, Levrero M, Mantovani A. The human toll signaling pathway: divergence of nuclear factor kB and JNK/SAPK activation upstream of tumor necrosis factor receptor-associated factor 6 (TRAF6). J Exp Med 1998; 187:2097–2101.
91. Burnsm K, Martinon F, Esslinger C, et al. MyD88, an adaptor protein involved in interleukin-1, signaling. J Biol Chem 1998;273:12203–12209.
92. Medzhitov R, Preston-Hurlburt P, Kopp E, et al. MyD88, is an adaptor protein in the hToll/IL-1, receptor family signaling pathways. Moll Cell 1998;2:253–258.
93. Adachi O, Kawai T, Takeda K, et al. Targeted disruption of the MyD88, gene results in loss of IL-1- and IL-18-mediated function. Immunity 1998;9:143–150.
94. Kawai T, Adachi O, Ogawa T, Takeda K, Akira S. Unresponsiveness of MyD88-deficient mice to endotoxin. Immunity 1999;11:115–122.
95. Takeuchi O, Takeda K, Hoshino K, Adachi O, Ogawa T, Akira S. Cellular responses to bacterial cell wall components are mediated through MyD88-dependent signaling cascades. Int. Immunol 2000;12:113–117.
96. Hacker H, Vabulas RM, Takeuchi O, Hoshino K, Akira S, Wagner H. Immune cell activation by bacterial CpG-DNA through myeloid differentiation marker 88, and tumor necrosis factor receptor-associated factor (TRAF) 6. J Exp Med 2000; 192:595–600.
97. Schnare M, Holt AC, Takeda K, Akira S, Medzhitov R. Recognition of CpG DNA is mediated by signaling pathways dependent on the adaptor protein MyD88. Curr Biol 2000;10:1139–1142.
98. Hemmi H, Takeuchi O, Kawai T, et al. A Toll-like receptor recognizes bacterial DNA. Nature 2000;408:740–745.
99. Shimazu R, Akashi S, Ogata H, et al. MD-2, a molecule that confers lipopolysaccharide responsiveness on Toll-like receptor 4. J Exp Med 1999;189:1777–1782.
100. Yang R-B, Mark MR, Gurney AL, Godowski PJ. Signaling events induced by lipopolysaccharide-activated Toll-like receptor 2. J Immunol 1999;163:639–643.
101. Akashi S, Shimazu R, Ogata H, et al. Cutting edge: cell surface expression and lipo-plysaccharide signaling via the Toll-like receptor 4-MD-2, complex on mouse peritoneal macrophages. J Immunol 2000;164:3471–3475.
102. Nomura F, Akashi S, Sakao Y, et al. Endotoxin tolerance in mouse peritoneal macrophages correlates with downregulation of surface Toll-like receptor 4 expression. J Immunol 2000;164:3476–3479.
103. Chu W-M, Gong X, Li Z-W, et al. DNA-PKcs is required for activation of innate immunity by immunostimulatory DNA Cell 2000;103:909–918.
104. Gottlieb TM, Jackson SP. The DNA-dependent protein kinase: requirement for DNA ends and association with Ku antigen. Cell 1993;72:131–142.

105. Hartley KO, Gell D, Smith GC, et al. DNA-dependent proein kinase catalytic subunit: a relative of phosphatidylinositol 3-kinase and ataxia telangiectasia gene product. Cell 1995;82:849–856.
106. Kirchgessner CU, Patil CK, Evans JW, et al. DNA-dependent proteins kinase (p350) as a candidate gene for the murine defect CID. Science 1995;267:1178–1183.
107. Chace JH, Hooker NA, Mildenstein KL, Krieg AM, Cowdery JS. Bacterial DNA-induced NK cell IFN-γ production is dependent on macrophage secretion of IL-12. Clin Immunol Immunopathol 1997;84:185–193.

# 6

# Cpg ODN As a Th1 Immune Enhancer
# for Prophylactic and Therapeutic Vaccines

## Arthur M. Krieg and Heather L. Davis

### INTRODUCTION

Adaptive immunity, which comes about through highly specific recognition of antigenic epitopes on B and T cells, results in the development of antigen-specific antibodies and cytotoxic T-cell responses. However, these processes rely very heavily on simultaneous activation of cells of the innate immune system including dendritic cells (DCs), macrophages, and monocytes. Cells of the innate immune system lack highly specific antigen receptors, but rather rely on a set of pattern recognition receptors (PRRs), which have a general ability to detect pathogen-associated molecular patterns (PAMPs) that are specific molecular structures found in pathogens, but not in self tissues *(1,2)*. Many of the PRRs are found in the family of Toll-like receptors (TLR), of which at least 10 types have been identified. Examples of PAMPs that PRRs detect include endotoxins, flagellin, high mannose proteins, single- and double-stranded viral ribonucleic acids (RNAs) and the unmethylated CpG dinucleotides in particular base contexts (CpG motifs) that are prevalent in bacterial and many viral deoxyribonucleic acids (DNAs), but are heavily suppressed and methylated in vertebrate genomes *(1–5)*. The immune system appears to use the presence of these PAMPs as a "danger signal" that indicates the presence of infection and activates appropriate defense pathways. Recently there has been broad interest in testing and developing such "danger signal" ligands of PRRs for immune stimulation, including use as adjuvants to enhance antigen-specific responses. Oligodeoxynucleotides containing CpG motifs (CpG ODN), which are ligands for TLR9, are being developed for, among other purposes, enhancement of adaptive immune responses; in other words, as vaccine adjuvants.

This review will provide an overview of the immune effects and mechanisms of CpG ODN, and specifically how they can be used to enhance prophylactic and therapeutic vaccines against infectious diseases, cancer, and allergies. We will also review the contribution of CpG ODN to vaccination through nontraditional

From: *Vaccine Adjuvants: Immunological and Clinical Principles*
Edited by: C. J. Hackett and D. A. Harn, Jr. © Humana Press Inc., Totowa, NJ

routes, for example, mucosal vaccines, in immune-compromised hosts such as neonates, and as a component of DNA vaccines.

## IMMUNE RECOGNITION OF CpG MOTIFS

It has long been known that bacterial DNA could effectively activate vertebrate immune defenses (6). In 1995, through seminal work carried out by Arthur Krieg and colleagues, it became clear that the mechanism of this immunostimulatory effect involves the recognition of unmethylated CpG dinucleotides, in particular base contexts that are prevalent in bacterial DNA, but rare in vertebrate DNA (4). In bacterial DNA, CpG dinucleotides are typically present at their expected random frequency of approx 1 in 1 6 bases, and are unmethylated, and many of these are immune-stimulatory CpG motifs. However, in vertebrate DNA, CpG dinucleotides are suppressed to about one-fourth of this frequency, and are usually methylated on the cytosine, which renders them nonimmune stimulatory (3). CpG DNA has direct stimulatory and mitogenic effects on murine and human B cells, and triggers cytokine production, immunoglobulin secretion, and resistance to apoptosis (4,7–11). CpG DNA also directly activates DCs to produce proinflammatory cytokines such as interleukin (IL)-12, to express increased levels of costimulatory molecules such as B7-1 and B7-2, and to stimulate more actively antigen-specific T cells in vitro and in vivo (12–16). Macrophages are also stimulated by CpG DNA, but with delayed kinetics (17–19). CpG DNA activates human and murine natural killer (NK) cells to produce increased interferon (IFN)γ and to have increased lytic activity (20–22).

Not just any unmethylated CpG will be immune stimulatory. Rather, the base context of the CpG dinucleotides is extremely important in establishing whether or not they will be a CpG motif and cause immune-stimulatory effects, and furthermore, what type of immune-stimulatory effects they will have. If the CpG is preceded by an A, G, or T, and if it is followed by an A, C, or T, then it is likely to trigger immune-stimulatory effects (8). In vertebrate genomes, CpG dinucleotides are most frequently preceded by a C and/or followed by a G, which severely reduces their immune-stimulatory effects, and the cytosine is almost always methylated, which abolishes any potential stimulatory effect (23). The immune-stimulatory effects of bacterial DNA can be mimicked by synthetic CpG ODN.

Based on specific immune-stimulatory properties, we have identified three main families of CpG ODN with distinct structural and biological characteristics. The A class is a potent activator of NK cells and IFNα secretion from DC, but is a poor stimulator of B cells. The B class is a strong B-cell stimulator, but weaker for induction of NK activity or IFNα. Otherwise, both classes induce Th1-type cytokines (24). The most recently discovered C class has properties of both the A and B classes (25). Almost all published studies to date using CpG

ODN as a vaccine adjuvant have been carried out with B class CpG ODN, thus the following sections refer to "CpG ODN" generically but this is actually referring to the B class. We have unpublished results, however, that the A and C classes may be superior to the B class for induction of cytotoxic T-lymphocyte (CTL) responses, hence it will be interesting to see how this develops. If this remains true in humans, the A and C classes may prove particularly effective for therapeutic vaccines.

Although optimal B class CpG motifs for driving murine B-cell proliferation have the general formula, purine-purine-CG-pyrimidine-pyrimidine, there are some species-specific differences regarding what is the optimal hexamer. For example, the optimal immune-stimulatory ODN CpG motif is GACGTT for mice *(4,8,26)*, but GTCGTT for humans *(11)* and many other vertebrate species, including cow, sheep, cat, dog, goat, horse, pig, and chicken *(26,27)*. The immune-stimulatory activity of an ODN is determined not only by the activity of a given hexamer CpG motif, but also by several other factors including (a) the number of CpG motifs in an ODN, in which two or three are optimal; (b) the spacing of the CpG motifs, which are best separated by at least two intervening bases, preferably Ts; (c) the presence of poly G sequences or other flanking sequences in the ODN; and (d) the ODN backbone, in which a nuclease-resistant phosphorothioate backbone is best for in vivo use *(4,8,10,11,20,28)*. Additionally, the immune-stimulatory effects of the ODN are enhanced if it has a TpC dinucleotide on the 5' end and is pyrimidine rich on the 3' side *(8,10,11)*.

## MECHANISM OF ACTION

Alum, the most commonly used adjuvant at present, has been used for a very long time without actually understanding its mechanism. That being said, the development of a new generation of adjuvants will require a more comprehensive knowledge of how they exert their immune-enhancement effects. A considerable body of knowledge about the mechanism of CpG ODN has been been elucidated, and owing to the intense research interest in CpGODN, it is probably the best understood immune stimulant to date. This has recently been extensively reviewed by Krieg *(24)*. In brief, it appears that the CpG ODN enters the lymphocyte after binding to cell surface DNA-binding proteins that are not CpG sequence-specific, to end up within the endosomal compartment *(29,30)*. It appears that the endosome may be the site of CpG-induced signal initiation *(31–36)* and this is initiated through the TLR9, which specifically recognizes CpG motifs.

TLRs function as PRRs to initiate innate immune activation in response to infection by detecting pathogen-specific molecular structures *(2,5)*. Other examples in which natural ligands have been identified include TLR2 and TLR6 that detect proteoglycans, TLR3 that detects double-stranded DNA of RNA viruses, TLR4, that detects endotoxin of Gram-negative bacteria and TLR5 that detects flagellin. TLR7 and TLR8 have been found to be activated by imidazoquin-olines (e.g., Imiquimod, Resiquimod = R848), however, these are not natural ligands *(37,38)*.

Among human cell types, TLR9 expression is highest in B cells and plasma-cytoid DCs, which are also the only cell types to be directly activated by CpG ODN *(31,39)*. TLR9 knockout mice show no CpG-induced activation of B cells, DCs, or NK cells *(40)*. The TLR9 protein appears to determine the species specificity of CpG motifs because 293 cells transfected to express the mouse TLR9 protein become optimally responsive to the preferred mouse CpG motif, GACGTT, whereas 293 cells transfected to express the human TLR9 protein become optimally responsive to the preferred human CpG motif, GTCGTT *(31)*. The current view is that TLR9 is an essential component of the postulated CpG DNA receptor that acts upstream of the adapter protein MyD88, and links CpG motif recognition to the TLR/IL-1R signaling pathway *(41)*. Several differ-ent pathways are activated by CpG ODN to bring about signal transduction, including activation of NFκB and at least two of the mitogen-activated protein kinases, namely the p38 and c-Jun $NH_2$-terminal kinase pathways, but appar-ently not extracellular receptor kinase pathways *(11,18,19,35,42)*. A role of DNA-PK in mediating immune activation by CpG DNA has been suggested by Raz and coworkers *(43)*, but this is inconsistent with previous reports that CpG DNA is a highly effective immune stimulator in SCID mice, which do not have DNA-PK catalytic function *(44)*.

Among the genes whose RNA expression is increased in B cells are *myc, myn, EGR-1, Jun, Bcl-2, Bcl-x$_L$, IL-6, IL-10*, and *IL-12, (8,9,42,45,46)*. CpG DNA also has potent transcription-activating effects on macrophages, leading to the increased transcription of TNF-α, IL-1β, plasminogen activator inhibitor-2, IL-6, IL-12, type 1 interferons, and several costimulatory and antigen-present-ing molecules such as class II major histocompatability complex (MHC), CD80, CD86, and CD40, *(12,18,19,44,47,48)*. As reviewed above, NK cells are induced by CpG DNA to produce IFNγ. Other cytokines whose expression is induced by CpG DNA, but for whom the cellular sources have not yet been conclusively determined, include IL-1RA, MIP-1β, MCP-1, and IL-18, *(49–51)*.

CpG DNA does not appear to have direct stimulatory effects on NK cells or resting T cells *(21,48,52,53)*. An initial report suggesting that CpG DNA directly stimulated cytokine secretion from T cells *(54)* now appears to have drawn an incorrect conclusion because of the use of inadequately purified cell popula-tions. However, in murine mixed cell populations, the type I IFNs produced by CpG-stimulated adherent cells stimulate T cells to produce some activation and costimulatory molecules, but also inhibit their proliferative response to TCR ligation *(48)*. Hence, indirect effects on T cells are possible, and certainly the Th1 cytokine milieu should aid the development of CD8+ T-cell responses.

The predominant effects of CpG DNA in vitro and in vivo are Th1-like. Local subcutaneous (SC) injection of CpG ODN, creates a systemic or regional Th1-like response in the draining lymph node that includes production of IL-12 and IFNγ *(54,55)* and lymphadenopathy that peaks at 7 to 10 days *(56)*. DC become a more prominent population in the lymph node, and exhibit an activated phenotype with increased expression of costimulatory molecules *(57)*. Remarkably, this local Th1-like environment appears to be sustained for several weeks because mice can respond to an antigen injection with a Th1-biased response, including CTL, even 5 weeks later *(56)*. This localized state of Th1 predisposition has also been observed following intradermal or intranasal delivery of the CpG *(58)*.

## CpG ODN AS A VACCINE ADJUVANT

Many direct and indirect effects of CpG ODN on immune cells have now been identified *(24)*, and several of these suggest potential efficacy as a vaccine adjuvant. First, purified B cells are synergistically activated when stimulated by CpG ODN in the presence of antigen, indicating cross-talk between the B-cell receptor and CpG signaling pathways *(4)*. Although CpG DNA can activate essentially any B cell without regard to its antigen specificity, the synergy observed in B-cell activation through CpG and the BCR suggests that antigen-specific B cells will be preferentially activated. Second, the induction of increased costimulatory molecule expression on B cells and other antigen-presenting cells (APCs) suggests that these should be more effective at promoting antigen-specific immune responses. Third, CpG ODN inhibit B-cell apoptosis, contributing to a more sustained immune response *(8,9)*. Fourth, the CpG-induced activation of DCs creates a Th1-like cytokine and chemokine environment in the secondary lymphoid organs *(18,56)*. CpG ODN promote cross-priming with strong cytolytic T-cell and antibody responses to peptides and protein antigens independently of T-cell help *(14,15,53,59–62)*.

The utility of CpG ODN as a vaccine adjuvant has been confirmed in studies using model antigens, such as hen egg lysozyme *(62)*, ovalbumin *(56)*, heterologous gammaglobulin *(63)*, or β-galactosidase *(49)*. Remarkably, these studies all confirmed that CpG ODN is a stronger Th1-like adjuvant than the "gold standard," complete Freund's adjuvant (CFA) as measured by its ability to drive the differentiation of CTL and IFNγ-secreting T cells. Moreover, CpG ODN accomplished this level of antigen-specific activation without inducing any of the harsh local inflammatory effects seen with CFA. The generation of CD8$^+$ CTL to purified protein antigens classically requires a specialized "immunological synapse" between an APC presenting an antigen and an antigen-specific helper CD4$^+$ T cells. The initial interaction triggers the expression of CD40L on the helper T cell that allows it to activate the APC sufficiently so that it can now

induce the differentiation of naïve CD8⁺ T cells of the appropriate antigen specificity into effector cells, such as CTL. By contrast to the general requirement
for T-cell help with protein antigens, the priming of CTL to an infectious pathogen is frequently CD4-independent.

To improve the generation of protective and therapeutic vaccine responses, it
would be highly desirable to identify adjuvants that could allow APC to prime
CD8⁺ T-cell responses in the absence of T-cell help. CpG ODN appears to be such
an adjuvant. Mice depleted of CD4⁺ T cells by treatment with depleting antibodies mounted efficient CTL responses to the hepatitis B virus (HBV) surface antigen (HBsAg) only if it was delivered together with CpG ODN *(15)*.
Although IL-12 has been proposed to play a crucial role in the generation and
maintenance of CTL responses, IL-12 unresponsive STAT 4 knockout mice
developed strong CTL responses when immunized with CpG ODN, even if the
mice had also been depleted of CD4⁺ T cells *(15)*.

## CpG ODN As Adjuvant to Infectious Disease Vaccines

CpG ODN has been shown to be very potent for augmenting humoral and
cellular responses to infectious disease antigens including the HBsAg *(15,59,
64)*, hepatitis C virus (HCV) envelope protein *(65)*, herpes-simplex virus (HSV)-
2 gD *(66)*, influenza *(67)*, rotavirus VP6 *(68)*, human immunodeficiency virus
(HIV) gp160 *(69)*, gp120-depleted HIV particles *(70)*, whole killed mycobacterium *(71)*, and leishmanial protein *(60)*. It was also possible to show protection against lethal challenge against HSV-2 *(66)*, influenza *(67)*, and rotavirus
*(68)*. Interestingly, CpG ODN was able to enhance immunogenicity and protective efficacy from challenge with the BCG vaccine against *Mycobacterium
tuberculosis*, which presumably already contains immune-stimulatory BCG-
derived immunostimulatory CpG motifs *(71)*. Using infectious disease antigens in mice, it has also been shown that CpG ODN brings about an earlier
appearance of immune responses, which in turn allows earlier boosting and
still obtaining the full boosting effect. Also, it is possible to reduce the dose of
antigen by up to 100-fold and still induce an equivalent humoral response to
that with antigen alone *(72)*. A typical dose of CpG ODN used in these mouse
vaccine studies is 10 to 50 µg.

The efficacy of CpG as an adjuvant to promote Th1-like immune responses
may be further enhanced by coadministration with other adjuvants, especially
adjuvants that may provide some depot function, such as alum or emulsions
*(59,73)*. Combinations of CpG with QS21, Titermax, and MPL also have shown
strong synergistic activity *(74)*.

The adjuvant effects of CpG ODN are not limited to mice. They have also
been shown to enhance antibody responses in Aotus monkeys against peptide
sequences derived from the circumsporozoite protein from *Plasmodium falcip-*

*arum* in a mineral oil emulsion *(75)* and for a HBV vaccine in chimpanzees *(10)*, orangutans *(76)*, and humans *(77,78)*.

A large number of orangutans were vaccinated as part of a rehabilitation program to reintroduce them to the wild. The findings are particularly interesting because they are otherwise hyporesponders to the commercial HBV vaccine that contains only alum as an adjuvant *(76)*. This hyporesponse is likely because of a genetic restriction at the T-help level (as can also occur for humans) and results in less than 15% seroconversion after two doses. However, addition of CpG ODN (50 μg) increased seroconversion rates after two doses to 100%, with much higher levels of antibodies, and no apparent adverse effects *(76)*. A human clinical study has shown that addition of CpG ODN to an HBV vaccine containing alum can also improve its efficacy in hyporesponsive humans, namely HIV-infected individuals who had failed to respond to a previous 3+ dose course of standard HBV vaccine *(79)*.

An interesting insight into the evolutionary history of immune recognition of CpG DNA is provided by the finding that fish not only respond to CpG DNA, but also may recognize different CpG motifs than do mice *(80)*. This result may be important in the further development of improved vaccination strategies for fish *(81)*.

Polysaccharide antigens represent a special problem in vaccination. Because they cannot be presented in the groove of the MHC molecules, polysaccharides can only activate B cells through crosslinking the surface receptor, which is inefficient at triggering isotype switching. Although high levels of immunoglobin M (IgM) antibodies can be induced by polysaccharide vaccines, these are generally relatively short-lived and are less efficient at fixing complement than some immunoglobin G (IgG) isotypes. Moreover, polysaccharide antigens tend to be very weakly or nonantigenic in the very young and very old populations, which are most at risk of infection. An early report concluded that CpG ODN was not an effective adjuvant for a polysaccharide vaccine *(82)*. However, these investigators only measured the IgM response, and used a nearly toxic dose of CpG ODN, 500 μg. Other investigators have found that although CpG ODN are not effective adjuvants for many pure polysaccharide antigens, they are quite effective if a protein carrier is conjugated to the polysaccharide *(83,84)*. CpG ODN does not have a great effect on the serum level of IgM antibodies, but causes profound isotype switching. Notably, these humoral responses are Th1-like, with high levels of IgG2a and IgG3 antibody in mice. Importantly, the adjuvant effect of CpG ODN for polysaccharide antigens is also prominent in neonatal and very old mice (2 years old) and can be demonstrated in vitro *(85)*.

## Mucosal Adjuvant Activity

Because most pathogens enter the body through one of the vast mucosal surfaces, there is a great deal of interest in effective adjuvants for mucosal immunization. Although effective mucosal adjuvants such as cholera toxin (CT) and the heat-labile enterotoxin (LT) have been identified, these are considered too toxic for human use and require mutagenesis to reduce the severe adverse effects. On the other hand, CpG ODN has been shown in mice to be extremely effective as an adjuvant when given by intranasal or oral routes. Indeed, CpG ODN is equally effective as CT and LT holotoxins but without the toxic effects; even doses 100-fold more than those required for optimal effect are well tolerated (67,86–91). Given mucosally, CpG ODN still induces Th1 immune responses both at systemic and mucosal immune surfaces, and also drives strong mucosal IgA responses at local and distant mucosal sites (88). A particularly potent method to induce very strong mucosal immunity was to prime systemically (intramuscular [IM]) and boost mucosally (intranasal [IN]) or vice versa; this gave even higher IgA than having both prime and boost IN (92). Surprisingly, control non-CpG ODN with a phosphorothioate backbone, which is essentially ineffective when given with antigen IM, also showed adjuvant activity through mucosal routes, but these responses were more Th2-like (88).

### Adjuvant Activity in Early Life

Inducing immunity during the early postnatal period is extremely important from the public health standpoint, but extremely difficult to attain because of the immaturity of the immune system at birth. Even with repeated vaccination, immune responses are generally modest in neonatal mice or humans. As such, vaccines are often postponed until the age of 3 months. Moreover, the neonatal immune system tends to be skewed more toward the generation of Th2 responses rather than the more desirable Th1 responses. CpG ODN may help overcome these problems if results obtained in neonatal mice translate to humans, as has been demonstrated with HBsAg (93,94), tetanus toxoid, live measles virus, and recombinant canary-pox expressing measles HA (95). In those studies, it was shown that newborn mice developed earlier and stronger immune responses that included very strong CTL responses. Furthermore, CpG was able to prime humoral and cellular immunity against HBsAg even in the presence of high levels of maternal antibodies (93,94). Before this, successful immunization of newborn mice in the presence of maternal antibodies had been restricted to DNA vaccines.

### Role of CpG Motifs in DNA Vaccine Efficacy

DNA vaccines, which were first described in 1993, raised a lot of hope for the possibility to develop simple, effective, and inexpensive vaccines against virtually any diseases, and furthermore that these vaccines that could induce, with a single dose, potent Th1-type immune responses by virtue of sustained in vivo antigen synthesis (96). Although all of this was realized in mice, results in humans have been more disappointing. The problem is likely related in large part to delivery, but that being said, it should also be possible to improve DNA vaccines in other ways such as vector design to improve antigen expression/ localization and optimizing the CpG content to increase immunogenicity.

DNA vaccines are plasmids that contain a eukaryotic promoter such as the cytomegalovirus (CMV) promoter driving expression of a cDNA encoding the antigen of interest. These plasmids are grown in bacteria, hence CpG dinucleotides are unmethylated. The average plasmid contains several hundred CpG motifs, and recent studies have reported that these motifs are required for the function of the DNA vaccine *(97–99)*. Plasmid DNA also has Th1 adjuvant activity for a protein antigen when they are mixed together *(100)*. Thus, DNA vaccines have two essential components: (a) the transcriptional unit that encodes the antigen, directing the specificity of the response, and (b) the CpG motifs in the backbone that acts as a built-in adjuvant. In vivo injection of DNA vaccines transfects only a very small fraction of APC to express the encoded antigen, but the CpG motifs in the vaccine activate a large majority of the DCs in the draining lymph nodes *(57)*. The vast majority (99%) of injected plasmid is degraded into ODN by tissue nucleases within 90 minutes after in vivo injection *(101)*.

The identification of the importance of CpG motifs in DNA vaccine efficacy suggests possible ways to further improve their activity by increasing CpG content. It was reported that simply cloning an extra two stimulatory CpG motifs into a plasmid was sufficient to dramatically enhance its efficacy *(98)*, but other groups have not reproduced this result *(102,103)*. It would certainly be unexpected for minor changes in the CpG content of a DNA vaccine to alter its efficacy, considering the large number of other stimulatory CpG motifs already present in the plasmid. On the other hand, the quantity of CpG motifs in a DNA vaccine seems to be somewhat limiting because addition of *Escherichia coli* DNA or additional noncoding vector DNA to a DNA vaccine dramatically enhances its efficacy in mice *(104,105)* and primates *(106)*. Likewise, addition of plasmid DNA to a suboptimal dose of a DNA vaccine enhances the Th1-like immune response *(96,99)*. We have demonstrated that more extensive mutagenesis of plasmids, affecting scores of CpG motifs, can significantly enhance the ability of a DNA vaccine to induce antigen-specific B- and T-cell responses *(23)*. However, addition of too many CpG motifs to a plasmid (50 or more) suppresses the humoral response, possibly because CpG-induced cytokines, such as IFNs, suppress expression of antigen from the commonly used CMV promotor *(23)*.

Although some investigators have simply added CpG ODN to DNA vaccines, this approach is generally unsuccessful because of the dose-dependent interference of the phosphorothioate ODN backbone with the uptake and expression of the plasmid *(106–108)*. Use of a gene gun, which should directly transfect

APCs, might avoid such uptake inhibition. Fensterle and associates have reported that individual dose (ID) administration of a CpG ODN at the site of gene gun delivery of a DNA vaccine against two immunodominant proteins from *Listeria monocytogenes* caused increased differentiation of antigen-specific IFNγ-secreting T cells, and improved protection against a bacterial challenge *(109)*. However, the co-injection of CpG ODN did not enhance the DNA vaccine-induced antibody or CTL responses *(109)*. Consistent with these results, immunization against an LCMV CTL epitope did not give increased levels of CTL after coating the beads with CpG ODN *(110)*. This failure of CpG to enhance these DNA vaccine responses must not be because of insufficient uptake, as the CpG was delivered via gene gun. Perhaps the requirement for CpG to be within the endosomal compartment is not met with it is introduced directly into the cell via gene gun. Alternatively, the failure to enhance all DNA vaccine responses could be secondary to CpG-induced interferons and other factors that inhibit expression of the DNA vaccine.

Another factor that affects the CpG optimization of DNA vaccines is the discovery of neutralizing CpG motifs. If immune recognition of CpG DNA has evolved as an effective defense against intracellular infections, then it seems likely that pathogens using this route of infection would evolve counter strategies to block or evade the defense. Some pathogens have reduced the number of CpGs in their genome to decrease its immune stimulatory effects. In principle, this mechanism should be much easier for pathogens with small genomes than for those with large genomes, and indeed, analyses of the genomes of small DNA viruses and retroviruses have revealed that these all have very low CpG content *(111–113)*. Large genome viruses are much less consistent in exhibiting CpG suppression, but some have evolved neutralizing CpG motifs (CpG-N) that can actually block the effects of a stimulatory CpG motif. All adenoviruses have the expected random content of approximately one CpG dinucleotide per 16 bases, but different serotypes show striking differences in the base context of their CpG motifs. Serotype 12 adenovirus, which causes an acute infection, has a similar distribution of CpG motifs to *E. coli* DNA and is immune stimulatory *(23)*. By contrast, serotypes 2 and 5 adenovirus, which cause more chronic infections, show a marked skewing in their CpG motifs with a dramatic overrepresentation of immune-neutralizing CpG-N motifs, which most typically contain CCG and CGG sequences. While on their own, ODN with CpG-N motifs have neither stimulatory nor inhibitory effects on the immune system. When mixed together with ODN-containing stimulatory CpG motifs, they prevent the stimulatory activity that would otherwise be noted *(114)*. The presence of such CpG-N motifs in a plasmid DNA backbone could reduce the adjuvant effect of the backbone. Indeed, when we eliminated 52 of the 134 putative CpG-N motifs from a plasmid vector by site-directed mutagenesis, this alone augmented both humoral and cell-mediated immune responses compared to the parent vector *(23)*. The vector showed progressively increasing immune stimulatory effects with the further addition of 16 CpG-S motifs, but addition of 6 4 CpG-S motifs actually resulted in a fall of the antibody response to the DNA vaccine *(23)*. We hypothesize that the addition of too many CpG-S motifs to a DNA vaccine may actually lead to the production of high levels of type I interferons, with resultant inhibition of plasmid expression from its viral promoter, and loss of immunogenicity. If this is the case, then optimization of CpG content in DNA vaccines can only be taken so far, unless a promoter is identified that has high levels of expression and that is further upregulated by IFNs.

## CpG ODN WITH THERAPEUTIC VACCINES

To date, there has not been a therapeutic vaccine licensed, but this may be owing more to the lack of an appropriate Th1-type adjuvant to induce the types of responses required, than it is to a "failure" of the theory. There are three main indications in which therapeutic vaccines may be applied: (a) vaccines to treat chronic infectious diseases such as HBV and HCV, HIV, HSV, and tuberculosis; (b) cancer vaccines that include tumor-specific antigens; and (c) vaccines to treat specific allergies. In the first two cases, the main goal of the vaccine would be to induce antigen-specific cell-mediated immunity to clear infected cells and kill tumor cells respectively. In the case of an allergy vaccine, the goal would be to redirect pre-existing Th2 responses to Th1 responses. In all cases, a strong Th1 bias is essential.

There are several factors that are responsible for the ability of CpG ODN to promote Th1-biased antigen-specific Ab and CTL immune responses. In fact, CpG DNA is a more effective Th1-like adjuvant than CFA *(62)*, and in a recent direct head-to-head comparison of 19 different adjuvants, a CpG ODN was found to be the strongest for inducing Th1-like immune responses against a tumor antigen *(115)*. In contrast to many vaccine adjuvants that have been extremely effective in mice but disappointing in humans, CpG ODN is highly effective in higher nonhuman primates *(10,11,75,116)* and in a recent human phase I/II clinical trial, the addition of a CpG ODN to a commercial HBV vaccine gave a seroconversion rate at 2 weeks of 93%, compared to 0% for subjects immunized without CpG *(76)*.

### CpG ODN in Therapeutic Infectious Disease Vaccines

The strong Th1-like adjuvant effects of CpG ODN along with the ability to provide T-help and to overcome hypo- and nonresponsiveness to antigens, make it an ideal candidate as an immune enhancer in therapeutic vaccines to treat chronic infections. Likely target indications are chronic infections of hepatitis B and C in which antigenic tolerance (HBV) and insufficient Th1-type T-cell responses (HBV and HCV) are thought to be a primary contributor to chronicity. There are no suitable small animal models for either of these diseases, but we have tested the ability of CpG ODN to break tolerance in HBsAg mice transgenic that express the protein principally in the liver under the control of the endogenous HBV promoter (117). These mice have high circulating levels of HBsAg, but no accumulation in the liver and no pathology. B- and T-cell tolerance in these Tg mice can be overcome by immunization with an HBsAg-expressing DNA vaccine (117), or with recombinant HBsAg plus CpG ODN (118). Surprisingly, the resulting immune response clears circulating HBsAg and markedly reduces HBsAg mRNA expression in the liver without causing a cytopathic effect (117). Adoptive transfer experiments showed that both CD4 and CD8 T cells are responsible for the noncytolytic control of viral expression, and that this required IFNγ, suggesting a Th1 type of response (119). To better ascertain the potential of CpG to overcome chronic viral infections in HBV and HCV, studies will have to be undertaken in chimpanzees, or humans themselves.

Other chronic diseases that might benefit from treatment with a CpG-containing vaccine that would induce Th1-type cell-mediated immunity include HSV, HIV, and tuberculosis.

## CpG ODN As Adjuvant for Cancer Vaccines

The strong Th1 adjuvant effects of CpG ODN also make them ideal candidates to use with tumor antigens in cancer vaccines. The antitumor adjuvant properties of CpG ODN have been shown effective in various murine tumor models with several types of vaccines including: (a) tumor derived peptide in a melanoma model (120) and cervical carcinoma model (121); (b) tumor-specific antigen in a B-cell lymphoma model (see below); (c) an adenoviral vector expressing tumor-specific antigen in a prostate tumor model (122); (d) irradiated whole cell tumor vaccine in neuroblastoma (123) and renal cell carcinoma (Renca) model (124); (e) pulsed DC vaccine in the Renca model (125); (f) DC cocultured with irradiated tumor cells in a murine colon cancer model (126); and (g) adoptive transfer of T cells primed in vivo and restimulated ex vivo against the tumor cells in an A20 lymphoma model (127).

In the 38C13 murine B-cell lymphoma model, which was originally developed by Ron Levy and colleagues (128), the idiotype (Id) of the 38C13 surface IgM serves as a highly specific tumor-associated antigen. The Id was conjugated to keyhole limpet hemocyanin (KLH) to improve antigenicity, and when mice were immunized with this together with CpG ODN (optimally 50–100 μg) or CFA, similar high levels of Id-specific antibody are detected (129). Control mice challenged with a lethal dose of tumor cells all died within 1 month of challenge, but mice immunized with Id-KLH together with CFA or CpG ODN had prolonged survival including 20 or 40% long-term survival, respectively

*(129)*. This slightly higher efficacy of the CpG adjuvant compared to CFA may be related to the fact that CpG induced more than twice as much of the IgG 2 a anti-Id isotype although CFA induced higher levels of IgG1. The efficacy of CpG ODN was further improved when the Id was conjugated to GMCSF *(130)*. The GMCSF-Id fusion protein on its own induced high levels of anti-Id antibodies, but these were mostly IgG1 isotype (Th2), and only 30% of mice were long-term survivors of a tumor challenge given 3 days after a single immunization. By contrast, when a CpG ODN was combined with the GMCSF-Id fusion protein, the antibody response was fivefold stronger and largely IgG2a, and the long-term survival of the mice was improved from 30 to 70% *(130)*. This is consistent with the strong synergy that these two immune activators show in in vitro experiments with murine or human DCs *(16)*.

## CpG ODN AS AN ADJUVANT FOR ALLERGY VACCINES

Allergic diseases result from Th2-type immune responses against otherwise harmless environmental antigens. Such responses lead to the generation of Th2 T cells that produce IL-4 and IL-5 and promote the differentiation of B cells into IgE-secreting cells. This IgE binds to the high affinity IgE Fc receptor on the surface of mast cells and basophils. Subsequent exposure of these cells to an allergen results in the binding of the allergen by surface IgE, crosslinking of the IgE Fc receptors, and activation and degranulation of the mast cells or basophils. These cells release a variety of preformed proinflammatory and vasoactive compounds including histamine, prostaglandins, leukotrienes, and cytokines. This results in immediate inflammatory response within 15 minutes, followed by a secondary late phase reaction several hours later.

Almost all current therapeutic efforts against allergic disease have been aimed at the control of the symptoms that are triggered by mast cell or basophil degranulation. However, a more fundamental approach to disease therapy would be to induce a Th1-like response against the allergen. Because Th1 and Th2 immune responses are typically mutually inhibitory, the induction of a Th1-like immune response to an allergen should suppress the Th2-like response that is responsible for the allergy-type symptoms. This has been tested in a murine model of respiratory asthma. Mice were first sensitized to a strong Th2-like stimulus, schistosome eggs, by intraperitoneal (IP) injection. On subsequent inhalation challenge with schistosome egg antigen (SEA), the presensitized mice developed severe eosinophilic airways disease with high levels of Th2-like cytokines in the airways, eosinophilic infiltrates, and evidence of broncho-constriction *(131)*. When such mice were then treated by parenteral immunization using SEA and CpG ODN, the eosinophilic airways disease was completely reversed and was no longer present on subsequent airway challenge. In fact, treatment with CpG ODN alone (i.e., without the allergen) was also able to reverse the allergic disease, but this took somewhat longer to occur *(131)*. Mice treated with CpG ODN immunotherapy developed a Th1-like immune response to the SEA instead of the Th2-like immune response, but this was not associated with any apparent airways pathology.

## USE OF CpG ODN WITH VACCINES IN HUMANS AND SAFETY ISSUES

CpG ODN has been tested in combination with Engerix-B® (GlaxoSmith Kline), a commercial HBV vaccine that contains HBsAg adsorbed to alum. In a double-blind phase I study, healthy adult volunteers were vaccinated at 0, 1, and 6 months by IM injection with the vaccine, with or without added CpG ODN (125 µg, 500 µg, or 1 mg). HBsAg-specific antibody responses (anti-HBs) appeared significantly earlier and were significantly higher at all time points up to the third dose in CpG than control subjects. Remarkably, a single vaccine dose induced 75% seroprotection (anti-HBs greater than or equal to 10 mIU/mL) if 500 µg of CpG ODN were added compared to 13% for the control vaccine. The experimental vaccines, like the control vaccine, to be well-tolerated, both locally and systemically *(76)*.

For any new drug, potential safety issues are of foremost concern in early-phase human trials. Effects of the ODN backbone *per se* were not expected to pose problems because chemically similar molecules had been given in doses orders of magnitude higher and much more frequently in antisense trials. Rather, the greatest perceived risk with CpG ODN was that by virtue of its strong Th1 immune stimulatory effects that it might induce autoimmunity, especially against DNA. Natural environmental exposures to CpG ODN in the form of infections are quite frequent and have not been shown to lead to an increased risk of autoimmune disease in humans, although viral infections may induce anti-double-stranded DNA (anti-dsDNA) antibody production *(132)*. The risk for developing lupus or other autoimmune diseases generally is not increased among patients with chronic infections who are presumably chronically exposed to high concentrations of CpG DNA. Thus, any added risk from injection of low dose CpG ODN for therapeutic purposes appears likely to be small.

More recently, many humans have received DNA vaccines in clinical trials, with no reports of autoimmune disease, to our knowledge. Patients who have received nonviral vectors that contained CpG DNA in gene therapy clinical trials have shown signs of immune activation with flu-like symptoms, but have not been described to develop autoimmune diseases *(133,134)*. These data suggest that administration of phosphodiester DNA containing CpG motifs to humans induces immune activation, but not autoimmune disease.

Hundreds of humans have received antisense ODN, which are made with the same synthetic backbone as CpG ODN. Many of these antisense drugs happen to have immune stimulatory CpG motifs, with no reports to date of association with appearance of anti-DNA antibodies or other forms of autoimmunity *(135)*. As mentioned above, antisense ODN are given at much higher doses and much more frequently than would ever be envisioned for using CpG ODN as a vaccine adjuvant, even in a therapeutic setting.

A number of potential safety concerns have been addressed in a wide range of studies. These have been extensively reviewed by Krieg *(24)*, but collectively they indicate that CpG DNA does not generally abrogate B- or T-cell tolerance, or induce autoantibody production or autoimmune disease, even in genetically predisposed individuals.

## CONCLUSION

CpG ODN is a potential Th1-type immune stimulant that has the potential to be highly effective in vaccines against infectious diseases, cancer, and allergies. For infectious diseases, it may allow the induction of protective immune responses with fewer and lower doses of antigen, even in neonates and hyporesponders. Most important is the possibility to produce therapeutic vaccines (pharmaccines) to treat chronic infections such as HBV and HCV, conditions that have been resistant to such treatments in the past, largely because of the failure to induce sufficient cell-mediated immunity. The same principles apply to cancer vaccines, in which numerous approaches are being tried in clinical trials. Finally the Th1 effects and the ability of CpG to redirect pre-existing Th2 responses to Th1 makes them ideal in allergy vaccines. CpG ODN have been shown to be highly effective and generally well-tolerated in human clinical studies of a prophylactic vaccine in normal volunteers. Only through additional clinical studies in actual patient populations will the true potential of CpG ODN as an enhancer of therapeutic vaccines be realized.

## REFERENCES

1. Dempsey PW, Allison ME, Akkaraju S, Goodnow CC, Fearon DT. C3d of complement as a molecular adjuvant: bridging innate and acquired immunity. Science 1996;271:348–350.
2. Kumar A, Yang YL, Flati V, et al. Deficient cytokine signaling in mouse embryo fibroblasts with a targeted deletion in the PKR gene: role of IRF-1 and NF-kappaB EMBO J 1997;16:406–416.
3. Bird A. CpG Islands as gene markers in the vertebrate nucleus. Trends Genet 1987; 3:342–347.
4. Krieg AM, Yi AK, Matson S, et al. CpG motifs in bacterial DNA trigger direct B-cell activation. Nature 1995;374:546–549.
5. Medzhitov R, Janeway CA Jr. Innate immunity: impact on the adaptive immune response. Curr Opin Immunol 1997;9:4–9.

6. Tokunaga T, Yamamoto H, Shimada S, et al. (1984) Antitumor activity of deoxy-ribonucleic acid fraction from mycobacterium bovis BCG isolation, physicochem-ical characterization, and antitumor activity. J Natl Cancer Inst 1984;72:955–962.

7. Liang H, Nishioka Y, Reich CF, Pisetsky DS, Lipsky PE. (1996) Activation of human B cells by phosphorothioate oligodeoxynucleotides. J Clin Invest 1996; 98:1119–1129.

8. Yi AK, Chang M, Peckham DW, Krieg AM, Ashman RF. CpG oligodeoxy-ribonucleotides rescue mature spleen B cells from spontaneous apoptosis and promote cell cycle entry. J Immunol 1998;160:5898–5906.

9. Yi AK, Hornbeck P, Lafrenz DE, Krieg AM. CpG DNA rescue of murine B lymphoma cells from anti-IgM-induced growth arrest and programmed cell death is associated with increased expression of c-myc and bcl-xL. J Immunol 1996; 157:4918–4925.

10. Hartmann G, Weeratna RD, Ballas ZK, et al. Delineation of a CpG phosphoro-thioate oligodeoxynucleotide for activating primate immune responses in vitro and in vivo. J Immunol 2000;164:1617–1624.

11. Hartmann G, Krieg AM. Mechanism and function of a newly identified CpG DNA motif in human primary B cells. J Immunol 2000;164:944–953.

12. Jakob T, Walker PS, Krieg AM, Udey MC, Vogel JC. (1998) Activation of cuta-neous dendritic cells by CpG-containing oligodeoxynucleotides: a role for den-dritic cells in the augmentation of Th1 responses by immunostimulatory DNA. J Immunol 1998;161:3042–3049.

13. Sparwasser T, Koch ES, Vabulas RM, et al. Bacterial DNA and immunostim-ulatory CpG oligonucleotides trigger maturation and activation of murine den-dritic cells. Eur J Immunol 1998;28:2045–2054.

14. Sparwasser T, Vabulas RM, Villmow B, Lipford GB, Wagner H. Bacterial CpG-DNA activates dendritic cells in vivo: T helper cell-independent cytotoxic T cell responses to soluble proteins. Eur J Immunol 2000;30:3591–3597.

15. Wild J, Grusby MJ, Schirmbeck R, Reimann J. Priming MHC-I-restricted cyto-toxic T lymphocyte responses to exogenous hepatitis B surface antigen is CD41 T cell dependent. J Immunol 1999;163:1880–1887.

16. Hartmann G, Weiner GJ, Krieg AM. CpG DNA: a potent signal for growth, acti-vation, and maturation of human dendritic cells. Proc Natl Acad Sci USA 1999; 96:9305–9310.

17. Hartmann G, Krieg AM. CpG DNA and LPS induce distinct patterns of activa-tion in human monocytes. Gene Ther 1999;6:893–903.

18. Sparwasser T, Miethke T, Lipford G, Erdmann A, Hacker H, Heeg K, Wagner H. Macrophages sense pathogens via DNA motifs: induction of tumor necrosis fac-tor-alpha-mediated shock. Eur J Immunol 1997;27:1671–1679.

19. Stacey KJ, Sweet MJ, Hume DA. Macrophages ingest and are activated by bacte-rial DNA. J Immunol 1996;157:2116–2122.

20. Ballas ZK, Rasmussen WL, Krieg AM. Induction of NK activity in murine and human cells by CpG motifs in oligodeoxynucleotides and bacterial DNA. J Immu-nol 1996;157:1840–1845.

21. Iho S, Yamamoto T, Takahashi T, Yamamoto S. Oligodeoxynucleotides contain-ing palindrome sequences with internal 5'-CpG-3' act directly on human NK and

activated T cells to induce IFN-gamma production in vitro. J Immunol 1999;163: 3642–3652.

22. Yamamoto T, Yamamoto S, Kataoka T, Tokunaga T. Lipofection of synthetic oligodeoxyribonucleotide having a palindromic sequence of AACGTT to murine splenocytes enhances interferon production and natural killer activity. Microbiol Immunol 1999;38:831–836.
23. Krieg AM, Wu T, Weeratna R, Efler SM, Love-Homan L, Yang L, Yi AK, Short D, Davis HL. Sequence motifs in adenoviral DNA block immune activation by stimulatory CpG motifs. Proc Natl Acad Sci USA 1998;95:12631–12636.
24. Krieg AM. CpG motifs in bacterial DNA and their immune effects. Annu Rev Immunol 2000;20:709–760.
25. Vollmer J, Weeratna R, Payette P, et al. (2004) Characterization of three CpG oligodeoxynucleotide classes with distinct immunostimulatory activities. Eur J Immunol 2004;34:251–262.
26. Rankin R, Pontarollo R, Ioannou X, et al. CpG motif identification for veterinary and laboratory species demonstrates that sequence recognition is highly conserved. Antisense Nucleic Acid Drug Dev 2001;11:333–340.
27. Brown WC, Estes DM, Chantler SE, Kegerreis KA, Suarez CE. DNA and a CpG oligonucleotide derived from Babesia bovis are mitogenic for bovine B cells. Infect Immun 1998;66:5423–5432.
28. Pisetsky DS, Reich CF, III. The influence of base sequence on the immunological properties of defined oligonucleotides. Immunopharmacology 1998;40:199–208.
29. Nicklin PS, Craig SJ, Phillips JA. Pharmacokinetic properties of phosphoro-thioates in animals—absorption, distribution, metabolism and elimination. In: Crooke ST, ed. Antisense Research and Application, Vol. 131. Berlin Heidelberg Germany, New York, NY: Springer-Verlag, 1998, pp. 141–168.
30. Zhao Q, Waldschmidt T, Fisher E, Herrera CJ, Krieg AM. Stage-specific oligo-nucleotide uptake in murine bone marrow B-cell precursors. Blood 1994;84: 3660–3666.
31. Bauer S, Kirschning CJ, Hacker H, Redecke V, Hausmann S, Akira S, Wagner H, Lipford GB. Human TLR9 confers responsiveness to bacterial DNA via species-specific CpG motif recognition. Proc Natl Acad Sci USA 2001;98:9237–9242.
32. Hacker H, Mischak H, Miethke T, et al. CpG-DNA-specific activation of anti-gen-presenting cells requires stress kinase activity and is preceded by non-spe-cific endocytosis and endosomal maturation. EMBO J 1998;17:6230–6240.
33. Macfarlane DE, Manzel L. Antagonism of immunostimulatory CpG-oligodeoxy-nucleotides by quinacrine, chloroquine, and structurally related compounds. J Immunol 1998;160:1122–1131.
34. Strekowski L, Zegrocka O, Henary M, et al. Structure-activity relationship analy-sis of substituted 4-quinolinamines, antagonists of immunostimulatory CpG-oli-godeoxynucleotides. Bioorg Med Chem Lett 1999;9:1819–1824.
35. Yi AK, Krieg AM. Rapid induction of mitogen-activated protein kinases by immune stimulatory CpG DNA. J Immunol 1998;161:4493–4497.
36. Yi AK, Tuetken R, Redford T, Waldschmidt M, Kirsch J, Krieg AM. CpG motifs in bacterial DNA activate leukocytes through the pH-dependent generation of reactive oxygen species. J Immunol 1998;160:4755–4761.

37. Janeway CA Jr, Medzhitov R. Innate immune recognition. Annu Rev Immunol 2002;20:197–216.
38. Jurk M, Heil F, Vollmer J, Schetter C, Krieg AM, Wagner H, Lipford G, Bauer S. Human TLR7 or TLR8 independently confer responsiveness to the antiviral compound R-848. Nat Immunol 2002;3:499.
39. Krug A, Towarowski A, Britsch S, et al. Toll-like receptor expression reveals CpG DNA as a unique microbial stimulus for plasmacytoid dendritic cells which synergizes with CD40 ligand to induce high amounts of IL-12. Eur J Immunol 2001;31:3026–3037.
40. Hemmi H, Takeuchi O, Kawai T, et al. A Toll-like receptor recognizes bacterial DNA. Nature 2000;408:740–745.
41. Wagner H. Interactions between bacterial CpG-DNA and TLR9 bridge innate and adaptive immunity. Curr Opin Microbiol 2002;5:62–69.
42. Yi AK, Krieg AM. CpG DNA rescue from anti-IgM-induced WEHI-231 B lymphoma apoptosis via modulation of I kappa B alpha and I kappa B beta and sustained activation of nuclear factor-kappa B/c-Rel. J Immunol 1998;160:1240–1245.
43. Chu W, Gong X, Li Z, et al. DNA-PKcs is required for activation of innate immunity by immunostimulatory DNA. Cell 2000;103:909–918.
44. Chace JH, Hooker NA, Mildenstein KL, Krieg AM, Cowdery JS. Bacterial DNA-induced NK cell IFN-gamma production is dependent on macrophage secretion of IL-12. Clin Immunol Immunopathol 1997;84:185–193.
45. Redford TW, Yi AK, Ward CT, Krieg AM. Cyclosporin A enhances IL-12 production by CpG motifs in bacterial DNA and synthetic oligodeoxynucleotides. J Immunol 1998;161:3930–3935.
46. Yi AK, Klinman DM, Martin TL, Matson S, Krieg AM. Rapid immune activation by CpG motifs in bacterial DNASy. stemic induction of IL-6 transcription through an antioxidant-sensitive pathway. J Immunol 1996;157:5394–5402.
47. Anitescu M, Chace JH, Tuetken R, Yi AK, Berg DJ, Krieg AM, Cowdery JS. Interleukin-10 functions in vitro and in vivo to inhibit bacterial DNA-induced secretion of interleukin-12. J Interferon Cytokine Res 1997;17:781–788.
48. Sun S, Zhang X, Tough DF, Sprent J. Type I interferon-mediated stimulation of T cells by CpG DNA. J Exp Med 1998;188:2335–2342.
49. Roman M, Martin-Orozco E, Goodman JS, et al. Immunostimulatory DNA sequences function as T helper-1-promoting adjuvants [see comments]. Nat Med 1997;3:849–854.
50. Schwartz DA, Quinn TJ, Thorne PS, Sayeed S, Yi AK, Krieg AM. CpG motifs in bacterial DNA cause inflammation in the lower respiratory tract. J Clin Invest 1997;100:68–73.
51. Zhao Q, Temsamani J, Zhou RZ, Agrawal S. Pattern and kinetics of cytokine production following administration of phosphorothioate oligonucleotides in mice. Antisense Nucleic Acid Drug Dev 1997;7:495–502.
52. Wagner H. Bacterial CpG DNA activates immune cells to signal infectious danger. Adv Immunol 1999;73:329–368.
53. Lipford GB, Bauer M, Blank C, Reiter R, Wagner H, Heeg K. CpG-containing synthetic oligonucleotides promote B and cytotoxic T cell responses to protein antigen: a new class of vaccine adjuvants. Eur J Immunol 1997;27:2340–2344.

54. Klinman DM, Yi AK, Beaucage SL, Conover J, Krieg AM. CpG motifs present in bacteria DNA rapidly induce lymphocytes to secrete interleukin 6, interleukin 12, and interferon gamma. Proc Natl Acad Sci USA 1996;93:2879–2883.

55. Krieg AM, Love-Homan L, Yi AK, Harty JT. CpG DNA induces sustained IL-12 expression in vivo and resistance to Listeria monocytogenes challenge. J Immunol 1998;161:2428–2434.

56. Lipford GB, Sparwasser T, Zimmermann S, Heeg K, Wagner H. CpG-DNA-mediated transient lymphadenopathy is associated with a state of Th1 predisposition to antigen-driven responses. J Immunol 2000;165:1228–1235.

57. Akbari O, Panjwani N, Garcia S, Tascon R, Lowrie D, Stockinger B. DNA vaccination: transfection and activation of dendritic cells as key events for immunity. J Exp Med 1999;189:169–178.

58. Kobayashi H, Horner AA, Takabayashi K, et al. Immunostimulatory DNA pre-priming: a novel approach for prolonged Th1-biased immunity. Cell Immunol 1999;198:69–75.

59. Davis HL, Weeratna R, Waldschmidt TJ, et al. CpG DNA is a potent enhancer of specific immunity in mice immunized with recombinant hepatitis B surface antigen. J Immunol 1998;160:870–876.

60. Rhee EG, Mendez S, Shah JA, et al. Vaccination with heat-killed leishmania antigen or recombinant leishmanial protein and CpG oligodeoxynucleotides induces long-term memory CD41 and CD81 T cell responses and protection against leishmania major infection. J Exp Med 2002;195:1565–1573.

61. Vabulas RM, Pircher H, Lipford GB, Hacker H, Wagner H. CpG-DNA activates in vivo T cell epitope presenting dendritic cells to trigger protective antiviral cytotoxic T cell responses. J Immunol 2000;164:2372–2378.

62. Chu RS, Targoni OS, Krieg AM, Lehmann PV, Harding CV. CpG oligodeoxynucleotides act as adjuvants that switch on T helper 1 (Th1) immunity. J Exp Med 1997;186:1623–1631.

63. Sun S, Kishimoto H, Sprent J. DNA as an adjuvant: capacity of insect DNA and synthetic oligodeoxynucleotides to augment T cell responses to specific antigen. J Exp Med 1998;187:1145–1150.

64. Schirmbeck R, Melber K, Reimann J. Adjuvants that enhance priming of cytotoxic T cells to a Kb-restricted epitope processed from exogenous but not endogenous hepatitis B surface antigen. Int Immunol 1999;11:1093–1102.

65. Ma X, Forns X, Gutierrex R, et al. DNA-based vaccination against hepatitis C virus (HCV): effect of expressing different forms of HCV E2 protein and use of CpG-optimized vectors in mice. Vaccine 2002;20:3263–3271.

66. Gallichan WS, Woolstencroft RN, Guarasci T, McCluskie MJ, Davis HL, Rosenthal KL. Intranasal immunization with CpG oligodeoxynucleotides as an adjuvant dramatically increases IgA and protection against herpes simplex virus-2 in the genital tract. J Immunol 2001;166:3451–3457.

67. Moldoveanu Z, Love-Homan L, Huang WQ, Krieg AM. CpGDNA, a novel immune enhancer for systemic and mucosal immunization with influenza virus. Vaccine 1998;16:1216–1224.

68. Choi AH, McNeal MM, Flint JA, et al. The level of protection against rotavirus shedding in mice following immunization with a chimeric VP6 protein is dependent on the route and the coadministered adjuvant. Vaccine 2002;20:1733–1740.

69. Deml L, Schirmbeck R, Reimann J, Wolf H, Wagner R. Immunostimulatory CpG motifs trigger a T helper-1 immune response to human immunodeficiency virus type-1 (HIV-1) gp 1 60 envelope proteins. Clin Chem Lab Med 1999;37:199–204.
70. Moss RB, Diveley J, Jensen F, Carlo DJ. In vitro immune function after vaccination with an inactivated, gp120-depleted HIV-1 antigen with immunostimulatory oligodeoxynucleotides. Vaccine 2000;8:1081–1087.
71. Freidag BL, Melton GB, Collins F, et al. CpG oligodeoxynucleotides and interleukin-12 improve the efficacy of Mycobacterium bovis BCG vaccination in mice challenged with M. tuberculosis. Infect Immun 2000;68:2948–2953.
72. Weeratna R, Comanita L, Davis HL. (2003) CPG ODN allows lower dose of antigen against hepatitis B surface antigen in BALB/c mice. Immunol Cell Biol 2003; 81:59–62.
73. Davis HL. Use of CpG DNA for enhancing specific immune responses. Curr Top Microbiol Immunol 2000;247:171–183.
74. Kim SK, Ragupathi G, Cappello S, Kagan E, Livingston PO. Effect of immunological adjuvant combinations on the antibody and T-cell response to vaccination with MUC1-KLH and GD3-KLH conjugates. Vaccine 2001;19:530–537.
75. Jones TR, Obaldia N, III, Gramzinski RA, et al. Synthetic oligodeoxynucleotides containing CpG motifs enhance immunogenicity of a peptide malaria vaccine in Aotus monkeys. Vaccine 1999;17:3065–3071.
76. Davis HL. DNA vaccines for prophylactic or therapeutic immunization against hepatitis B virus. Mt Sinai J Med 1999;66:84–90.
77. Cooper CL, Davis H, Morris ML, et al. CpG 7 909, an immunostimulatory TLR9 agonist oligodeoxynucleotide, as adjuvant to Engerix-B HBV vaccine in healthy adults: a double-blind Phase I/II study. J Clin Immunol 2004;24:693–702.
78. Siegrist C-A, Pihlgren M, Tougne C, et al. Co-administraction of CpG oligonucleotides enhances the late affinity maturation process of human anti-hepatitis B vaccine response. Vaccine 2004;23:615–622.
79. Cooper CL, Davis HL, Angel JB, et al. CpG 7909 is safe and highly effective as an adjuvant to HBV vaccine in HIV seropositive adults. AIDS 2005 (in press).
80. Kanellos TS, Sylvester ID, Butler VL, et al. Mammalian granulocyte-macrophage colony-stimulating factor and some CpG motifs have an effect on the immunogenicity of DNA and subunit vaccines in fish. Immunology 1999;96:507–510.
81. Lorenzen N, Lorenzen E, Einer-Jensen K, Heppell J, Wu T, Davis HL. Protective immunity to VHS in rainbow trout (Oncorhynchus mykiss, Walbaum) following DNA vaccination. Fish Shellfish Immunol 1998;8:261–270.
82. Threadgill DS, McCormick LL, McCool TL, Greenspan NS, Schreiber JR. Mitogenic synthetic polynucleotides suppress the antibody response to a bacterial polysaccharide. Vaccine 1998;16:76–82.
83. Chu RS, McCool T, Greenspan NS, Schreiber JR, Harding CV. CpG oligodeoxynucleotides act as adjuvants for pneumococcal polysaccharide-protein conjugate vaccines and enhance antipolysaccharide immunoglobulin G2a (IgG2a) and IgG3 antibodies. Infect Immun 2000;68:1450–1456.
84. Kovarik J, Bozzotti P, Tougne C, et al. Adjuvant effects of CpG oligodeoxynucleotides on responses against T-independent type 2 antigens. Immunology 2001; 102:67–76.

85. Chelvarajan RL, Raithatha R, Venkataraman C, et al. CpG oligodeoxynucleotides overcome the unresponsiveness of neonatal B cells to stimulation with the thymus-independent stimuli anti-IgM and TNP-Ficoll. Eur J Immunol 1999;29: 2808–2818.

86. Horner AA, Ronaghy A, Cheng PM, et al. Immunostimulatory DNA is a potent mucosal adjuvant. Cell Immunol 1998;190:77–82.

87. McCluskie MJ, Davis HL. CpG DNA is a potent enhancer of systemic and mucosal immune responses against hepatitis B surface antigen with intranasal administration to mice. J Immunol 1998;161:4463–4466.

88. McCluskie MJ, Davis HL. Oral, intrarectal and intranasal immunizations using CpG and non-CpG oligodeoxynucleotides as adjuvants. Vaccine 2000;19:413–422.

89. McCluskie MJ, Weeratna RD, Clements JD, Davis HL. Mucosal immunization of mice using CpG DNA and/or mutants of the heat- labile enterotoxin of Escherichia coli as adjuvants. Vaccine 2001;19:3759–3768.

90. McCluskie MJ, Weeratna RD, Davis HL. The potential of oligodeoxynucleotides as mucosal and parenteral adjuvants. Vaccine 2001;19:2657–2660.

91. McCluskie MJ, Weeratna RD, Krieg AM, Davis HL. CpG DNA is an effective oral adjuvant to protein antigens in mice. Vaccine 2000;19:950–957.

92. McCluskie MJ, Weeratna RD, Payette PJ, Davis HL. Parenteral and mucosal prime-boost immunization strategies in mice with hepatitis B surface antigen and CpG DNA FEMS Immunol Med Microbiol 2002;32:179–185.

93. Brazolot Millan CL, Weeratna R, Krieg AM, Siegrist CA, Davis HL. CpG DNA can induce strong Th1 humoral and cell-mediated immune responses against hepatitis B surface antigen in young mice. Proc Natl Acad Sci USA 1998;95:15553–15558.

94. Weeratna RD, Brazolot Millan CL, McCluskie MJ, Siegrist CA, Davis HL. Priming of immune responses to hepatitis B surface antigen in young mice immunized in the presence of maternally derived antibodies. FEMS Immunol Med Microbiol 2001;30:241–247.

95. Kovarik J, Bozzotti P, Love-Homan L, et al. CpG oligodeoxynucleotides can circumvent the Th2 polarization of neonatal responses to vaccines but may fail to fully redirect Th2 responses established by neonatal priming. J Immunol 1999; 162:1611–1617.

96. Donnelly JJ, Ulmer JB, Shiver JW, Liu MA. DNA vaccines. Annu Rev Immunol 1997;15:617–648.

97. Klinman DM, Yamshchikov G, Ishigatsubo Y. Contribution of CpG motifs to the immunogenicity of DNA vaccines. J Immunol 1997;158:3635–3639.

98. Sato Y, Roman M, Tighe H, et al. Immunostimulatory DNA sequences necessary for effective intradermal gene immunization. Science 1996;273:352–354.

99. Porter KR, Kochel TJ, Wu SJ, Raviprakash K, Phillips I, Hayes CG. Protective efficacy of a dengue 2 DNA vaccine in mice and the effect of CpG immunostimulatory motifs on antibody responses. Arch Virol 1998;143:997–1003.

100. Gursel M, Tunca S, Ozkan M, Ozcengiz G, Alaeddinoglu G. Immunoadjuvant action of plasmid DNA in liposomes. Vaccine 1999;17:1376–1383.

101. Barry ME, Pinto-Gonzalez D, Orson FM, McKenzie GJ, Petry GR, Barry MA. Role of endogenous endonucleases and tissue site in transfection and CpG-medi-

ated immune activation after naked DNA injection. Hum Gene Ther 1999;10: 2461–2480.

102. Biswas S, Ashok MS, Reddy GS, Srinivasan VA, Rangarajan PN. Evaluation of the protective efficacy of rabies DNA vaccine in mice using an intracerebral challenge model. Curr Sci 1999:6:1012–1016.

103. Vinner L, Nielsen HV, Bryder K, Corbet S, Nielsen C, Fomsgaard A. Gene gun DNA vaccination with Rev-independent synthetic HIV-1 gp160 envelope gene using mammalian codons. Vaccine 1999;17:2166–2175.

104. Grifantini R, Finco O, Bartolini E, et al. Multi-plasmid DNA vaccination avoids antigenic competition and enhances immunogenicity of a poorly immunogenic plasmid. Eur J Immunol 1998;28:1225–1232.

105. Lee SW, Sung YC. Immuno-stimulatory effects of bacterial-derived plasmids depend on the nature of the antigen in intramuscular DNA inoculations. Immunology 1998;94:285–289.

106. Gramzinski RA, Millan CL, Obaldia N, Hoffman SL, Davis HL. Immune response to a hepatitis B DNA vaccine in Aotus monkeys: a comparison of vaccine formulation, route, and method of administration. Mol Med 1998;4:109–118.

107. Hartl A, Kiesslich J, Weiss R, et al. Isoforms of the major allergen of birch pollen induce different immune responses after genetic immunization. Int Arch Allergy Immunol 1999;120:17–29.

108. Weeratna R, Brazolot Millan CL, Krieg AM, Davis HL. Reduction of antigen expression from DNA vaccines by coadministered oligodeoxynucleotides. Antisense Nucleic Acid Drug Dev 1998;8:351–356.

109. Fensterle J, Grode L, Hess J, Kaufmann SH. Effective DNA vaccination against listeriosis by prime/boost inoculation with the gene gun. J Immunol 1999;163: 4510–4518.

110. Oehen S, Junt T, Lopez-Macias C, Kramps TA. Antiviral protection after DNA vaccination is short lived and not enhanced by CpG DNA. Immunology 2000;99: 163–169.

111. Karlin S, Ladunga I, Blaisdell BE. Heterogeneity of genomes: measures and values. Proc Natl Acad Sci USA 1994;91:12837–12841.

112. Krieg AM. Lymphocyte activation by CpG dinucleotide motifs in prokaryotic DNA. Trends Microbiol 1996;4:73–76.

113. Shpaer EG, Mullins JI. Selection against CpG dinucleotides in lentiviral genes: a possible role of methylation in regulation of viral expression. Nucleic Acids Res 1990;18:5793–5797.

114. Han J, Zhu Z, Hsu C, Finley WH. Selection of antisense oligonucleotides on the basis of genomic frequency of the target sequence. Antisense Res Dev 1994;4: 53–65.

115. Kim SK, Ragupathi G, Musselli C, Choi SJ, Park YS, Livingston PO. Comparison of the effect of different immunological adjuvants on the antibody and T-cell response to immunization with MUC1-KLH and GD3-KLH conjugate cancer vaccines. Vaccine 2000;18:597–603.

116. Davis HL, Suparto II, Weeratna RR, et al. CpG DNA overcomes hyporesponsiveness to hepatitis B vaccine in orangutans. Vaccine 2000;18:1920–1924.

117. Mancini M, Hadchouel M, Davis HL, Whalen RG, Tiollais P, Michel ML. DNA-mediated immunization in a transgenic mouse model of the hepatitis B surface antigen chronic carrier state. Proc Natl Acad Sci USA 1996;93:12496–12501.
118. Malanchère-Brès E, Payette PJ, Mancini M, Tiollais P, Davis HL, Michel ML. CpG oligodeoxynucleotides with hepatitis B surface antigen (HBsAg) for vaccination in HBsAg in transgenic mice. J Virol 2001;75:6482–6491.
119. Mancini M, Hadchouel M, Tiollais P, Michel ML. Regulation of hepatitis B virus mRNA expression in a hepatitis B surface antigen transgenic mouse model by IFN-γ-secreting T cells after DNA-based immunization. J Immunol 1998;161: 5564–5570.
120. Miconnet I, Koenig S, Speiser D, et al. CpG are efficient adjuvants for specific CTL induction against tumor antigen-derived peptide. J Immunol 2002;168: 1212–1218.
121. Davila E, Kennedy R, Celis E. Generation of antitumor immunity by cytotoxic T lymphocyte epitope peptide vaccination, CpG-oligodeoxynucleotide adjuvant, and CTLA-4 blockade. Cancer Res 2003;63:3281–3288.
122. Lubaroff D, personal communication, June 2005.
123. Sandler AD, Chihara H, Kobayashi G, et al. CpG Oligonucleotides enhance the tumor antigen-specific immune response of a granulocyte macrophage colony-stimulating factor-based vaccine strategy in neuroblastoma. Cancer Res 2003;63: 394–399.
124. Weeratna RD, Davis HL, Medynski L, Krieg AM. Potential use of CpG for cancer immunotherapy. Cancer Chemotherapy and Biological Response Modifiers, Elsevier (in press).
125. Chagnon F, Tanguay S, Ozdal OL, et al. Potentiation of a dendritic cell vaccine for murine renal cell carcinoma by CpG oligonucleotides. Clin Can Res 2005;11: 1302–1311.
126. Brunner C, Seiderer J, Schlamp A, et al. Enhanced dendritic cell maturation by TNF-α or cytidine-phosphate-guanosine DNA drives T cell activation in vitro and therapeutic anti-tumor immune responses in vivo. J Immunol 2000;165: 6278–6286.
127. Egeter O, Mocikat R, Ghoreschi K, Dieckmann A, Rocken M. Eradication of disseminated lymphomas with CpG-DNA activated T helper type 1 cells from nontransgenic mice. Cancer Res 2000;60:1515–1520.
128. Campbell MJ, Esserman L, Byars NE, Allison AC, Levy R. Idiotype vaccination against murine B cell lymphoma. Humoral and cellular requirements for the full expression of antitumor immunity. J Immunol 1990;145:1029–1036.
129. Weiner GJ, Liu HM, Wooldridge JE, Dahle CE, Krieg AM. Immunostimulatory oligodeoxynucleotides containing the CpG motif are effective as immune adjuvants in tumor antigen immunization. Proc Natl Acad Sci USA 1997;94:10833–10837.
130. Liu HM, Newbrough SE, Bhatia SK, Dahle CE, Krieg AM, Weiner GJ. Immunostimulatory CpG oligodeoxynucleotides enhance the immune response to vaccine strategies involving granulocyte-macrophage colony-stimulating factor. Blood 1998;92:3730–3736.

131. Kline JN, Waldschmidt TJ, Businga TR, Lemish JE, Weinstock JV, Thorne PS, Krieg AM. Modulation of airway inflammation by CpG oligodeoxynucleotides in a murine model of asthma. J Immunol 1998;160:2555–2559.

132. Fredriksen K, Skogsholm A, Flaegstad T, Traavik T, Rekvig OP. Antibodies to dsDNA are produced during primary BK virus infection in man, indicating that anti-dsDNA antibodies may be related to virus replication in vivo. Scand J Immunol 1993;38:401–406.

133. Krieg AM. Direct immunologic activities of CpG DNA and implications for gene therapy. J Gene Med 1999;1:56–63.

134. Krieg AM. Minding the Cs and Gs [comment]. Mol Ther 2000;1:209–210.

135. Glover JM, Leeds JM, Mant TG, et al. Phase I safety and pharmacokinetic profile of an intercellular adhesion molecule-1 antisense oligodeoxynucleotide (ISIS 2 302). J Pharmacol Exp Ther 1997;282:1173–1180.

# 7

# Modified Bacterial Toxins

## Ed C. Lavelle, Olive Leavy, and Kingston H. G. Mills

### INTRODUCTION

Bacteria produce a range of virulence factors that allow them to invade, colonize, and cause disease in humans and other hosts. Bacterial toxins are harmful virulence factors that can kill or damage host cells and have powerful immunomodulatory that can subvert immune responses of the host. Immune responses against these toxins, in particular the production of antitoxin antibodies, are often a key component of the protective immunity against the bacteria and modified bacterial toxins, inactivated by chemically or genetic means, have formed the basis of several successful antibacterial vaccines. However, because of their immunomodulatory properties, bacterial toxins can also enhance immune responses to unrelated antigens, especially when administered by mucosal routes. Therefore bacterial toxins and nontoxic derivatives are also developed as mucosal adjuvant for subunit vaccines against a range of infectious diseases.

### BACTERIAL TOXINS

Toxin production has evolved as a strategy to confer virulence on bacteria and much of the pathology during bacterial infections can be attributed to the effect of toxins either directly on host tissues or indirectly as a result of immunological responses induced by the toxin. Bacterial toxins include exotoxins of most Gram-positive and many Gram-negative bacteria, released extracellularly during multiplication of the organism and endotoxin or lipopolysaccharide (LPS), which forms part of the outer layer of the Gram-negative bacterial cell wall and are only released in large amounts on lysis of the cell. Bacterial toxins target surface receptors on host cells, causing tissue damage and modulating signaling events in cells involved in multiple physiological functions, including immune responses. However, the host has also evolved a range of strategies to counteract the effects of bacterial toxins, the most effective of which is the production of toxin-neutralizing antibodies. Because this adaptive immune response is very effective in a primed host, it has been exploited in the development of antibacterial vaccines based on detoxified bacterial toxins.

From: *Vaccine Adjuvants: Immunological and Clinical Principles*
Edited by: C. J. Hackett and D. A. Harn, Jr. © Humana Press Inc., Totowa, NJ

In addition to activating antigen-specific T and B cells of the acquired immune system, bacterial toxins can have more immediate effects on cells of the innate immune system. Local and systemic inflammation is probably the best-characterized immunological response to bacterial toxins and although not desirable in terms of vaccine safety, if properly controlled this does provide a powerful means of augmenting immune responses to co-administered antigens, especially when delivered by mucosal routes. Indeed the immunogenicity of killed and attenuated bacterial vaccines can be attributed, at least in part, to the adjuvant activity of toxins, together with other cell wall components of the bacteria. For example, killed *Bordetella pertussis* is a powerful adjuvant used experimentally for decades to boost immune responses to unrelated antigens. It now appears that its adjuvanticity may be attributed at least in part to residual active toxins, including LPS, pertussis toxin (PT), and adenylate cyclase toxin (CyaA). Unlike killed or attenuated bacteria and viruses, purified native or recombinant protein or polysaccharide vaccines are poorly immunogenic, but their immunogenicity can be restored to that of the live or killed bacteria by the addition of bacterial toxins, which provide the danger signals to stimulate the innate immune responses. However, the reactogenicity of killed vaccines can be largely attributed to contaminating toxin. Therefore, a major goal has been to modify these toxins in such a way that reduces their toxicity but retains their adjuvant properties.

## BACTERIAL TOXINS AND THE IMMUNE RESPONSE

### The Innate Immune Response: A Primary Target for Bacterial Toxins

The first line of immunological defense against infection with pathogenic microbes is the innate immune system. Innate immune responses not only help to prevent colonization and infection but also help to shape the subsequent adaptive immune responses *(1)*. Recognition and activation of cells of the innate immune system by microbial pathogens involves interaction of invariant molecular structures, termed pathogen-associated molecular patterns, with pattern recognition receptors (PRRs) on macrophages and dendritic cells (DCs), which function as antigen-presenting cells (APCs) for T cells. These nonclonal receptors, which bind to conserved structures associated with microbial pathogens, include CD14, Toll-like receptors (TLRs), mannose binding protein, serum amyloid P, complement receptors, C-reactive protein, Fc receptors, CD11b/CD18, and collectins. PRRs are strategically expressed on cells that are the first to encounter pathogens during infection, such as surface epithelial cells and APCs *(1)*. The PRRs that recognize a number of bacterial products have been identified. For example, TLR4 recognizes the Gram-negative bacterial product LPS, TLR2 recognizes bacterial lipopeptide, TLR5 recognizes bacterial flagellin, and TLR9 recognizes CpG motifs in bacterial DNA *(1–3)*. Binding of certain microbial molecules, such as LPS to TLRs, transduces signals through the adaptor protein, myeloid differentiation factor 88 and the transcription factor NFκB, leading to transcription of several immune response genes including interleukin (IL)-1, tumor necrosis factor (TNF)-α, IL-12 at variable levels, [L1] and costimulatory molecules, including CD80, CD86, and CD40 *(1–3)*. Ligation of PRRs on APCs increases the potency of the cell in antigen presentation and stimulation of T-cell responses. LPS from different bacteria signal through TLR4 or TLR2, and a range of other bacterial toxins bind to other receptors on innate cells, which may also be considered as PPRs.

## *Role of Microbial Molecules in Polarizing Th Cell Subtypes Through DC Maturation*

Protective immunity against certain diseases is dependent on the differential induction of T helper (Th)1 or Th2 responses. The induction of Th1 responses is desirable for immunization against many intracellular pathogens; Th1 cells mediate cellular immunity against viruses, many bacteria and small parasites *(4)*, but also provide helper function for B-cell production of opsonizing and complement fixing antibodies of the immunoglobin (Ig)G2a subclass in mice *(5)*. Th2 cells are induced in response to helminth parasites, but are also induced by allergens and by immunization with soluble or alum-adsorbed antigens *(4,6)*. Th2 cells mediate immunity to extracellular parasites and bacteria and provide helper function for the production of IgE, IgA, and neutralizing IgG antibodies against bacterial toxins. Recent evidence has suggested that most pathogens also generate a population of T cells with regulatory or suppressive activity called regulatory T (Tr) cells. These function to maintain tolerance and prevent autoimmune disease but also control Th1/Th2 and inflammatory responses during infection *(7)*. Induction of an immune response by adjuvants generally results in its polarization to a certain subtype, which is influenced by the APC and the cytokine environment at the site of immunization.

Recent evidence suggests that the differentiation of Th cells from naïve precursors is regulated by the activation status of the DC *(7,8)*. Macrophages and DCs secrete the Th1 polarizing cytokines IL-12, IL-18, IL-23, and IL-27 in response to certain microbial products, notably LPS from Gram-negative bacteria *(4,9,10)*. IL-4 and IL-6 play a role in driving the Th2 pathway; DCs may secrete IL-4 in responses to certain pathogen-derived molecules *(11)*, but the cellular source of this early IL-4 remains to be fully defined. Other pathogen derived products including several bacterial toxins, promote IL-10 and inhibit IL-12 production from DC and consequently promote the induction of IL-10-secreting Tr cells *(7)*. The initiation of T-cell responses is dependent on maturation of the DC and the signal for maturation can be provided by interaction of microbial products, including bacterial toxins, with surface PRR and activation of signaling pathways that result in transcription of immune responses genes. When immature DCs encounter antigen in the tissues, they express the chemokine receptors CCR5 and CCR6 and low levels of class II major histocompatability complex (MHC), CD80 and CD86, the cells are highly phagocytic and readily take up foreign antigen. After antigen acquisition, CCR5 and CCR6 expression is downregulated and CCR7 upregulated, and the DCs migrate to the lymph nodes and undergo maturation *(12)*. The maturation of DCs is accompanied by a decreased ability to acquire and process antigen, but an increased ability to present antigen as a consequence of enhanced expression of CD80, CD86, and class II MHC molecules *(8,12)*. Maturation signals can be provided by conserved molecules from microbial pathogens, such as LPS, CpG motifs on bacterial DNA, CD40L expressed on T cells or IL-1 and TNF-α secreted by macrophages in response to pathogen-derived molecules. Furthermore, the ability of DCs to function as APCs for Th1, Th2, or Tr cells appears to depend on distinct activation signals provided by different pathogens. LPS from Gram-negative bacteria promotes maturation of DC that selectively activate Th1 cells, whereas phosphorylcholine-containing glycoproteins derived from nematode parasites and cholera toxin (CT) activate DC, which direct the induction of Th2 cells *(13,14)*. Recent evidence suggests that bacterial products can also promote the activation of DC into a semimature phenotype, which promote the polarization of type 1 Tr (Tr1) cells *(14,15)*.

Therefore, pathogen-derived immunomodulatory molecules have the capacity to activate acquired immune responses and to control T-cell differentiation by differentially regulating the cytokine production and maturation of DCs.

## Costimulation and Activation of T Cells by Bacterial Toxins

Activation of T cells is dependent on two signals, one provided by the interaction of the antigen-specific T-cell receptor with peptide-MHC and the other between costimulatory molecules, such as CD28 on T cells and CD80 or CD86 on the APC. Following engagement of T-cell receptor and CD28, the T cell receives signals through the associated CD3 complex, which eventually leads to transcription of several activation-associated and cytokine genes, including IL-2 *(16)*. In contrast to these stimulatory interactions, the engagement of CTLA-4, another costimulatory molecule on T cells, can result in anergy or unresponsiveness. The costimulatory molecule ICOS (inducible costimulator) is expressed only on activated T cells and binds to B7-H2 on APCs, this interaction is important for IL-10 production and for polarization of Th2 responses *(16)*. Additional interactions, such as those between CD40 and CD40L, LFA-1, or DC-Sign with ICAM-3 and LFA-3 with CD2, help to build the "immunological synapse" between the APCs and T cells *(17)*. Certain pathogen-derived immunomodulatory molecules function by enhancing or disrupting the costimulation of T cells by APCs, and this property can be exploited in vaccine development by employing nontoxic microbial products that act as adjuvants to enhance innate and hence acquired immune responses. Furthermore bacterial toxins can bind directly to and activate T cells in a polyclonal fashion. For example, PT induces proliferation and cytokine production by naïve T cells in vitro *(18)*. This may contribute to its adjuvant activity by expanding or augmenting the induction of T cells specific for unrelated antigens administered with the toxin in vivo. Furthermore there is evidence that AB toxins, such as CT and PT, may directly interact with T cells and selectively modulate cytokine secretion *(19)*.

## Targeting Antigens to the Endogenous Route of Antigen Processing for the Induction of Class I-Restricted MHC CTL

Cytotoxic T lymphocytes (CTLs) represent an important immune effector mechanism for clearance of many intracellular viruses and bacteria. Following recognition of processed viral and bacterial fragments presented on the infected cell surface, CTLs destroy the infected cells. Additionally, as CTLs target all viral gene products that are expressed during viral replication, specific CTL responses may help to lower the viral load by interfering with viral assembly *(20)*. Unlike $CD4^+$ T cells that recognize exogenous antigen in association with class II MHC molecules and are readily generated by soluble antigens, $CD8^+$ CTL recognize endogenous antigen in association with class I MHC molecules. Therefore, to generate an effective CTL response, an exogenous antigen has to be directed to the endogenous pathway of processing, for presentation to class I-restricted T cells. Vaccines based on attenuated bacteria or viruses or live vectors are effective at generating class I-restricted CTL responses, whereas recombinant proteins in conventional adjuvants, such as alum, are effective at generating antibody and $CD4^+$ T-cell responses, but generally fail to generate $CD8^+$ CTL responses *(6,21)*. However it has been demonstrated that incorporation of antigens into particles or lipid structures, such as liposomes, PLG microparticles, immune-stimulating complexes (ISCOMs), or saponins/QS21 can allow antigens to escape from endosomes into the cytoplasm of the APC, thus allowing access to the endogenous route of antigen processing *(21)*. More recently, it has been demonstrated that bacterial toxins, fused to or mixed with foreign antigens, can direct the antigens to the class I processing pathway *(22,23)*.

## Mucosal Immunity: The Role of Bacterial Toxins in Overcoming Tolerance

Because the majority of human pathogens initially infect the host through the mucosal tissues, nasal or oral delivery of vaccines may facilitate the prevention of certain infectious diseases through the induction of local immunity at the site of infection. Local immune responses are not generated following parenteral immunization, but can be induced when the antigen is delivered to a mucosal surface. Therefore mucosal vaccination may improve the efficacy of current parenterally delivered vaccines and may provide a basis for preventing a range of infectious diseases for which successful vaccines have yet to be developed. Additionally, mucosal immunization abrogates the need for injections and may reduce certain of the adverse reactions seen when the vaccines are administered by parenteral routes. Mucosal defense against pathogens consists of physical barriers, such as the epithelium and mucus, innate immune responses, and adaptive immune responses. Mucosal antibodies, in particular secretory IgA, may provide an early defense against invading pathogens, although serum IgG may be required for prevention of systemic infection, but also functions at mucosal surfaces after transudation from the serum *(20)*. Secretory IgA is induced when antigens are transported across mucosal surfaces and into mucosal lymphoid tissue. Processing of the antigens leads to homing of specific IgA producing cells to various mucosal effector sites. Secretory IgA may protect against pathogens that replicate on or enter via mucosal surfaces by blocking their attachment or colonization and by neutralizing surface acting toxins.

A major obstacle to the development of mucosal vaccines is the poor immunogenicity of protein antigens when delivered mucosally, especially by the oral route. Because mucosal surfaces are constantly exposed to foreign material (inhaled antigens and food), mucosal tolerance or unresponsiveness has evolved to prevent unwanted inflammation to harmless soluble antigens *(24)*. Therefore the development of effective mucosal vaccines is dependent on the use of antigen delivery systems that will protect the antigen from enzymatic digestion and promote uptake by M cells and epithelial cells at mucosal surfaces and the inclusion of adjuvants that will stimulate innate immune responses and direct the appropriate adaptive immune responses. The most promising immunomodulatory molecules assessed as mucosal adjuvants to date are bacterial toxins. However, most toxins are too toxic for human use and must be modified to reduce their toxicity but retain the beneficial immunomodulatory activity.

## MODIFIED BACTERIAL TOXINS AS VACCINE ANTIGENS

Potent immune responses are generated against bacterial toxins, during infection or following vaccination and these responses can often protect against diseases caused by the toxin-producing bacteria. Chemically modified toxoids of diphtheria toxin and tetanus toxin can prevent diseases caused by *Corynebacterium diphtheria* or *Clostridium tetani* respectively and genetically or chemically inactivated PT in combination with other virulence factors of *B. pertussis* can protect against whooping cough *(25,26)*. All pertussis acellular vaccines (Pa) licensed to date include modified PT as a component. A monocomponent Pa, based on hydrogen peroxide-treated PT protected 71% of children in a placebo-controlled trial carried out in Gothenburg, Sweden *(27)*. Two, three, or five component Pa, comprising aldehyde or genetically detoxified PT and filamentous hemagglutinin, with or without pertactin and fimbrae, had efficacies of 84 to 85% *(25,26)*. The genetically detoxified PT used by one vaccine manufacturer was created using site directed mutagenesis of amino acids in the A subunit involved in ADP-ribosylating activity *(28)*. Substitution of $Arg_9$ to Lys and $Glu_{129}$ to Gly created the mutant PT-9K/129G, which was nontoxic but fully immunogenic. The PT mutant was highly effective at inducing functionally relevant antibody responses at lower doses than those required for the chemically treated PT *(29)* and also induced T-cell responses *(30,31)*. The reduced immunogenicity of the chemically compared with genetically detoxified PT may reflect loss of conformational antibody binding sites and receptor interaction sites and difficulties of antigen processing of the cross-linked protein *(32,33)*. Although the mutant toxin was not assessed as a mono-component vaccine in placebo-controlled efficacy trials in humans, it conferred a high level of protection without additional pertussis antigens in mice *(30)*.

Several nontoxic or partially toxic mutants of diphtheria toxin that cross-react immunologically with it, and hence are called cross-reacting materials (CRM), have been produced and elicit strong immune responses against diphtheria toxin. Diphtheria toxin is composed of two disulfide-linked fragments, an enzymatically active A fragment, and a B fragment, that is responsible for binding and entry of the toxin into sensitive eukaryotic cells. Protein synthesis in these cells is inhibited by inactivation of the ribosomal elongation factor 2, caused by the specific ADP-ribosylating activity of fragment A, resulting in cell death *(34)*. One mutant of diphtheria toxin, $CRM_{197}$, contains a glycine to glutamic acid mutation at position 52 in the A subunit, rendering it enzymatically inactive and therefore nontoxic *(35)*. Because $CRM_{197}$ is naturally nontoxic it does not require formaldehyde detoxification and can be obtained at close to 100% purity, avoiding the cross-linking to accessory antigens that occurs during formaldehyde treatment of diphtheria toxin. It would therefore appear to be an ideal candidate as a vaccine against diphtheria. Studies have shown that $CRM_{197}$ is less immunogenic than conventional diphtheria toxoid, but that its immunogenicity can be increased after stabilization with formaldehyde *(36–38)*. Intranasal immunization with $CRM_{197}$ formulated with chitosan, a cationic polysaccharide derived from chitin with potential for vaccine delivery and as an adjuvant, induced high levels of antigen-specific IgG, secretory IgA and toxin-neutralizing antibodies in mice and protective antibodies against the toxin in a guinea pig passive challenge model *(38)*. Furthermore, this formulation induced T-cell responses, predominately of Th2 subtype, whereas native and mildly formaldehyde-treated $CRM_{197}$ and conventional diphtheria toxoid (DT) induced mixed

Th1/Th2 responses and similar levels of anti-DT serum IgG following parenteral immunization. Priming parenterally with DT in alum and boosting intranasally with $CRM_{197}$ was shown to be a very effective method of immunization in mice, capable of inducing high levels of anti-DT IgG and neutralizing antibodies in the serum and secretory IgA in the respiratory tract (38). In a clinical trial, nasal delivery of $CRM_{197}$ with chitosan as a powder was well tolerated, without any serious side effects, induced local IgA and boosted diphtheria toxin-specific serum antibodies in adult human volunteers (39). The immune responses were significantly higher when $CRM_{197}$ was administered in combination with chitosan. Furthermore, formulation of the nasal diphtheria vaccine with chitosan significantly augmented Th2-type responses, which correlated with protective levels of toxin-neutralizing antibodies in intranasally boosted individuals (40). Therefore intranasal administration of $CRM_{197}$ antigen may be very effective booster vaccination approach in adolescents or adults who have previously been parenterally immunized with a conventional diphtheria toxoid vaccine.

## BACTERIAL TOXINS AS ADJUVANTS

The realization that adjuvants are capable of altering cytokine production and costimulatory molecule expression on cells of the innate immune system, including APCs, which determine the induction of T-cell subtypes in a nonantigen specific manner has opened a new approach to vaccine design. Bacterial molecules, and detoxified forms of these molecules, provide the major source of immune-stimulating adjuvants, because these molecules are the key microbial structures that have provided the infectious danger signals to the immune system. Modified bacterial toxins with immunomodulatory properties, in particular the ability to enhance or suppress distinct T-cell subtypes or inflammatory responses also have the potential to act as immuno-therapeutic agents for the treatment of immune-mediated diseases.

## CHOLERA TOXIN AND *ESCHERICHIA COLI* LT

### Structure and Function

The enterotoxins CT from *Vibrio cholerae* and LT from enterotoxigenic strains of *E. coli* are members of the AB class of bacterial toxins. Both toxins are composed of an enzymatically active A subunit with adenosine-diphosphate (ADP)-ribosyltransferase activity, that is responsible for toxicity, and a pentameric B oligomer that binds to receptors on the eukaryotic cell surface (41–45). The B-subunits of LT (LTB) and CT (CTB) are formed by five monomers that are arranged in a cylinder-like structure with a central cavity. The B-subunits are stable as pentamers in trypsin or proteinase K and at acidic pH (pH 2.0 and above for LTB and pH 3.9 and above for CTB). Interaction of LTB and CTB with their cell surface receptors is necessary for internalization of the globular A subunit *(46)*. When administered mucosally, the specific interaction of the B subunit with its receptor on epithelial cells is necessary for uptake from the lumen of the gastrointestinal tract (oral delivery) or the respiratory tract (intranasal delivery). The receptor binding site is specific for galactose-containing molecules; CTB and LTB bind with high affinity to the glycosphingolipid, GM1-ganglioside [Gal($\beta$1-3)GalNAc ($\beta$1-4)(NeuAc($\alpha$2-3))Gal($\beta$1-4)Glc($\beta$1-1) ceramide], present on the surfaces of mammalian cells *(47)*. CTB and LTB can also bind to GD1b-ganglioside, but with a lower affinity than to GM1 *(46)*. Additionally, LTB may bind to other glycosphingolipids (asialo-GM1), to glycoprotein receptors, polyglycosilceramides and to paragloboside *(44)*. This broader binding specificity of LT may explain the differences in the type of immune response induced by the toxins.

The A subunit is composed of a globular enzymatically active $A_1$ domain and an $A_2$ domain formed by a long $\alpha$ helix. The two domains are attached via a trypsin-sensitive loop and a disulphide bridge between $A_1$–$cys_{187}$ and $A_2$–$cys_{199}$. To become activated, the loop must be proteolytically cleaved and the disulphide bond reduced *(47)*. The A1 fragment enters the cell cytosol and ADP-ribosylates the stimulatory $\alpha$-subunit of a guanosine 5'-triphosphate (GTP)-binding protein ($G_s$) that causes permanent activation of adenylate cyclase resulting in an elevation in intracellular cyclic AMP (cAMP) concentration *(41,48)*. This triggers a number of events including the phosphorylation of protein kinase A leading to opening of the cystic fibrosis transmembrane conductance regulator Cl⁻ channel, and osmotic movement of water into the gut lumen and diarrhea. The major function of the $A_2$-fragment is interaction with the B-subunits. However, the C-terminus of the $A_2$-fragment also contains a sequence motif associated with retrieval of proteins from the *trans*-Golgi network to the endoplasmic reticulum *(49)*. It has been suggested that this may be important in delivery of the $A_1$-fragment to the correct cellular compartment *(46)*. The basal ADP-ribosyltransferase activity of CT and LT is enhanced by interaction with GTP-binding proteins, known as ADP-ribosylation factors or ARFs *(50)*. ARFs play a crucial role in vesicular membrane trafficking and contribute to the maintenance of organelle integrity and the assembly of coat proteins in eukaryotic cells.

### Immunogenicity and Adjuvanticity of CT, LT, and Their B-Subunits

CT and LT are powerful mucosal immunogens; low doses induce strong antitoxin secretory and systemic antibody responses *(43–45,51,52)*. These antitoxin responses are so potent that immune responses are also generated against foreign bystander molecules that are present simultaneously at the mucosal surfaces. Consequently, CT and LT have been extensively used as mucosal adjuvants with a wide variety of antigens in animal models and more recently in clinical trials.

Co-administration of CT and LT with antigen via the nasal, oral, and other mucosal routes results in substantial enhancement of antigen-specific mucosal IgA
and serum IgG responses. The adjuvant effects of CT and LT have also been
demonstrated in studies involving immunization via the subcutaneous, intraperitoneal, intravenous, intradermal and transcutaneous routes *(43–45).*

In addition to enhancing humoral immunity, CT and LT also augment cellular immune responses to co-administered antigens. Most studies indicate that
CT induces a Th2 biased response to itself and to bystander antigens (Table 1).
This is based on the findings that IL-4, IL-5, and IL-10 are produced with little
interferon (IFN)$\gamma$ *(53–59)* and supported by evidence that IgE *(54,55,58)* and
higher titers of IgG1 than IgG2a *(54,55,58,60–65)* are induced by antigens co-
administered with CT by mucosal routes. However, mixed Th1/Th2 responses
have also been reported following oral immunization with CT and KLH *(66),*
human immunodeficiency virus (HIV) reverse transcriptase *(67), Helicobacter
pylori (68),* or hen egg lysozyme *(69),* and intranasal immunization with fimbrial protein from *Porphyromonas gingivalis (70).* We have recently demonstrated that although CT does elicit a population of Th1 cells, the response is
Th2-biased and the toxin also induces a population of IL-10-producing Tr1 cells
*(14,71).* On the other hand, most studies have demonstrated that LT strongly
enhances the induction of Th1 and Th2 cells to antigens delivered by oral or
nasal routes *(72–74),* but unlike CT may not enhance IgE responses *(74).* Analysis of IgG antibody subclasses against the third-party antigens demonstrated
an enhancement of both IgG1 and IgG2a with a dominance of IgG1 or IgG2a
in different studies *(60,63,73–78)* (Table 2). In a comparison of CT with type
II LT (serogroup I heat labile toxins consist of CT and LT-1 and serogroup II
enterotoxins include *E. coli* type II LT, with two antigenic variants (LT-IIa and
LTIIb), LTIIa was found to enhance IL-4 and IFN$\gamma$ production, but significantly higher levels of IFN$\gamma$ were produced than with CT *(65).* Codelivery of
antigens with CT and LT can also induce antigen-specific class I restricted CTL
responses *(23,79,80).* Priming for ovalbumin (OVA)-specific CTL was demonstrated following oral delivery of OVA with CT *(79).*

The B-subunits of LT and CT have immunomodulatory activity independent
of the A subunit. Initial commercial preparations of CTB in which the B-subunit was purified from the active toxin had strong adjuvant activity; however it
was later found that much of this activity was derived from contamination
with active CT *(81).* Recombinant CTB and LTB have now become available,
and using these it has become clear that the B-subunits, especially LTB, have
activity as mucosal adjuvants but this is generally weaker than in the case of
the holotoxins *(55,57,60,73,78,81,82).* Additionally, the B-subunits of LT or
CT can enhance immune responses to directly conjugated antigens delivered

# Table 1
## Adjuvant Effect of CT and Its Derivatives on Th1/Th2, IgG1/IgG2a, and IgE Responses

| Toxin | Route | Dose (µg) | Antigen | Cytokines enhanced | Ab enhanced | Ref. |
|---|---|---|---|---|---|---|
| CT | IN | 3.3, 10 | TT | IL-5 | IgG1 > IgG2a, IgE | 58 |
| CT | IN | 1 | OVA | | IgG1 > IgG2a | 60 |
| CT | IN | 1 | P. gingivalis fimbrial | IL-2, IL-4, IL-5, IL-6, IL-10, IFNγ | IgG1 > IgG2a | 70 |
| CT + CTB | IN | 0.5 + 10 | HSV-1 Gp | IL-2, IL-4, IL-5, IFNγ | IgG1 > IgG2a, IgE | 64 |
| CT + CTB | IN | 0.5 > 10 | HSV-1 Gp | IL-4, IL-10 | IgG1 > IgG2a | 82 |
| RTCB | | 100 | | Little effect | Little effect | |
| CTS61F | IN | 0.5 | OVA | IL-4, IL-5, IL-6, IL-10 | IgG1 > IgG2a, IgE | 55 |
| RCTB | | 5 | | IL-4, IL-5, IL-6, IL-10 | IgG1 > IgG2a, IgE | |
| | | 10 | | No effect | No effect | |
| CT-E29H | IN | 0.1, 1.0 | RSV-F | | IgG1 > IgG2a | 95 |
| RCTB | IN | 10 | RHBs | | IgG1 = IgG2a | 84 |
| CT | IN | 2 | KLH | | IgG1 = IgG2a | 98 |
| CTA1-DD | IN | 20 | | | IgG1 = IgG2a | |
| CT | Oral | 10 | KLH | IL-2, IL-4 | IgG1 > IgG2a | 59 |
| CT | Oral | 10 | OVA | IL-4, IL-5 | | 61 |
| CT | Oral | 10 | TT | IL-4, IL-5 | | 53 |
| CT | Oral | 10 | OVA | IL-4 | | 57 |
| CT | Oral | 100 | TT | IL-4 | IgG1 > IgG2a, IgE | 54 |
| CTA2/B | Oral | 10 | SBR-CTA2/B | IL-2, IL-4, IL-5, IFNγ | | 83 |
| CT | Oral | 10 | KLH | IL-2, IL-4, IFNγ | | 66 |
| | IV | 1 | | IL-2, IL-4, IFNγ | | |
| CT | SC | 1 | OVA | IL-4, IL-5, IL-6, IL-10 | IgG1 > IgG2a, IgE | 56 |
| CTE112K | | 10 | | IL-4, IL-5, IL-6, IL-10 | IgG1 > IgG2a, IgE | |
| CTS61F | | 10 | | IL-4, IL-5, IL-6, IL-10 | IgG1 > IgG2a, IgE | |
| RCTB | | 10 | | IL-4, IL-5, IL-10 (IFNγ; weak) | No effect | |
| CT | SC | 1 | KLH | IL-4, IL-5, IL-10 | IgG1 > IgG2a | 14 |

This is not an exhaustive list of studies involving the adjuvant effect of CT.

RCTB, recombinant B-subunit of cholera toxin; IN, intranasal; IV, intravenous; TC, transcutaneous; TT, tetanus toxoid; OVA, ovalbumin; HSV-1 Gp, herpes virus-1 glycoprotein; P. gingivalis fimbrial; Porphyromonas gingivalis fimbrial protein; RSV-F, respiratory syncytial virus F protein; RHBs, recombinant hepatitis B surface antigen; KLH, keyhole limpet haemocyanin; SBR-CTA2/B, Streptococcus mutans Ag I/II genetically coupled to cholera toxin A2- and B-subunits.

**Table 2**
**Adjuvant Effect of LT and Its Derivatives on Th1/Th2, IgG1/IgG2a, and IgE Responses**

| Toxin | Route | Dose (μg) | Antigen | Cytokines enhanced | Ab enhanced | Ref. |
|---|---|---|---|---|---|---|
| LT | IN | 1 | OVA | | IgG2a > IgG1 | 60 |
| LT | IN | 1 | OVA | | IgG2a > IgG1 | 76 |
| LT | IN | 1 | OVA | | IgG1 > IgG2a | 197 |
| LT | Oral | 1 | H. pylori urease | | IgG2a > IgG1 | 77 |
| RLTB | | 50 | | | IgG2a > IgG1 | |
| LT | SC | 0.01 | | | IgG1 > IgG2a, IgE | |
| RLTB | | 5, 50 | | | IgG1 > IgG2a | |
| LTR192G | IN | 10 | C. albicans | | IgG2a > IgG1 | 92 |
| LT | IN | 1 | OVA | | IgG2a > IgG1 | 76 |
| LTK63 | | | | | IgG1 > IgG2a | |
| LTR72 | | | | | IgG1 > IgG2a | |
| RLTB | | | | | Low titres | |
| LTR72 | IN | 1 | B. pertussis Ag | IL-4, IL-5 | | 72 |
| | | 10 | | IFNγ, IL-4, IL-5 | | |
| LTK63 | | 1 | | IFNγ, IL-4, IL-5 | | |
| | | 10 | | IFNγ, IL-4, IL-5 | | |
| LTR72 | SC | 1 | KLH | IFNγ, IL-4, IL-5, IL-10 | IgG1 > IgG2a | Unpub. |
| LTK63 | | | | IFNγ, IL-4, IL-5, IL-10 | IgG1 > IgG2a | |
| LTR72 | IN | 10, 25 | Influenza HA | | IgG2a > IgG1 | 97 |
| LT-IIa | IN | 1 | Smutans Ag | IFNγ, IL-4 | IgG1 > IgG2a | 65 |
| LT-IIb | | | | | IgG2a > IgG1 | |
| RLTB | IN | 10–100 | HSV-1 Gp | IL-4, IL-10 | IgG1 > IgG2a | 82 |
| LT | IN | 5 | TT | IFNγ, IL-6, IL-10 | | 73 |
| LTS61F | | | | IL-10 | | |
| LTA69G | | | | IFNγ, IL-6, IL-10 | | |

| | Route | Dose | Antigen | Cytokines | Antibody | |
|---|---|---|---|---|---|---|
| LTE112K | | | | IL-10 | | |
| LTR192G | | | | IFNγ, IL-6, IL-10 | | |
| RLTB | | | | Little effect | | |
| LT | Oral | 25 | | IFNγ, IL-6, IL-10 | | |
| LTS61F | | | | IL-6 | | |
| LTA69G | | | | IFNγ, IL-6, IL-10 | | |
| LTE112K | | | | IL-6 | | |
| LTR192G | | | | IFNγ, IL-6, IL-10 | | |
| RLTB | | | | IL-6 | | |
| LT | Oral | 10 | TT | IFNγ, IL-4, IL-5, IL-10 | IgG1 > IgG2a | 74 |
| LTR192G | Oral | 25 | Salmonella | IL-2, IFNγ, | | 94 |
| LT | Oral | 50 | KLH | IFNγ, IL-5 | IgG1 > IgG2a | 75 |
| LTH192 | | | | IFNγ, IL-5 | IgG1 > IgG2a | |
| RLTB | | | | Little effect | IgG1 (no IgG2a) | |

RLTB, recombinant B-subunit of *E coli* heat labile enterotoxin; IN, intranasal; SC, subcutaneous; OVA, ovalbumin; *C. albicans*, killed *Candida albicans*, *B. pertussis* Ag, *Bordetella pertussis* antigens (recombinant PT, FHA and pertactin); KLH, keyhole limpet haemocyanin; influenza HA, influenza virus haemagglutinin; *S. mutans* Ag; *streptococcus mutans* Ag I/Ii; Herpes virus-1 glycoprotein; TT, tetanus toxoid; Salmonella, killed *Salmonella* spp, Unpub, Lavelle, McNeela and Mills, unpublished.

by mucosal or parenteral routes *(76,77,82–84)*. There is little consistency amongst reported studies on the Th1 or Th2 bias of the immune responses generated with native or recombinant B-subunits. Some studies have demonstrated enhanced IFNγ and/or elevated IgG2a over IgG1 *(56,77)*; others have reported enhancement of either Th1 and Th2-type responses or IgG1 and IgG2a to the co-administered antigen or the toxin *(77,78,84)*. By contrast, one group has documented enhanced type 2 cytokines and increased IgG1 over IgG2a with LTB *(82)*. These differences may reflect variations in the nature and dose of antigen used, the route of delivery and possibly levels of contaminating LPS in the different toxin preparations.

CTB and LTB can also suppress immune responses and induce tolerance to orally or nasally delivered antigens and can prevent experimental autoimmune diseases *(45,85–89)*. Both Th1 and Th2 and IgG1 and IgG2a antibody responses to CTB-conjugated OVA were suppressed, but type 1 and type 2 responses were enhanced to birch pollen allergen Bet v 1, suggesting that induction of tolerance is dependent on the nature of the coupled antigen *(89)*. Antigen-specific class I-restricted CTL can also be generated in mice immunized with a soluble antigen mixed with CTB *(82)*.

## CT and LT Mutants

A number of successful attempts have been made to reduce the toxicity of LT and CT, without removing the adjuvanticity, most of which have focused on eliminating or attenuating the enzyme activity of the A subunit *(53,60,76,90–95)*. Site-directed mutagenesis has been used to target amino acids in the active site of the toxins that are critical for enzymatic activity. Some of the mutant derivatives obtained are efficiently assembled into the AB structure, are stable on storage and have either greatly reduced or undetectable toxicity. These CT and LT mutants have opened up the possibility of using AB toxins for clinical use and have also provided ideal tools to examine the role of the enzyme and binding domains in their adjuvanticity.

Initially it was thought that ADP-ribosylation and accumulation of cAMP were essential for adjuvanticity of LT and CT. It was reported that mice immunized orally with KLH and recombinant CTB or mutated LT, devoid of enzymatic activity (LTE112K), as the adjuvant generated very weak antibody responses *(96)*. However, more recently, mutants lacking ADP-ribosyltransferase activity have been shown to retain the ability to act as mucosal adjuvants *(53,56,60,76, 90–95)*. Two CT-A subunit mutants, CTS61F and CTE112K, constructed by site-directed mutagenesis had no ADP-ribosylation activity and did not promote cAMP production, or fluid accumulation in ligated mouse ileal loops *(55)*. However, both molecules retained adjuvant properties; co-administration with ovalbumin by the subcutaneous route induced significantly higher serum IgG titers than when the antigen was delivered alone. LTR72 and CTS106, which retain residual enzyme activity and toxicity in vitro and in vivo, appear to exert the strongest mucosal adjuvanticity of mutant toxins, with properties similar to those of wild-type LT or CT *(60,76)*. These two mutant toxins may have their toxicity sufficiently reduced to be safe in humans, but maintain some enzymatic activity that significantly enhances their adjuvanticity, especially for oral immunization.

Mutations have also been constructed in the protease sensitive loop of the toxins, rendering the loop insensitive to proteases and hence eliminating the susceptibility of the toxins to the cleavage required for activation of the enzymatic activity and toxicity *(92–94)*. Like the parent toxins, the mutant toxins enhance antibody and T-cell responses to co-administered antigens. The CT mutants CTS61F, CTE112K and CTE29H selectively enhanced Th2 responses and IgG1 and IgE *(55,56,95)*. However the subtype of T cells induced with certain LT mutants differed from that induced by the wild-type toxin and appears to be affected by its enzyme activity. The completely nontoxic mutant, LTK63, enhanced Th2 responses to a protein from serogroup B *Neisseria meningitidis* and at high doses Th1 and Th2 responses, whereas LTR72, which retains 1% of the ADP-ribosyltransferase activity, had a more potent enhancing effect on Th1 responses, although both mutants enhanced IgG1 and IgG2a antibody responses *(95a)*. By contrast, IgG2a was the dominant subclass of antibody induced following intranasal immunization with killed *Candida albicans* and LTR192G *(92)* or influenza virus hemagglutinin and LTR72 *(97)*. However, mixed Th1/Th2 responses have also been demonstrated following oral or nasal immunization with tetanus toxoid and LTA69G and LTR192G *(73)*. As in the case of the holotoxins, these variable results likely reflect the influence of the different antigens and routes used and the possible contribution of contaminating LPS. However, this does not detract from the fact that both the partially active and inactive mutants of CT and particularly LT have considerable potential as mucosal adjuvants.

In addition to these approaches involving site-directed mutagenesis of the A1 subunit, a fusion of the intact CT A1 subunit with a dimer of an Ig-binding fragment D, of *Staphylococcus aureus* protein A (CTA1-DD) has been described. This was designed to target B cells in contrast to CT, which binds to multiple cell types. CTA1-DD is an effective parenteral and mucosal adjuvant, capable of enhancing IgG1 and IgG2a antibodies to co-administered antigens *(98,99)*.

The suggestion that the adjuvant action of CT or LT derives from a independent contributions of the A subunit, B subunit, enzyme activity, or the nontoxic AB complex might account for the wide diversity of results obtained using different LT or CT mutants (Tables 1 and 2). Furthermore, in addition to variation in the immunomodulatory molecules and the assay system employed, the findings of enhanced or suppressed Th1/Th2 responses are likely to be influenced by the toxin dose, form (conjugated vs mixed) and purity (LPS contamination was not ruled out in all studies), route of delivery and nature and dose of the third party antigen used to demonstrate modulation of the bystander immune response.

Mucosal immunizations with vaccines formulated with CT or LT mutant toxin as adjuvant have been shown to provide effective protective immunity in several animal models of infection. Mice were protected against infection with *Helicobacter pylori* following oral immunization with recombinant Vac A, urease, and CagA antigens formulated with LTK63 or LTR72 *(100)*. LTK7 has been shown to enhance levels of protection in mice immunized with tetanus toxin fragment C *(91)*. Intranasal immunization with polysaccharide or protein subunit vaccines formulated with LT mutants can protect against invasive pneumococcal *(101)* and *Bordetella pertussis (72)* infections respectively. Mucosal immunization with the LT mutant, LTR192G has induced protective immunity against viral and bacterial infections in murine models *(92–95)*.

*Mechanism of Adjuvant Action*

The mechanism of action of CT and LT has long been controversial, and a number of hypotheses have been put forward to explain the potent immunogenicity and adjuvanticity of these toxins. Enhanced uptake of antigen at mucosal surfaces is one mechanism whereby CT and LT may enhance the immunogenicity of coupled or co-administered antigens. When rabbit nasal mucosal membrane was exposed to CTB and CT in Using chambers, the short-circuit current and conductance of the mucosa increased with increasing concentration of toxin and these changes could be blocked by addition of the ganglioside GM1 *(102)*. Following oral delivery of KLH, dextran and CT, CT strongly increased the gut permeability for dextran concomitantly with a strong enhancing effect on the KLH-specific immune response in the lamina propria *(103)*. By contrast, CTB failed to increase gut permeability and KLH-specific immune responses. It was therefore proposed that the adenylate cyclase/cAMP system plays a regulatory role in gut permeability, facilitating access of luminal antigens to the gut mucosal immune system, and thereby enhancing mucosal immune responses *(103)*. To confirm the role of adenylate cyclase activation in increasing gut permeability, the effects of nontoxic CT and LT mutants on gut permeability should be assessed.

Activation of cells of the innate immune system leading to potentiation of APC function and T-cell responses are likely to be a key feature in the adjuvant action of CT and LT. CT enhances alloantigen presentation by cultured intestinal epithelial cells *(104)*. However it has also been demonstrated that antigen processing can be inhibited by the ADP-ribosyltransferase activity of AB toxins;

LT and CT, but not LTB, CTB, or nontoxic LT mutant LT-E112D, suppressed intracellular antigen processing in APCs *(105)*. This is consistent with the demonstration that wild-type LT or LTR72, but not LTK63, suppressed IFNγ production by a Th1 clone in vitro *(90)*. However APC pretreatment with LT or LTR72 or direct addition of these toxins to T cells in culture enhanced IL-5 production by a Th2 clone *(90)*. Pretreatment of APCs with CT or CTB can enhance IL-4 production by a T-cell clone, by direct interaction of CTB-associated APCs and non-GM1 receptors on T cells *(106)*.

Expression of the costimulatory molecule CD86 on bone marrow macrophages is enhanced by treatment with CT, but not CTB *(107)*. Furthermore, CD86 expression by Mac1+ Peyer's patch cells was increased after intraluminal exposure to CT. Treatment of mice with an anti-CD86 antibody inhibited both the mucosal adjuvanticity and immunogenicity of CT *(108)*. Conversely LT, LTR72, and LTK63 enhanced CD80 expression, whereas only LT enhanced CD86 *(90)*. CT has also been shown to induce upregulation of CD80 and CD86 on murine Flt3L-expanded DCs *(109)* and on human DCs *(110)*. We have shown that CT selectively alters costimulatory molecule expression on murine bone marrow-derived DC, leading to enhanced expression of CD80 and CD86 although suppressing the expression of CD40 and intercellular adhesion molecule-1 (ICAM-1) *(14)*. Furthermore, in the presence of LPS the expression of CD80 is further enhanced whereas the LPS-induced enhancement of CD40 and ICAM-1 expression is suppressed. Thus a selective enhancement of the costimulatory activity and maturation of mucosal DCs would appear to be important for the mucosal adjuvanticity and immunogenicity of this molecule.

The AB toxins can also modulate the production of regulatory cytokines and chemokines by cells of the innate immune system. CT inhibits the production of bioactive IL-12 (p70) and the expression of the β1 and β2 chains of the IL-12 receptor on human monocytes and DCs, leading to a suppression of Th1 cell differentiation and driving a Th2-type response *(111)*. Similarly, exposure of human DCs to CT inhibited IL-12 p70, TNF-α, but not IL-6, IL-8, or IL-10 secretion in response to LPS or CD40 ligand *(110)*. We have reported similar findings with murine DC; CT alone induced the production of the chemokine MIP-2, although the proinflammatory cytokines and chemokines IL-12, TNF-α, MIP-1α, and MIP-1β were inhibited *(14)*. By contrast, the toxin enhanced LPS induced production of IL-1, IL-6, and the anti-inflammatory cytokine IL-10. Forskolin, a direct activator of adenylate cyclase, mediated similar effects to CT implicating cAMP as a determining factor in these responses *(112,113)*. Furthermore we have demonstrated that the ADP-ribosyltransferase activity of the A-subunit of LT leads to the accumulation of intracellular cAMP, which has enhancing effects on Th2 cells and inhibitory effects on inflammatory responses and the development of Th1 cells *(90)*.

It has also been suggested that GM1-binding or ADP-ribosylation activity is not essential for the adjuvanticity of LT. Recombinant mutant LTA molecules, without enzymatic activity, enhanced immune responses to co-administered influenza subunit antigen when delivered by the nasal route in mice *(114)*. It was concluded that the adjuvanticity of LTB was directly related to GM1-binding whereas adjuvanticity of LT was independent of GM1-binding and ADP-ribosylation activity. Furthermore, studies with the CTA1-DD fusion protein *(98,99)* suggested that potent adjuvant activity could be mediated via a ganglioside-GM1 independent pathway. Therefore, the modulation of immune response by CT or LT may be dependent on distinct contributions of the enzyme activity, the B-subunit interaction with GM1, and other, non-enzymatic activities of A subunit, on biochemical signaling pathways in cells of the innate immune system and perhaps directly on T cells.

## Pertussis Toxin

### Structure and Function

PT is an AB exotoxin and one of the main virulence factors of *Bordetella pertussis*, playing a major role in its pathogenesis. The B-oligomer, which is composed of four noncovalently-linked subunits (S2 to S5), in a ratio of 1:1:2:1 *(115,116)*, mediates binding of the toxin to surface glycoproteins, including lactosylceramide and gangliosides, expressed on a variety of mammalian cells, including cilia, macrophages, and lymphocytes *(117,118)*. Additionally, a 43 kDa plasma-membrane protein *(119)* and CD14 *(120)* have been proposed as receptors for PT. Binding of the B-oligomer to host cells allows the A subunit to enter the cell, in which it ADP-ribosylates $G_i$ proteins, which transmit inhibitory signals to the adenylate cyclase complex, [L3] affecting signaling pathways in many cell types, including cells of the immune system *(121)*, thus contributing to immune dysfunction in infected patients. It has been shown that PT impairs the delivery of signals that promote the survival of B cells in vitro *(122)*. PT has been shown to inhibit macrophage chemotaxis in vivo *(123)* and neutrophil and lymphocyte chemotaxis in vitro by altering intracellular calcium levels *(124)*. PT is also responsible for many of the systemic effects of *B. pertussis* infection and mediates certain of the local and systemic inflammatory responses of Pw, in which it is also present at variable levels as an active toxin *(125,126)*. Lymphocytosis, histamine sensitization, and hypoglycemia and neurological responses have all been attributed to the active toxin *(121,126)*. Recent evidence has shown that the leukocytosis induced by PT may result from G protein-dependent chemokine regulated extraversion of leukocytes. PT inhibits the increase in intracellular $Ca^{+1}$ levels in $CD4^+$ and $CD8^+$ T cells, induced by the CC chemokines, MCP-1, MCP-2, MCP-3, MIP-1α, MIP-1β, and RANTES

*(127)*, Ca$^{+1}$ mediated activation of neutrophils by IL-8 *(128)* and MCP-I induced chemotaxis of NK cells *(129)*.

*Adjuvant Activity*

PT, like LT and CT, possesses adjuvant properties, boosting immune responses to unrelated bystander antigens co-administered by systemic or nasal routes in mice *(18,130–132)* (Table 3). There is also indirect evidence of an adjuvant effect of PT in humans; antibody responses to other components of combination vaccines are diminished in the absence of whole cell pertussis vaccines *(133,134)*. Although LPS is likely to play a dominant role, it appears that PT is responsible in part for the adjuvant effect of the vaccine *(18,135)*. PT induces both local and systemic antibody responses, increasing IgE, IgG and IgA to co-administered antigen *(130,132,136)*. PT also induces delayed type hypersensitivity (DTH) *(137)* and promotes certain organ-specific autoimmune diseases, such as experimental autoimmune encephalitis, in mice *(138,139)*.

It has been demonstrated that the adjuvant effect of PT for IgE responses is associated with augmented production of IL-4 *(131)*. Furthermore, the potentiation of DTH reactions by PT is associated with enhanced antigen driven IFNγ production by sensitized lymphoid cells *(131,140)*. These findings suggest that the adjuvanticity of PT may be associated with enhanced production of both Th1 and Th2 cytokines. Indeed independent studies have demonstrated that PT enhances antigen-specific IFNγ and IL-2 *(123)* or IFNγ and IL-4 and/or IL-5 *(18,131,141–143)* (Table 3). Work carried out in our laboratory has shown a mixed Th1/Th2 response with increases in T-cell proliferation, IFNγ, IL-2, IL-4 and IL-5 after co-injection with PT and the bystander antigens, KLH or *B. pertussis* FHA *(18)*. An increase in IgG1 and IgG2a subclasses also provides indirect evidence of enhancement of Th1 and Th2 responses *(18)*. However, it has been demonstrated that PT can enhance IgE, IgG1 and Th2 responses to tetanus toxoid and ovalbumin *(136)* and to increase the ratio of IgG1 to IgG2a induced in response to respiratory syncytial virus in mice *(141)*. Furthermore priming with PT followed by respiratory syncytial virus (RSV) infection induced IgE, IgG1 and a strong IL-4 response to RSV antigen *(143)*.

*PT Mutants*

Because of its toxicity and adverse effects on the immune system, PT cannot be used for clinical applications. Chemical-treatment can eliminate the undesirable toxic effects of PT, but has been shown to affect its antigenicity and immunogenicity and abrogates its adjuvant activities *(32,33)*. By contrast, recombinant PT molecules with mutations in the S-1 subunit, that abrogate ADP-ribosyltransferase activity are nontoxic and highly immunogenic *(28,118, 121)*, and may also retain beneficial immunopotentiating activities of the native

**Table 3**
**Adjuvant Effect of PT and Its Derivatives on Th1/Th2, IgG1/IgG2a, and IgE Responses**

| Toxin | Route | Dose (µg) | Antigen | Cytokines enhanced | Ab enhanced | Ref. |
|---|---|---|---|---|---|---|
| PT | IV | 0.4 | KLH + CFA | IL-2, IFNγ | | 140 |
| PT | IP | 0.4 | OVA + IFA | IL-4 | IgE | 198 |
| PT | IP | 0.4 | OVA + IFA | IL-4, IFNγ | IgE | 131 |
| PT | IP | 0.1 | TT | | IgG1, IgE | 136 |
| PT | IP | 0.1 | KLH | IL-2, IL-4, IL-5, IFNγ | | 18 |
| | | 1 | | IL-2, IL-4, IL-5, IFNγ | | |
| | | 5 | | IL-2, IL-4, IL-5, IFNγ | IgG2a > IgG1 | |
| PT | IP | 5 | FHA | IL-5, IFNγ | | 18 |
| PT-9K/129G | | 5 | | IL-5, IFNγ | | |
| PTX-RENK | | 5 | | No effect | | |
| PT | IM | 0.2 | RSV | IL-4, IFNγ | | 141 |
| PT-9K/129G | | 0.2 | | IL-4, IFNγ | | |
| PT | IN | 0.2 | RSV | IL-4, IFNγ | IgG1 > IgG2a, IgE | 143 |
| PT | IN | 3 | TT-C | | IgG1 > IgG2a, IgE | 130 |
| PT-9K/129G | | 3 | | | IgG1 > IgG2a | |
| PT | IP | 0.2 | HEL + IFA | IL-5, IFNγ | IgG2a | 142 |
| PT-B | | | | No effect | | |
| PT-A | | | | No effect | | |
| PT | IP | 1.0 | KLH | IL-2, IL-4, IL-5, IL-10 | IgG2a = IgG1, IFNγ | 19 |

PT-B, B-subunit of PT; PT-A, A subunit of PT; IV, intravenous, IP, intraperitoneal, IM, intramuscular, IN, intranasal; KLH, keyhole limpet hemocyanin; CFA, complete Freund's adjuvant; OVA, ovalbumin; IFA, incomplete Freund's adjuvant; FHA, filamentous hemagglutinin from *B. pertussis*; RSV, respiratory syncytial virus; TT-C, tetanus toxin fragment C; HEL, hen egg lysozyme.

toxin that are lost through chemical toxoiding. Several genetically engineered mutants of PT have been developed and compared to the native toxin for enzymatic activity and immunomodulatory characteristics *(28,118,121,144)*. Replacing one or two key amino acids within the enzymatically active S1 subunit resulted in well-assembled mutants, with indistinguishable subunit banding patterns from native toxin. Some of the mutants retained residual enzymatic activity and caused in vitro clustering of CHO cells. One double mutant, with substitutions at residues 9 (Arg to Lys) and 129 (Glu to Gly) in the S1 subunit (PT-9K/129G, did not show any detectable toxicity and ADP-ribosyltransferase activity could not be detected in vitro *(28)*. PT-9K/129G has been used as an antigen in a commercial, acellular pertussis vaccine *(25,28)* and has also been shown to be an effective adjuvant in mice *(18,130)*. PTX-RENK, a genetic mutant with substitutions/deletions in the S-1 and B-oligomer components is completely non-toxic, does not induce leukocytosis or clustering of CHO cells, but exhibits reduced binding to sialoglycoproteins and CHO cells and is not mitogenic for T cells *(118)*, whereas PT-9K/129G retains mitogenicity and the ability to bind to receptors on eukaryotic cells *(28)*.

These mutants have been used to help unravel the debate surrounding the mechanism of adjuvant action of PT and are useful antigens for pertussis vaccines and potential adjuvants for enhancing immune responses to unrelated antigens. It has been demonstrated that the S-1 mutants, that retain receptor-binding activity, can modulate immune responses to unrelated antigens. Although chemically treated PT does not retain adjuvant activity, mutants of PT with site-directed substitutions in the S-1 subunit that do not possess ADP-ribosyltransferase activity, but retain receptor binding, have adjuvant properties, including the ability to enhance specific serum IgG and Th1 and Th2 responses to co-administered antigen *(18)*. Ryan and associates *(18)* demonstrated that the mutant PT-9K/129G enhanced antigen-specific IFNγ, IL-2, and IL-5 production following co-injection with FHA from *B. pertussis*. However responses were more polarized to Th1 than observed with the wild-type toxin. Furthermore, priming with PT-9K/129G followed by RSV enhanced IFNγ-dominant memory response to both PT-9K/129G and RSV antigens *(141)*. By contrast, intranasal (IN) administration of tetanus toxin fragment C with PT-9K/129G induced high-titer antitoxin antibodies, predominantly IgG1 in serum and IgA in the lungs, whereas PT enhanced IgG1, IgG2a and IgE *(130)*.

In contrast to the S-1 mutant, a toxin with mutations in both the enzyme and binding domain had no adjuvant activity, suggesting that binding of PT to its receptor is an essential, but not necessarily the only, feature of adjuvanticity *(18)*. It has been reported that purified B-oligomer can enhance antibody responses to an influenza vaccine administered IN to mice *(145)*. It has also been demonstrated that certain of the immunomodulatory effects of PT, such as augmentation of IgE is dependent on the ADP-ribosyltransferase activity and mutants lacking enzymatic activity are unable to induce antigen-specific IgE *(146,147)*. Indeed, the B-oligomer alone can trigger phospholipase C and tyrosine kinase-dependent signal transduction through interaction with its cell surface receptor *(148)*. Thus, like CT and LT, both the enzyme activity and the nontoxic AB complex of PT appear to have immunomodulatory functions.

*Mechanisms of Adjuvant Activity*

Although the precise mechanism of action is not clear, it appears that PT functions as an adjuvant by activating both innate and adaptive immune responses and targets both APCs and T cells. Binding of the toxin to surface receptors on cells of the innate and acquired immune system activates signaling pathways involved in cytokine secretion and accessory molecule expression. PT and nontoxic mutants activate macrophages to secrete IL-1β, and to upregulate surface expression of the costimulatory molecules CD80 and CD86 on macrophages *(18)* and DCs *(19,149)*. It has also been suggested that the cellular signaling pathways linked to the inhibition of G proteins by PT in APCs results in their activation with increased expression of costimulatory molecules and class II MHC and the secretion of IL-1, IL-6, and IL-12 *(142)*. However, both PT and PT-9K/129G increase the expression of CD80 and CD86 on macrophages and B cells *(18)* and augment CD80, CD86, HLA-DR, and CD83 on human monocyte-derived DC *(149)*, which suggests that the ADP-ribosyltransferase activity of the toxin is not essential for the activation of APCs.

PT also induces proliferation, IL-2 and IFNγ secretion by T cells and enhances their surface expression of the costimulatory molecule CD28 *(18)*. Enhancement of experimental autoimmune encephalitis by PT appears to occur by interference with tolerance to self-proteins *(138)*. This may occur by antagonizing the delivery of negative signals to T cells, because active PT prevents superantigen-induced deletion of T cells in vivo *(150)*. Although the antitolerance effect was dependent on ADP-ribosyltransferase activity *(150)*, its effect on T-cell proliferation and cytokine production does not require enzyme activity *(14)*. Protein kinase C and tyrosine protein kinases are critical component in T-cell activation, and PT has been shown to activate these kinases in other cell types *(151)*. This mechanism of T-cell activation seems to be dependent on binding of the B oligomer to its receptor rather than its ADP-ribosyltransferase activity *(152)*. Additionally, the rapid increase in tyrosine phosphorylation indicates that it is a receptor-mediated event and does not rely on the ADP-ribosylation of a G protein *(151)*. PT also stimulates IL-2 production, which is not associated with the ADP-ribosyltransferase activity of the toxin *(18,153)*. Indeed, both PT and its B subunit can stably bind to the surface of DC, resulting in increased adherence of the DC to surrounding cells *(154)*.

Recent studies have shown that PT synergizes with LPS to enhance DC maturation and cytokine production, specifically IL-12 *(149)* and promotes the generation of DC that direct the differentiation of Th1 cells *(155)*. Augmentation of spleen cell IL-12 production in response to both microbial and non-microbial stimuli by PT has been linked to inhibition of $G_i$ protein signaling in leukocytes *(156)*, suggesting that the ADP-ribosyltransferase activity of the toxin promotes the induction of Th1 responses. Regardless of the selective effects on Th1 and Th2 cells, and there is evidence to suggest that both populations are augmented, the immunomodulatory effects of PT appear to be mediated by the independent contribution of the enzyme activity and the B oligomer or the nontoxic AB complex.

*Adenylate Cyclase Toxin*

Adenylate cyclase toxin (CyaA) from *B. pertussis* is a major virulence factor and plays a central role in the pathogenicity of *B. pertussis* *(157)*. CyaA, which is released by *B. pertussis* during growth, can be taken up by many cell types, in which it catalyses the conversion of cellular ATP to cAMP *(158)*. The toxin is a bifunctional protein, with a hemolysin enzyme domain that is critical for entry into cells and the adenylate cyclase domain that elevates intracellular cAMP *(159)*. Elevated intracellular cAMP interferes with intracellular signaling in cells of the immune system, and modulates a variety of immune effector functions, including oxidative responses and TNF-$\alpha$ production by monocytes or macrophages *(159,160)* and also induces apoptosis in macrophages *(161)* and DCs. CyaA inhibits production of the proinflammatory cytokines and chemokines IL-12, TNF-$\alpha$, CCL3, and CCL4 and enhances production of IL-10 in response to LPS *(162)*. Similar to cholera toxin *(14)*, CyaA enhances cell surface expression of CD80 and CD86 while inhibiting expression of CD40 and ICAM-1 *(162)*. However, LPS is closely associated with CyaA and the selective enhancing and inhibitory effects of LPS may complicate interpretation of certain studies with this toxin, which copurifies with the toxin. Recombinant CyaA mutants with disruptions in the adenylate cyclase catalytic domain, but with cell invasive activity, have been exploited to deliver unrelated foreign peptides and proteins to the cytosol, for the induction of class I-restricted CTL *(22)*. Immunization with recombinant CyaA hybrids expressing $CD8^+$ T-cell epitopes has been shown to induce class I-restricted CTL responses and protect against viruses and tumor in mice. Insertion of the foreign peptide in the adenylate cyclase domain, but not in the hemolysin moiety, appeared to target the antigens to the class I processing pathway *(22)*. Furthermore immunization with recombinant CyaA containing $CD4^+$ T-cell epitopes resulted in the induction of Th1 cells *(163)*.

The adenylate cyclase activity of the active toxin appears to have immunomodulatory activity and delivers antigens to the cytosol of the APC. Expression of the structural gene *cyaA* and *cyaC*, which is required for acylation of the toxin in *E. coli*, resulted in a recombinant protein that protected mice against *B. pertussis (164)*. This recombinant toxin also enhanced IgG responses to ovalbumin following co-administration by the subcutaneous route. In contrast, an inactive recombinant toxin prepared in the absence of *cyaC* had poor adjuvant activity. More recently we have demonstrated that CyaA is an effective parenteral adjuvant, principally inducing Th2 and Tr1 cells and an IgG1-dominated serum IgG response *(162)*. The adjuvant activity appears to be dependent, at least in part, on the enzymatic activity and is associated with an increase in intracellular cAMP concentrations in innate cells, but is independent of the acylation status *(165)*.

*Monophosphoryl Lipid A*

Monophosphoryl lipid A (MPL), a derivative of LPS, primarily from *Salmonella minnesota*, which retains much of the immunostimulatory properties of LPS without the inherent toxicity, has been used extensively as an adjuvant for parenteral administration of antigens. The parent molecule, LPS, a constituent of the outer surface of all Gram-negative bacteria is a powerful immunomodulator and stimulator of inflammatory responses. At submicromolar concentrations, LPS is capable of inducing dramatically elevated levels of the pro-inflammatory cytokines IL-1, IL-6, TNF-$\alpha$, and IL-12 *(166,167)*. However, LPS-induced disruption in the balance of pro- and anti-inflammatory mediators can result in endotoxic shock, which, depending on the severity of the reaction may be fatal. Consequently vaccine manufacturers go to great lengths to eliminate or reduce endotoxin contamination. Nevertheless, it is likely that the effectiveness of some traditional whole cell vaccines can be attributable, at least in part, to residual LPS contamination *(135)*. Although LPS is a potent immunomodulator and inducer of cytokines, including the Th1-promoting cytokine IL-12 *(167)*, it is too toxic for use in humans. Attempts to selectively reduce the toxic effects of LPS, although maintaining beneficial functions, led to the delineation of the structure–function relationship of analogues of chemically modified LPS. The lipid A portion of LPS was found to be the active moiety with respect to adjuvanticity and toxicity. Chemical modification of lipid A has resulted in the production of less toxic compounds. Mild acid hydrolysis of lipid A and removal of a base labile fatty acyl residue attached to carbon 3 of the diglucosamine backbone results in the production of MPL. MPL has subsequently been shown to exhibit dramatically reduced toxicity compared to LPS, although retaining potent adjuvant functions *(168,169)*.

Although the mechanism of action of MPL has not been defined clearly, it is probably similar to LPS, involving interaction with TLR4 and CD14 resulting in the activation of NF$\kappa$B and the production of proinflammatory cytokines. The adjuvant activity of MPL is primarily attributed to its ability to activate APCs and elicit cytokine production, in particular IL-12 by DCs and macrophages, resulting in the induction of antigen-specific cellular immunity and enhancement of complement fixing antibodies *(170)*. MPL induces the synthesis and release of cytokines by macrophages, particularly IFNγ and IL-12 and enhances CD80 expression *(170,171)*.

IN vaccination with MPL may be particularly beneficial in instances in which both systemic Th1-type responses and local secretory IgA are desired, as may be required for the elimination of many viruses and intracellular bacteria. Intranasal immunization with influenza virus antigens formulated with MPL induced antigen-specific IgA, CTL, and antibody responses suggestive of Th1-type immunity *(172)*. Furthermore, MPL enhanced local and systemic antibody responses to soluble or liposomal *Streptococcus mutans* crude glucosyltransferase delivered by the nasal or oral route *(173)*. Although MPL alone can augment humoral and cellular immune responses to foreign antigens, it has been found to be more effective when combined with other adjuvants or delivery systems. For example, MPL with QS21, a nontoxic derivative of saponin, significantly enhanced Th1 responses to a HIV gp120 recombinant glycoprotein *(170)*. This adjuvant combination also augmented cytotoxic responses of human CD8$^+$ T cells to herpes simplex virus in vitro, by enhancing IL-12 and IFNγ production *(174)*.

## CLINICAL EXPERIENCE
## WITH MODIFIED BACTERIAL TOXINS

Chemically detoxified diphtheria toxin, tetanus toxin, and chemically or genetically detoxified PT have been used in routine pediatric DTP vaccines for several decades. Additionally, tetanus toxoid and diphtheria toxoids, because of their acceptance for human use and availability, have been used as carriers for polysaccharide vaccines in humans *(175)*. Polysaccharides do not generate effective T-cell responses and the protein carriers enhance IgG responses and immunological memory, by providing targets for CD4$^+$ Th cells. Because bacterial toxins are highly effective stimulators of T cells, they fulfill this function very effectively. However, chemical treatment of toxins introduces batch-to-batch variation and affects the physiochemical properties and the immunogenicity of the toxin *(175)*. Recently CRM$_{197}$, a nontoxic analog of diphtheria toxin has been used as a carrier for the *Haemophilus influenzae* type b capsular polysaccharide vaccine in humans *(176)*.

Although mucosally administered vaccines that include native or modified bacterial toxins have been assessed in phase 1 clinical trials in human volunteers, there is limited data available on adjuvant effects in humans. CT and LT are clearly strong mucosal immunogens and adjuvants in animal models, but can cause side effects. Humans are exquisitely sensitive to these toxins; a diarrheagenic response may be triggered even at low doses that are nontoxic in mice.

Oral immunization of *H. pylori*-infected adult volunteers with *H. pylori* urease with LT-enhanced anti-urease IgA and reduced gastric *H. pylori* density, but also caused diarrhea in 66% of volunteers *(177)*. Clinical trials with an intranasally administered influenza virus vaccine formulated with LT showed that the vaccine stimulated local and systemic anti-influenza virus antibody *(178,179)*. Two nasal sprays with virosomal influenza vaccine and 1 µg LT as adjuvant were shown to induce antigen-specific immune responses comparable to those observed with a single parenteral vaccination in adult volunteers *(179)*. However, following licensing of the vaccine in Switzerland, a number of cases of Bells palsy was reported in vaccine recipients *(180)* and the vaccine was withdrawn from the market. In an unrelated study in mice, intranasal administration of CT has associated with retrograde transport of the toxin to the brain via the olfactory bulb *(181)*.

The potential side effects associated with native AB toxins has motivated the development and clinical testing of recombinant B-subunits of CT and LT mutants that retain adjuvant activity but with minimal toxicity. A number of clinical trials have been performed with CTB mixed with killed enterotoxigenic *E. coli* (ETEC) or inactivated *Vibrio cholerae* as oral vaccines against diarrheal diseases, including cholera *(182–184)*. In volunteers vaccinated with CTB by the route IN, toxin-specific IgG and IgA were elevated in secretions up to 6 months after immunization *(185)*. A nasally delivered influenza vaccine formulated with recombinant LTB mixed with trace amounts (0.5%) of LT enhanced hemagglutination-inhibiting antibodies in human volunteers *(186)*. The LT mutant, LTK63, which is completely devoid of toxicity, has exhibited an excellent safety profile in recent clinical trials with a nasally delivered influenza vaccine (Stephenson et al., manuscript in review).

An adjuvant formulation comprising MPL and QS21 in combination with an emulsion system has been evaluated in clinical trials with malaria *(187)* and HIV *(188)* vaccines. Although enzyme-linked immunoabsorbent assay (ELISA) antibody responses were detected in healthy HIV negative volunteers immunized with the HIV vaccine, sera did not neutralize primary isolates of HIV and HIV-specific class I-restricted CTL could not be detected *(188)*. In the malaria trial, antigen-specific T-cell proliferation and IFNγ production was detected in lymphocytes from immunized volunteers *(187)*. Although protection against malaria was reported, this was not sustained past 6 months and the immune responses evaluated did not correlate with protection *(187)*.

## SAFETY IMPLICATIONS
## FOR THE USE OF BACTERIAL TOXINS IN VACCINES

Parenteral immunization with bacterial toxins can result in a range of reactions from mild local inflammation to severe systemic and neurological reactions. Certain toxins such as tetanus toxin are neurotoxic and lethal to guinea pigs at nanogram concentrations. However these toxins are important protective antigens and antitoxin antibodies can prevent the bacterial disease caused by the parent bacteria. Modification of the toxins by treatment with aldehydes renders them non-toxic, but does not abrogate their capacity to generate toxin-neutralizing antibodies. However, the process used to prepare the toxoids involves the addition of glutaraldehyde or formaldehyde prior to purification and this results in a relatively impure preparation with other bacterial components, including cell wall components, cross-linked to the toxoids. These may contribute to the reactogenicity of the diphtheria, tetanus, and pertussis (DTP) combination vaccines. The DTP is highly reactogenic when the pertussis component is whole cell, and although it is significantly reduced with the introduction of the acellular pertussis vaccine, DT alone or DTPa vaccines still induce a significant number of local and systemic reactions.

The whole-cell pertussis vaccine is considered one of the most reactogenic vaccines in clinical use today. Centrally controlled responses, including fevers and seizures, are detected at a relatively high frequency following parenteral immunization with Pw and although controversial, there is also evidence of the more severe central nervous system complications in a small proportion of vaccinated children *(126,189,190)*. It has been suggested that active toxins present in the Pw may be responsible for the neurological responses *(126)*. Recent studies in our laboratory have shown that it is possible to induce fever, and seizure-like behavioral changes in mice following parenteral injection of Pw and exposure to high ambient temperature *(190,191)*. Certain neurological responses to vaccination appear to be mediated by inflammatory cytokines, which are produced not only locally and systemically but also in the brain in response to active bacterial toxins *(190,192)*. Systemic administration of Pw results in an elevation of IL-1$\beta$ protein and induction of IL-1$\beta$ mRNA transcripts in the hippocampus of mice 2 to 6 h after injection *(190,192)*. Because the expression is more persistent in the brain than in the circulation, it appears that the production is induced locally in the brain, either by activated macrophages, bacterial toxins, or other mediators that have crossed the blood–brain barrier. By contrast, IL-1$\beta$ levels were not significantly elevated in the brains of mice systemically immunized with a three-component Pa, comprising detoxified PT, FHA, and PRN *(190)*. Pw, but not Pa, are known to induce fever in a high proportion of immunized children *(25,26)*. In immunized mice, the kinetics of fever induction coincide with the elevated IL-1$\beta$ in the hypothalamus *(191)*. The elevated IL-1$\beta$ in the hippocampus induced with Pw, could be mimicked by injecting either purified PT or LPS and was associated with elevated c-jun N-terminal kinase and modulated neurotransmitter release in hippocampal synaptosomes *(192)*. Furthermore studies using IL-1 type 1 receptor defective mice provided direct evidence of a link between the seizure-like behavioral changes induced in mice immunized with Pw and toxin-induced IL-1β in the hippocampus *(190)*. These observations, together with reports of seizure activity with shigella toxin *(193)* provide direct evidence of a link between bacterial toxins and the neurological manifestations of the infection and vaccination and demonstrate that certain of the centrally controlled responses, such as fever and seizures, are mediated by toxin-induced proinflammatory cytokines.

Nasal immunization with vaccine formulations that include native or modified bacterial toxins as antigens or adjuvants may pose a risk of neurological side effects, associated with direct transport from the nose to the brain via the olfactory bulb. It has recently been demonstrated that CT can redirect vaccine proteins into olfactory tissue *(181)*. Radiolabeled CT or CT-B subunit were detected in the olfactory nerves/epithelium and olfactory bulbs and persisted for 6 days; however, neither molecule was present in nasal-associated lymphoreticular tissues beyond 24 h *(181)*. This uptake into olfactory regions was GM1-dependent. Intranasal vaccination with tetanus toxoid together with unlabeled CT as adjuvant resulted in antigen uptake into the olfactory nerve/epithelium, but not the olfactory bulb, whereas tetanus toxoid alone did not penetrate into the central nervous system. It was concluded that GM1-binding molecules like CT target the olfactory nerve/epithelium and are retrograde transported to the olfactory bulb and may promote uptake of vaccine proteins into olfactory neurons. However, a recent report has demonstrated that IN administration of CTB or LTB supplemented with trace amounts of holotoxin in mice did not localize to the brain or cause any histological changes in brain tissue *(181)*. Nevertheless, this is clearly a significant issue and raises safety concerns for $GM_1$-binding molecules or other bacterial toxins that might facilitate targeting of vaccines to neuronal tissues, especially when delivered by the nasal route. However, additional work is required to assess the functional implications of toxins in the central nervous system. Recent evidence from our laboratory suggests that neurological responses to bacterial toxins are dependent on delivery by the nasal route; CT induced pro-inflammatory cytokine production in the brain, when delivered nasally but not parenterally *(194)*. Therefore future clinical trials with vaccines that include bacterial toxins, whether native or modified and delivered by mucosal or parenteral routes, should be carefully monitored for potential neurological side effects.

In contrast to the proinflammatory effects associated with the induction of IL-1, TNF-α, and IFNγ, enhancement of IL-4, IL-5, and IgE responses by vaccines or adjuvants may also carry certain risks in relation to possible induction or enhancement of anaphylactic or allergic reactions. CT (but not LT) is known to enhance IgE responses *(54,55,58,74)* and the currently used adjuvant for most subunit vaccines in humans, alum, also enhances IgE production to the antigenic components of the vaccines. Significant local adverse reactions, including leg swelling, have also been reported with increasing booster doses of DTPa administered parenterally with alum as the adjuvant *(195)*. It was suggested that the leg swelling might result from IgE-mediated type I hypersensitivity. Children that received a fourth dose of Pa at 4 to 5 years of age developed potent PT-specific serum IgE responses and a highly polarized *B. pertussis*-specific Th2 response *(196)*. Because Th2 cell cytokines IL-4 and IL-5 enhance IgE production and IgE-dependent mast cell degranulation, the local reactions with Pa could be a type of anaphylactic reaction, which are significantly elevated after booster immunization with Pa. Therefore substitution of alum, which is know to enhance Th2 and IgE responses, with adjuvants that promote the induction of Th1 cells may not only reduce the incidence of these local reactions, but also improve the efficacy of the vaccines.

## AREAS FOR FUTURE REFINEMENT

Most vaccines based on attenuated or killed bacteria or viruses in use today are highly effective at preventing a number of life-threatening diseases. However, increasing concerns about safety has motivated a shift in emphasis to purified subunit protein and conjugated polysaccharide vaccines. Furthermore, the need to reduce the number of injected pediatric vaccines and the possibility of improving local immunity has motivated the assessment of mucosal routes of immunization. Although alum has gained universal approval for human use, it is often ineffective for purified or recombinant antigens; it cannot be used by mucosal routes and does not promote the induction of cellular immunity. Therefore new generation adjuvants and delivery systems are under evaluation and amongst the most promising candidates, especially for mucosal delivery, are modified bacterial toxins.

The identification of bacterial products with immunomodulatory activity capable of directing the immune responses to humoral or cell mediated immunity and that can selectively induce type 1 or type 2 T-cell responses should make it possible to design protective vaccines based on prior knowledge of the protective mechanism. For example, diseases like diphtheria and tetanus, which are largely mediated by bacterial toxins, can be prevented by toxin neutralizing antibodies. Therefore, new generation vaccines against these diseases should be possible using genetically detoxified recombinant toxins delivered parenterally or nasally with a delivery system or adjuvants, such AB toxins, that can enhance antibody and Th2 responses. More effective acellular vaccines against pertussis may be possible by replacing alum with adjuvants or delivery systems, such as PLG microparticles, LT or CT mutants or IL-12, that can stimulate Th1 responses, which function together with antibody in the rapid elimination of the bacteria from the lungs. Finally, CD8+ CTL and CD4+ Th1 cells appear to be critical in the prevention and control of viral infections, including HIV and hepatitis C virus, and protective vaccines against these viral infections may be possible using delivery systems such as naked DNA, live vectors, or CyaA that targets antigens to the class I processing pathway or immunomodulators that induce IL-12 production.

The use of delivery systems or immunomodulators to enhance immune responses to mucosally delivered vaccines should make it possible to design nasal or oral recombinant protein or DNA vaccines that can induce protective immune responses. The major obstacle to the development of nonreplicating oral vaccines is the poor immunogenicity of antigens delivered by this route and consequently the high dose of antigen required. However, the oral route ensures the greatest patient compliance and is considered to be the safest. Approaches to prevent degradation by encapsulation, to enhance uptake by targeting, and to improve immunogenicity by incorporating powerful mucosal adjuvants, such as CT or LT mutants, may bring further breakthroughs in oral vaccination. In the meantime the focus has turned to nasal vaccines, which are now showing considerable promise in preclinical studies and phase I clinical trials. Most of the trials have reported good immunogenicity and although there have been reports of adverse events, none have reported major side effects. Nevertheless, regulatory authority approval for the licensing of new adjuvants for routine use in humans will require a clear demonstration of a lack of reactogenicity. Therefore, future developments in vaccine formulation are dependent on identifying adjuvants, such as mutated bacterial toxins, in which it is possible to discriminate between beneficial immunomodulatory activity for enhanced immunogenity and the deleterious inflammatory effects that promote reactogenicity.

## ACKNOWLEDGMENTS

We would like to acknowledge the financial support of Science Foundation Ireland, the European Union, The Wellcome Trust, The Irish Health Research Board, Enterprise Ireland, and The Irish Higher Education Authority Programme for Research in Third Level Institutions.

## REFERENCES

1. Medzhitov R, Janeway C. Innate immunity: the virtues of a nonclonal system of recognition. Cell 1997;91:295–298.
2. Takeda K, Akira S. Toll-like receptors in innate immunity. Int Immunol 2005;17: 1–14.
3. Hemmi H, Takeuchi O, Kawai T, et al. A Toll-like receptor recognizes bacterial DNA. Nature 2000;408:740–745.

4. Mossman TR, Sad S. The expanding universe of T-cell subsets: Th1, Th2 and more. Immunol Today 1996;17:138–146.

5. Mahon BP, Katrak K, Nomoto A, Macadam AJ, Minor PD, Mills KHG. Poliovirus-specific Th1 clones with cytotoxic and helper activity mediate protective humoral immunity against a lethal poliovirus infection in a transgenic mouse model. J Exp Med 1995;181:1285–1292.

6. Moore A, McGuirk P, Adams S, Jones WC, McGee JP, O'Hagan D, Mills KHG. Induction of HIV-specific CD8+ CTL and CD4+ Th1 cells by immunization with recombinant gp120 entrapped in biodegradable microparticles. Vaccine 1995; 13:1741–1749.

7. Mills KHG. Regulatory T cells: friend or foe in immunity to infection? Nat Rev Immunol 2004;4:841–855.

8. Banchereau J, Briere F, Caux C, et al. Immunobiology of dendritic cells. Ann Rev Immunol 2000;18:767–811.

9. Trinchieri G, Pflanz S, and Kastelein RA. The IL-12 family of heterodimeric cytokines: new players in the regulation of T cell responses. Immunity 19:641–644.

10. Dinarello CA, Novick D, Puren AJ, et al. Overview of interleukin-18: more than an interferon-γ inducing factor. J Leuc Biol 1998;63:658–664.

11. d'Ostiani CF, Del Sero G, Bacci A, et al. Dendritic cells discriminate between yeasts and hyphae of the fungus Candida albicans. Implications for initiation of T helper cell immunity in vitro and in vivo. J Exp Med 2000;191:1661–1674.

12. Sallusto F, Palermo B, Lenig D, et al. Rapid and coordinated switch in chemokine receptor expression during dendritic cell maturation. Eur J Immunol 1998;28: 2760–2769.

13. Whelan M, Harnett MM, Houston KM, Patel V, Harnett W, Rigley KP. A filarial nematode secreted product signals dendritic cells to acquire a phenotype that drives development of Th2 cells. J Immunol 2000;164:6453–6260.

14. Lavelle EC, McNeela E, Armstrong ME, Leavy O, Higgins SC, Mills KH. Cholera toxin promotes the induction of regulatory T cells specific for bystander antigens by modulating dendritic cell activation. J Immunol 2003;171:2384–2392.

15. McGuirk P, McCann C, Mills KH. Pathogen-specific T regulatory 1, cells induced in the respiratory tract by a bacterial molecule that stimulates interleukin 10, production by dendritic cells: a novel strategy for evasion of protective T helper type 1, responses by Bordetella pertussis. J Exp Med 2002;195:221–231.

16. Chambers CA. The expanding world of co-stimulation: the two signal model revisited. Immunol Today 2001;22:217–223.

17. Friede P, Gunzer M. Interaction of T cells with APCs: the serial encounter model. Immunol Today 2001;22:187–191.

18. Ryan M, McCarthy L, Mahon B, Rappuoli R, Mills KHG. Pertussis toxin potentiates Th1, and Th2, responses to co-injected antigen: adjuvant action is associated with enhanced regulatory cytokine production and expression of the co-stimulatory molecules B7-1, B7-2, and CD28. Int Immunol 1998;10:651–662.

19. Leavy O. Mechanisms of immunomodulatory activity of cholera toxin. PhD thesis, Trinity College Dublin, 2005.

20. van Ginkel FW, Nguyen HH, McGhee JR Vaccines for mucosal immunity to combat emerging infectious diseases. Emerg Infect Dis 2000;6:123–132.
21. Raychaudhuri S, Morrow JW. Can soluble antigens induce CD8+ cytotoxic T-cell responses? A paradox revisited. Immunol Today 1993;14:344–348.
22. Osicka R, Osickova A, Basar T, et al. Delivery of CD8+ T-cell epitopes into major histocompatibility complex class I antigen presentation pathway by Bordetella pertussis adenylate cyclase: delineation of cell invasive structures and permissive insertion sites. Infect Immun 2000;68:247–256.
23. Simmons CP, Hussell T, Sparer T, Walzl G, Openshaw P, Dougan G. Mucosal delivery of a respiratory syncytial virus CTL peptide with enterotoxin-based adjuvants elicits protective, immunopathogenic, and immunoregulatory antiviral CD8+ T cell responses. Immunol J 2001;166:1106–1113.
24. Czerkinsky C, Anjuere F, McGhee JR, et al. Mucosal immunity and tolerance: relevance to vaccine development. Immunol Rev 1999;170:197–222.
25. Greco D, Salmaso S, Mastrantonio P, et al. A controlled trial of two acellular vaccines and one whole-cell vaccine against pertussis. Progetto Pertosse Working Group. N Engl J Med 1996;334:341–348.
26. Gustafsson L, Hallander HO, Olin P, Reizenstein E, Storsaeter J. A controlled trial of a two-component acellular, a five-component acellular, and a whole-cell pertussis vaccine. N Engl J Med 1996;334:349–355.
27. Trollofors B, Taranger J, Lagergard T, et al. A placebo-controlled trial of a pertussis-toxoid vaccine. N Engl J Med 1995;333:1045–1050.
28. Pizza M, Covacci A, Bartoloni A, et al. Mutants of pertussis toxin suitable for vaccine development. Science 1989;246:497–499.
29. Rappuoli R. Rational design of vaccines. Nat Med 1997;3:374–376.
30. Mills KHG, Ryan M, Ryan E, Mahon BP. A murine model in which protection correlates with pertussis vaccine efficacy in children reveals complementary roles for humoral and cell-mediated immunity in protection against Bordetella pertussis. Infect Immun 1998;66:594–602.
31. Ryan M, Mills KHG. The role of the S-1, and B-oligomer components of pertussis toxin in its adjuvant properties for Th1, and Th2, cells. Biochem Soc Trans 1997;25:126S.
32. Mills KHG, Barnard A, Watkins S, Redhead K. Specificity of the T cell response to Bordetella pertussis in aerosol infected mice. In: Manclarck CR, ed. Proceedings of the 6th International Symposium on Pertussis. Bethesda, MD: Department of Health and Human Services, United States Public Health Service, 1990, pp. 166–174.
33. Nencioni L, Volpini G, Peppoloni S, Bugnoli M, De Magistris T, Marsili I, Rappuoli R. Properties of pertussis toxin mutant PT-9K/129G after formaldehyde treatment. Infect Immun 1991;59:625–630.
34. Ratti G, Rappuoli R, Giannini G. The complete nucleotide sequence of the gene coding for diphtheria toxin in the corynephage omega (tox+) genome. Nuc Acids Res 1983;11:6589–6595.
35. Rappuoli R. (1997) New and improved vaccines against diphtheria and tetanus. In: Levine MM, Woodrow GC, Kaper JB, Cobon GS, ed. New generation vaccines (2nd edition). New York: Mercel Dekker, 1997, pp. 417–436.

36. Gupta RK, Collier RJ, Rappuoli R, Siber GR. Differences in the immunogenicity of native and formalinized cross reacting material ($CRM_{197}$) of diphtheria toxin in mice and guinea pigs and their implications on the development and control of diphtheria vaccine based on CRMs. Vaccine 1997;15:1341–1343.
37. Porro M, Saletti M, Nencioni L, Tagliaferri L, Marsili I. Immunogenic correlation between cross-reacting material (CRM197) produced by a mutant of Corynebacterium diphtheriae and diphtheria toxoid. J Infect Dis 1980;142:716–724.
38. McNeela EA, O'Connor D, Jabbal-Gill I, et al. A mucosal vaccine against diphtheria: Formulation of cross reacting material ($CRM_{197}$) of diphtheria toxin with chitosan enhances local and systemic antibody and Th2, responses following nasal delivery. Vaccine 2000;19:1188–1198.
39. Mills KH, Cosgrove C, McNeela EA, et al. Protective levels of diphtheria-neutralizing antibody induced in healthy volunteers by unilateral priming-boosting intranasal immunization associated with restricted ipsilateral mucosal secretory immunoglobulin a. Infect Immun 2003;71:726–732.
40. McNeela EA, Jabbal-Gill I, Illum L, et al. Intranasal immunization with genetically detoxified diphtheria toxin induces T cell responses in humans: enhancement of Th2, responses and toxin-neutralizing antibodies by formulation with chitosan. Vaccine 2004;22:909–914.
41. Spangler BD. Structure and function of cholera toxin and the related Escherichia coli heat-labile enterotoxin. Micbobiol Rev 1992;56:622–647.
42. Zhang RG, Scott DL, Westbrock ML, et al. The three-dimensional structure of cholera toxin. J Mol Biol 1995;251:563–573.
43. Rappuoli R, Pizza M, Douce G, Dougan G. Structure and mucosal adjuvanticity of cholera and Escherichia coli heat-labile enterotoxins. Immunol Today 1999; 20:493–500.
44. Pizza M, Giuliani MM, Fontana MR, et al. Mucosal vaccines: non toxic derivatives of LT and CT as mucosal adjuvants. Vaccine 2001;19:2534–2541.
45. Williams NA, Hirst TR, Nashar TO. Immune modulation by the cholera-like enterotoxins: from adjuvant to therapeutic. Immunol Today 1999;20:95–101.
46. Holmgren J, Lonroth I, Svennerholm L. Tissue receptor for cholera exotoxin: postulated structure from studies with GM1, ganglioside and related glycolipids. Infect Immun 1973;8:208–214.
47. Gill DM, Rappaport RS. Origin of the enzymatically active A1, fragment of cholera toxin. J Infect Dis 1979;139:674–680.
48. Field M, Rao MC, Chang EB. Intestinal electrolyte transport and diarrheal disease: Part 1. N Engl J Med 1989;321:800–806.
49. Pelham HR. The Florey Lecture. The secretion of proteins by cells. Proc R Soc Lond B Biol Sci 1992;22(250):1–10.
50. Tsai SC, Noda M, Adamik R, Moss J, Vaughan M. Stimulation of choleragen enzymatic activities by GTP and two soluble proteins purified from bovine brain. J Biol Chem 1988;263:1768–1772.
51. Lycke N, Lindholm L, Holmgren J. IgA isotype restriction in the mucosal but not in the extramucosal immune response after oral immunizations with cholera toxin or cholera subunit B. Int Archs Allergy Appl Immunol 1983;72:119–127.

144                                                                    *Lavelle et al.*

52. Lycke N, Holmgren J. Long-term mucosal memory to cholera toxin in mice after oral immunizations: antitoxin production from isolated lamina propria cells after in vivo or in vitro boosting. In: Strober W, Lamm ME, McGhee JR, James SP, eds. Mucosal Immunity and Infections at Mucosal Surfaces. New York: Oxford University Press, 1988, pp. 401–404.
53. Xu-Amano J, Kiyono H, Jackson RL, et al. Helper T cell subsets for immunoglobulin responses A, oral immunization with tetanus toxoid and cholera toxin as adjuvant selectively induces Th2, cells in mucosa-associated tissues. J Exp Med 1993;178:1309–1320.
54. Marinaro M, Staats HF, Hiroi T, et al. Mucosal adjuvant effect of cholera toxin in mice results from induction of T helper 2, (Th2) cells and IL-4. J Immunol 1995; 155:4621–4629.
55. Yamamoto S, Kiyono H, Yamamoto M, et al. A non toxic mutant of cholera toxin elicits Th2-type responses for enhanced mucosal immunity. Proc Natl Acad Sci USA 1997;94:5267–5272.
56. Yamamoto S, Yoshifumi K, Yamamoto M, et al. Mutants in the ADP-ribosyltransferase cleft of cholera toxin lack diarrheagenicity but retain adjuvanticity. J Exp Med 1997;185:1203–1210.
57. Yamamoto M, Rennert P, McGhee, RJ, et al. Alternate mucosal immune system: organized Peyer's patches are not required for IgA responses in the gastrointestinal tract. J Immunol 2000;164:5184–5191.
58. Simecka JW, Jackson RJ, Kiyono H, McGhee JR. Mucosally induced immunoglobulin E-associated inflammation in the respiratory tract. Infect Immun 2000; 68:672–679.
59. Clarke CJ, Wilson AD, Williams NA, Stokes CR. Mucosal priming of T-lymphocyte responses to fed protein antigens using cholera toxin as adjuvant. Immunology 19991;72:232–328.
60. Douce G, Fontana M, Pizza M, Rappuoli R, Dougan G. Intranasal immunogenicity and adjuvanticity of site-directed mutant derivatives of cholera toxin. Infect Immun 1997;65:2821–2828.
61. Pierre P, Denis O, Bazin H, Mbella EM, Vaerman J-P. Modulation of oral tolerance to ovalbumin by cholera toxin and its subunit B. Eur J Immunol 1992;22:3127–3128.
62. Glenn G, Scharton-Kersten T, Vassell R, Mallet CP, Hale TL, Alving CR. Cutting edge: transcutaneous immunization with cholera toxin protects mice against lethal mucosal toxin challenge. J Immunol 1998;161:3211–3214.
63. Reudel C, Rieser C, Kofler N, Wick G, Wolf H. Humoral and cellular immune responses in the murine respiratory tract following oral immunization with cholera toxin or *Escherichia coli* heat-labile enterotoxin. Vaccine 1996;14:792–798.
64. Richards, CM, Shimeld C, Williams NA, Hill TJ. Induction of mucosal immunity against herpes simplex virus type 1, in the mouse protects against ocular infection and establishment of latency. J Infect Dis 1998;177:1451–1457.
65. Martin M, Metzger DJ, Michalek SM, Connell TD, Russell MW. Comparative analysis of the mucosal adjuvanticity of the type II heat-labile enterotoxins LT-IIa and LTIIb. Infect Immun 2000;68:281–287.
66. Hornquist E, Lycke N. Cholera toxin adjuvant greatly promotes antigen priming of cells T. Eur J Immunol 1993;23:2136–2143.

67. Pacheco SE, Gibbs RA, Ansari-Lari A, Rogers P. Intranasal immunization with HIV reverse transcriptase: effect of dose in the induction of helper type 1, and 2, immunity. AIDS Res Hum Retroviruses 2000;16:2009–2017.
68. Akhiani AA, Schon K, Lycke N. Vaccine-induced immunity against Helicobacter pylori infection is impaired in IL-18-deficient mice. J Immunol 2004;173:3348–3356.
69. Schaffeler MP, Brokenshire JS, Snider DP. Detection of precursor Th cells in mesenteric lymph nodes after oral immunization with protein antigen and cholera toxin. Int Immunol 1997;9:1555–1562.
70. Yanagita M, Hiroi T, Kitagaki N, et al. Nasopharyngeal-associated lympho-reticular tissue (NALT) immunity: fimbriae-specific Th1, and Th2, cell-regulated IgA responses for the inhibition of bacterial attachment to epithelial cells and subsequent inflammatory cytokine production. J Immunol 1999;162:3559–3565.
71. Lavelle EC, Jarnicki A, McNeela E, et al. Effects of cholera toxin on innate and adaptive immunity and its application as an immunomodulatory agent. J Leukoc Biol 2004;75:756–763.
72. Ryan EJ, McNeela E, Murphy G, et al. Mutants of Eesherichia coli heat labile toxin act as effective mucosal adjuvants for nasal delivery of an acellular pertussis vaccine: differential effects of the non-toxic AB complex and enzyme activity on Th1, and Th2, cells. Infect Immun 1999;67:6270–6280.
73. Cheng E, Cárdenas-Freytag L, Clements JD. The role of cAMP in mucosal advuvanticity of Escherichia coli heat-labile enterotoxin (LT). Vaccine 1999;18:38–49.
74. Takahashi I, Kiyono H, Marinaro M, et al. Mechanisms for mucosal immunogenicity and adjuvanticity of Escherichia coli labile toxin. J Infect Dis 1996;173:627–635
75. Douce G, Giannelli V, Pizza M, Lewis D, Everest P, Rappuoli R, Dougan G. Genetically detoxified mutants of heat-labile toxin from Escherichia coli are able to act as oral adjuvant. Infect Immun 1999;67:4400–4406.
76. Giuliani MM, Del Giudice G, Giannelli V, Dougan G, Douce G, Rappuoli R, Pizza M. Mucosal adjuvanticity and immunogenicity of LTR72, a novel mutant of Escherichia coli heat-labile enterotoxin with partial knockout of ADP-ribo-syltransferase activity. J Exp Med 1998;187:1123–1132.
77. Weltzin R, Guy B, Thomas WD, Giannasca PJ, Monath TP. Parenteral adjuvant activities of Escherichia coli heat-labile toxin and its subunit for immunization of mice against gastric Helicobacter pylori infection. Infect Immun 2000;68:2775–2782.
78. Douce G, Giuliani MM, Giannelli V, Pizza MG, Rappuoli R, Dougan G. Mucosal immunogenicity of genetically detoxified derivatives of heat labile toxin from *Escherichia coli*. Vaccine 1998;16:1065–1073.
79. Bowen JC, Nair SK, Reddy R, Rouse BT. Cholera toxin acts as a potent adjuvant for the induction of cytotoxic T-lymphocyte responses with non-replicating antigens. Immunology 1994;81:338–342.
80. Simmons CP, Mastroeni P, Fowler R, Ghaem-maghami M, Lycke N, Pizza M, Rappuoli R, Dougan G. MHC class I-restricted cytotoxic lymphocyte responses induced by enterotoxin-based. J Immunol 1999;163:6502–6510.

81. Tamura S, Yamanaka A, Shimohara M, et al. Synergistic action of cholera toxin B subunit (and Escherichia coli heat-labile toxin B subunit) and a trace amount of cholera whole toxin as an adjuvant for nasal influenza vaccine. Vaccine 1994; 12:419–426.
82. Richards CM, Aman AT, Hirst TR, Hill TJ, and Williams NA. Protective mucosal immunity to ocular herpes simplex virus type 1, infection in mice by using *Escherichia coli* heat-labile enterotoxin B subunit as an adjuvant. J Virol 2001;75: 1664–16671.
83. Toida N, Hajishengallis G, Wu HY, Russell MW. Oral immunization with the saliva-binding region of Streptococcus mutans AgI/II genetically coupled to the cholera toxin B subunit elicit T-helper-cell responses in gut-associated lymphoid tissues. Infect Immun 1997;65:909–915.
84. Isaka M, Yasuda Y, Mizokami M, et al. Mucoosal immunization against hepatitis B virus by intranasal co-administration of recombinant hepatitis B surface antigen and recombinant cholera toxin B subunit as an adjuvant. Vaccine 2001;19: 1460–1466.
85. Sun JB, Mielcarek N, Lakew M, et al. Intranasal administration of a Schistosoma mansoni glutathione S-transferase-cholera toxoid conjugate vaccine evokes antiparasitic and antipathological immunity in mice. J Immunol 1999;15:1045–1052.
86. Sun J-B, Rask C, Olsson T, Holmgren J, Czerkinsky C. Treatment of experimental autoimmune encephalomyelitis by feeding myelin basic protein conjugated to cholera toxin subunit B. Proc Natl Acad Sci USA 1996;93:7196–7201.
87. Williams NA, Stasiuk LM, Nashar TO, et al. Prevention of autoimmune disease due to lymphocyte modulation by the B-subunit of Escherichia coli heat-labile enterotoxin. Proc Natl Acad Sci USA 1997;94:5290–5295.
88. Ploix C, Bergerot I, Durand A, Czerkinsky C, Holmgren J, Thivolet C. Oral administration of cholera toxin B-insulin conjugates protects NOD mice from autoimmune diabetes by inducing CD4+ regulatory T-cells. Diabetes 1999;48:2150–2156.
89. Widermann U, Jahn-Schmid B, Repa A, Kraft D, Ebner C. Modulation of an allergic immune response via the mucosal route in a murine model of inhalative type-1, allergy. Int. Arch. Allergy Immunol 1999;118:129–132.
90. Ryan EJ, McNeela E, Pizza M, Rappuoli R, O'Neill L, Mills KHG. Modulation of innate and acquired immune responses by Escherichia coli heat-labile toxin: distinct pro- and anti- inflammatory effects of the nontoxic AB complex and the enzyme activity. J Immunol 2000;165:5750–5759.
91. Douce G, Turcotte C, Cropley I, et al. Mutants of Escherichia coli heat-labile toxin lacking ADP-ribosyltransferase activity act as nontoxic, mucosal adjuvants. Proc Natl Acad Sci USA 1995;92:1644–1648.
92. Cárdenes-Freytag L, Cheng E, Mayeux P, Domer JE, Clements JD. Effectiveness of heat-killed Candida albicans and a novel mucosal adjuvant, LT(R192G), against systemic candidiasis. Infect Immun 1999;67:826–833.
93. O'Neal CM, Clements JD, Estes MK, Conner ME. Rotavirus 2/6, viruslike particles administered intranasally with cholera toxin, Escherichia coli heat-labile toxin (LT), and LT-R192G induce protection from rotavirus challenge. J Virol 1998;72:3390–3393.

Modified Bacterial Toxins                                                                    147

94. Chong C, Friberg M, Clements JD. LT(R192G), a non-toxic mutant of the heat-labile enterotoxin of Escherichia coli, elicits enhanced humoral and cellular immune responses associated with protection against lethal oral challenge with Salmonella spp. Vaccine 1998;16:732–740.
95. Tebby PW, Scheuer CA, Peek JA, et al. Effective mucosal immunization against respiratory syncytial virus using purified F protein and a genetically detoxified cholera holotoxin, CT-E29H. Vaccine 2000;18:1223–2734.
95a. Bowe F, Lavelle EC, McNeela EA, et al. Mucosal vaccination against serogroup B meningococcus: induction of bactericidal antibodies and cellular immunity following intranasal immunization with NadA of *Neisseria meningitidis* and mutants of *Escherichia coli* heat-labile enterotoxin. Infect Immun 2004;72:4052–4060.
96. Lycke N, Tsuji T, Holmgren J. The adjuvant effect of Vibrio cholerae and *Escherichia coli* heat-labile enterotoxins is linked to their ADP-ribosyltransferase activity. Eur J Immunol 1992;22:2277–2281.
97. Barakman JD, Ott G, O'Hagan DT. Intranasal immunization of mice with influenza virus vaccine in combination with the adjuvant LT-R72, induces potent mucosal and serum immunity which is stronger than that with traditional intramuscular immunization. Infect Immun 1999;67:4276–4279.
98. Agren LC, Ekman L, Lowenadler B, Lycke N. Genetically engineered nontoxic vaccine adjuvant that combines B cell targeting with immunomodulation by cholera toxin A1, subunit. J Immunol 1997;158:3936–3946.
99. Lycke N, Schon K. The B cell targeted adjuvant, CTA1-DD, exhibits potent mucosal immunoenhancing activity despite pre-existing anti-toxin immunity. Vaccine 2001;19:2542–2548.
100. Marchetti M, Rossi M, Giannelli V, et al. Protection against Helicobacter pylori infection in mice by intragastric vaccination with H pylori antigens is achieved using a non-toxic mutant of E coli heat-labile enterotoxin (LT) as adjuvant. Vaccine 1998;16:33–37.
101. Jakobsen H, Schulz D, Pizza M, Rappuoli R, Jonsdottir I. Intranasal immunization with pneumococcal polysaccharide conjugate vaccines with nontoxic mutants of Escherichia coli heat-labile enterotoxins as adjuvants protects mice against invasive pneumococcal infection. Infect Immun 1999;67:5892–5897.
102. Gizurarson S, Tamura S, Kurata T, Hasiguchi K, Ogawa H. The effect of cholera toxin and cholera toxin B subunit on the nasal mucosal membrane. Vaccine 1991; 9:825–832.
103. Lycke N, Karlsson U, Sjolander A, Magnusson KE. (1991) The adjuvant action of cholera toxin is associated with an increased intestinal permeability for luminal antigens. Scand J Immunol 1991;33:691–698.
104. Bromander AK, Kjerrulf M, Holmgren J, Lycke N. Cholera toxin enhances alloantigen presentation by cultured intestinal epithelial. Scand J Immunol 1993;37: 452–458.
105. Matousek MP, Nedrud JG, Cieplak W, Harding CV. Inhibition of class II histocompatability complex antigen processing by Escherichia coli heat-labile enterotoxin requires an enzymatically active subunit A. Infect Immun 1998;66:3480–3484.
106. Li TK, Fox BS. Cholera toxin B subunit binding to an antigen-presenting cell directly co-stimulates cytokine production from a T cell clone. Int Immunol 1996; 8:1849–1856.

107. Cong Y, Weaver CT, Elson CO. The mucosal adjuvanticity of cholera toxin involves enhancement of costimulatory activity by selective up-regulation of B72 expression. J Immunol 1997;159:5201–5208.
108. Yamamoto M, Kiyono H, Yamamoto S, et al. Direct effects on antigen-presenting cells and T lymphocytes explain the adjuvanticity of a nontoxic cholera toxin mutant. J Immunol 1999;162:7015–7021.
109. Williamson E, Westrich GM, Viney JL. Modulating dendritic cells to optimize mucosal immunization protocols. J Immunol 1999;163:3668–3675.
110. Gagliardi MC, Sallusto F, Marinaro M, Langenkamp A, Lanzavecchia A, DeMagistris MT. Cholera toxin induces maturation of human dendritic cells and licences them for Th2, priming. Eur J Immunol 2000;30:2394–2403.
111. Braun MC, He J, Wu CY, Kelsall BL. Cholera toxin suppresses interleukin (IL)-12, production and IL-12, receptor β1, and β2, chain expression. J Exp Med 1999; 189:541–552.
112. Panina-Bordignon P, Mazzeo D, Lucia PD, et al. Beta2-agonists prevent Th1, development by selective inhibition of interleukin 12. J Clin Invest 1997;100: 1513–1519.
113. Munoz E, Zubiaga AM, Merrow M, Sauter NP, Huber BT. Cholera toxin discriminates between T helper 1, and 2, cells in T cell receptor-mediated activation: role of cAMP in T cell proliferation. J Exp Med 1990;172:95–103.
114. De Haan L, Holtrop M, Verweij WR, Agsteribbe E, Wilschut J. Mucosal immunogenicity and adjuvant activity of recombinant A subunit of the Escherichia coli heat-labile enterotoxin. Immunology 1999;97:706–713.
115. Tamura M, Nogimori A, Murai A, et al. Subunit structure of islet-activation protein, pertussis toxin, in conformity with the A-model B, Biochemistry 1982;21: 5516–5522.
116. Kaslow HR, Burns DL. Pertussis toxin and target eurkaryotic cells: binding, entry and activation. FASEB J 1992;6:2684–2690.
117. Saukkonen K, Burnette WN, Mar VL, Masure HR, Tuomanen EI. Pertussis toxin has eukaryotic-like carbohydrate recognition domains. Proc Natl Acad Sci USA 1992;89:118–122.
118. Lobet Y, Feron C, Dequesne G, Simoen E, Hauser P, Locht C. Site-specific alterations in the B oligomer that affect receptor-binding activities and mitogenicity of pertussis toxin. J Exp Med 1993;177:79–87.
119. Zhang XM, Berland R, Rosoff PM. Differential regulation of accessory mitogenic signaling receptors by the T cell antigen receptor. Mol Immunol 1995;32:323–332.
120. Li H, Wong WS. Mechanisms of pertussis toxin-induced myelomonocytic cell adhesion: role of CD14, and urokinase receptor. Immunology 2000;100:502–509.
121. Burnette WN. Perspectives in recombinant pertussis toxoid development. In: Koff W, Six HR, eds. Vaccine Research and Development. New York: Marcel Dekker, 1992, pp. 143–193.
122. Lyons AB. Pertussis toxin pretreatment alters the in vivo cell division behaviour and survival of B lymphocytes after intravenous transfer. Immunol Cell Biol 1997; 75:7–12.
123. Meade BD, Kind PD, Manclark CR. Altered mononuclear phagocyte function in mice treated with the lymphocytosis promoting factor of Bordetella pertussis. Dev Biol Stand 1985;61:63–74.

124. Spangrude GJ, Sacchi F, Hill HR, Van Epps DE, Daynes RA. Inhibition of lymphocyte and neutrophil chemotaxis by pertussis toxin. J Immunol 1985;135:4135–4143.
125. Sidey FM, Furman BL, Wardlaw AC. Effect of hyperreactivity to endotoxin on the toxicity of pertussis vaccine and pertussis toxin in mice. Vaccine 1989;7:237–241.
126. Cherry JD, Brunel PA, Golden GS, Karzon DT. Report of the task force on pertussis immunization–1988. Pediatrics 1988;81:939–984.
127. Loetscher P, Seitz M, Clark-Lewis I, Baggiolini M, Moser B. Monocyte chemotactic proteins MCP-1, MCP-2, and MCP-3, are major attractants for human CD4$^+$ and CD8$^+$ lymphocytes T. FASEB J 1994;8:1055–1060.
128. Schorr W, Swandulla D, Zeilhofer HU. Mechanisms of IL-8-induced Ca$^{2+}$ signaling in human neutrophil granulocytes. Eur Immunol 1999;29:897–904.
129. Allavena P, Bianchi G, Zhou D, et al. Induction of natural killer cell migration by monocyte chemotactic protein-1, -2, and -3. Eur J Immunol 1994;24:3233–3236.
130. Roberts M, Bacon A, Rappuoli R, et al. A mutant toxin molecule that lacks ADP-ribosyltransferase activity, PT-9K/129G, is an effective mucosal adjuvant for intranasally delivered proteins. Infect Immun 1995;63:2100–2108.
131. Mu H-H, Sewell WA. Regulation of DTH and IgE responses by IL-4, and IFN-γ in immunized mice given pertussis toxin. Immunology 1994;83:639–645.
132. Munoz JJ, Peacock MG. Action of Pertussigen (pertussis toxin) on serum IgE and on Fcε receptors on lymphocytes. Cell Immunol 1990;127:327–336.
133. Bell F, Heath P, MacLennan J, et al. Adverse effects and sero-responses to an acellular pertussis/diphtheria/tetanus vaccine when combined with Haemophilus influenzae type b vaccine in an accelerated schedule. Eur J Pediatr 1999;158:329–336.
134. Richie E, Punjabi NH, Harjanto SJ, et al. Safety and immunogenicity of combined diphtheria-tetanus-pertussis (whole cell and acellular)-Haemophilus influenzae-b conjugate vaccines administered to Indonesian children. Vaccine 1999;17:1384–1393.
135. Mahon BP, Ryan M, Griffin F, Mills KHG. Interleukin-12, is produced by macrophages in response to live or killed Bordetella pertussis and enhances the efficacy of an acellular pertussis vaccine by promoting the induction of Th1 cells. Infect Immun 1996;64:5295–5301.
136. Samore MH, Siber GR. Pertussis toxin enhanced IgG1, and IgE responses to primary tetanus immunization are mediated by interleukin-4, and persist during secondary responses to tetanus alone. Vaccine 1996;14:290–297.
137. Tamura S-I, Tanaka H, Takayama R, Sato H, Sato Y, Uchida N. Break of unresponsiveness of delayed-type hypersensitivity to sheep red blood cells by pertussis toxin. Cell Immunol 1985;92:376–390.
138. Kamradt T, Soloway PD, Perkins DL, Gefter ML. Pertussis toxin prevents the induction of peripheral T cell anergy and enhances the T cell response to an encephalitogenic peptide of myelin basic protein. J Immunol 1991;147:3296–3302.
139. Zou LP, Ljunggren HG, Levi M, et al. P0, protein peptide 180-199, together with pertussis toxin induces experimental autoimmune neuritis in resistant C57BL/6, mice. J Neurosci Res 2000;62:717–721.
140. Sewell WA, De Moerloose PA, Hamilton JA, Schrader JW, Mackay IR, Vadas MA. Potentiation of delayed-type hypersensitivity by pertussigen or cyclohosphamide with release of different lymphokines. J Immunol 1987;61:483–488.

141. Fischer JE, Johnson JE, Johnson TR, Graham BS. Pertussis toxin sensitization alters the pathogenesis of subsequent respiratory syncytial virus infection. J Infect Dis 2000;182:1029–1038.
142. Shive CL, Hofstetter H, Arredondo L, Shaw C, Forsthuber TG. The enhanced antigen-specific production of cytokines induced by pertussis toxin is due to clonal expansion of T cells and not to altered effector functions of long-term memory cells. Eur J Immunol 2000;30:2422–2431.
143. Fischer JE, Johnson TR, Peebles RS, Graham BS. Vaccination with pertussis toxin alters the antibody response to simultaneous respiratory syncytial virus challenge. J Infect Dis 1999;180:714–719.
144. Loosmore S, Zealey G, Cockle S, Boux H, Chong P, Yacoob R, Klein M. Characterization of pertussis toxin analogs containing mutations in B-oligomer subunits. Infect Immun 1993;61:2316–2324.
145. Oka T, Honda T, Morokuma K, Ginnaga A, Ohkuma K, Sakoh M. Enhancing effects of pertussis toxin B oligomer on the immunogenicity of influenza vaccine administered intranasally. Vaccine 1994;12:1255–1258.
146. Van der Pouw-Kraan CTM, Rensink HJAM, Rappuoli R, Aarden LA. Co-stimulation of T cells via CD28, inhibits human IgE production; reversal by pertussis toxin. Clin Exp Immunol 1995;99:473–478.
147. Black WJ, Munoz JJ, Peacock MG, et al. ADP-ribosyltransferase activity of pertussis toxin and immunomodulation by Bordetella pertussis. Science 1988;240: 656–658.
148. Wong WS, Rosoff PM. Pharmacology of pertussis toxin B-oligomer. Can J Physiol Pharmacol 1996;74:559–564.
149. Ausiello CM, Fedele G, Urbani F, Lande R, Di Carlo B, Cassone A. Native and genetically inactivated pertussis toxins induce human dendritic cell maturation and synergize with lipopolysaccharide in promoting T helper type 1, responses. J Infect Dis 2002;186:351–60.
150. Gonzalo JA, Gonzalez-Garcia A, Baixeras E, et al. Pertussis toxin interferes with superantigen-induced deletion of peripheral T cells without affecting T cell activation in vivo. Inhibition of deletion and associated programmed cell death depends on ADP-ribosyltransferase. J Immunol 1994;152:4291–4219.
151. Thom RE, Casnellie JE. Pertussis toxin activates protein kinase C and a tyrosine protein kinase in the human T cell line Jurkat. FEBS Letts 1989;244:181–184.
152. Sommermeyer H, Resch K. Pertussis toxin B-subunit-induced $Ca^{2+}$-fluxes in jurkat human lymphoma cells: the action of long-term pre-treatment with cholera and pertussis holotoxins. Cell Signal 1990;2:115–128.
153. Grenier-Brossette N, Bourget I, Breittmayer JP, Ferrua B, Fehlmann M, Cousin JL. Pertussis toxin-induced mitogenesis in human lymphocytes T. Immunopharmacology 1991;21:109–119.
154. Wakatsuki A, Borrow P, Rigley K, Beverley PC. Cell-surface bound pertussis toxin induces polyclonal T cell responses with high levels of interferon-gamma in the absence of interleukin-12. Eur J Immunol 2003;33:1859–1868.
155. de Jong EC, Vieira PL, Kalinski P, et al. Microbial compounds selectively induce Th1, cell-promoting or Th2, cell-promoting dendritic cells in vitro with diverse th cell-polarizing signals. J Immunol 2002;168:1704–1709.

156. He J, Gurunathan S, Iwasaki A, Ash-Shaheed B, Kelsall BL. Primary role for Gi protein signaling in the regulation of interleukin 12, production and the induction of T helper cell type 1, responses. J Exp Med 2000;191:1605–1610.
157. Gross MK, Au DC, Smith AL, Storm DR. Targeted mutations that ablate either the adenylate cyclase or hemolysin function of the bifunctional cyaA toxin of Bordetella pertussis abolish virulence. Proc Natl Acad Sci USA 1992;89:4898–4902.
158. Mouallem M, Farfel Z, Hanski E. Bordetella pertussis adenylate cyclase toxin: intoxication of host cells by bacterial invasion, Infect Immun 1990;58:3759–3764.
159. Pearson RD, Symes P, Conboy M, Weiss AA, Hewlett EL. Inhibition of monocyte oxidative responses by Bordetella pertussis adenylate cyclase toxin. J Immunol 1987;139:2749–2754.
160. Njamkepo E, Pinot F, Francois D, Guiso N, Polla BS, Bachelet M. Adaptive responses of human monocytes infected by Bordetella pertussis: the role of adenylate cyclase hemolysin. J Cell Physiol 2000;183:91–99.
161. Gueirard P, Druilhe A, Pretolani M, Guiso N. Role of adenylate cyclase-hemolysin in alveolar macrophage apoptosis during Bordetella pertussis infection in vivo. Infect Immun 1998;66:1718–1725.
162. Ross PJ, Lavelle EC, Mills KH, Boyd AP. Adenylate cyclase toxin from Bordetella pertussis synergizes with lipopolysaccharide to promote innate interleukin-10, production and enhances the induction of Th2, and regulatory cells T. Infect Immun 2004;72:1568–1579.
163. Dadaglio G, Moukrim Z, Lo-Man R, Sheshko V, Sebo P, Leclerc C. Induction of a polarized Th1, response by insertion of multiple copies of a viral T-cell epitope into adenylate cyclase of Bordetella pertussis. Infect Immun 2000;68:3867–3872.
164. Hormozi K, Parton R, Coote J. Adjuvant and protective properties of native and recombinant Bordetella pertussis adenylate cyclase toxin preparations in mice. Med Microbiol 1999;23:273–282.
165. Boyd AP, Ross PJ, Conroy H, Mahon N, Lavelle EC, Mills KHG. (2004) *Bordetella pertussis* adenylate cyclase toxin modulates innate and adaptive immune responses: distinct roles for acylation and enzymatic activity in immunomodulation and cell death. J Immunol 2005;175:731–738.
166. Dinarello CA. The proinflammatory cytokines interleukin-1, and tumour necrosis factor and treatment of the septic shock syndrome. J Infect Dis 1991;163:1177–1184.
167. Higgins SC, Lavelle EC, McCann C, et al. Toll-like receptor 4-mediated innate IL-10, activates antigen-specific regulatory T cells and confers resistance to Bordetella pertussis by inhibiting inflammatory pathology. J Immunol 2003;171:3119–3127.
168. Ribi E. Beneficial modification of the endotoxin molecule. J Biol Response Mod 1984;3:1–9.
169. Ulrich JT, Myers KB. Monophosphoryl lipid A as an adjuvant past experiences and new directions. In: Powell MF, Newman JM, eds. Vaccine Design: The Subunit and Adjuvant Approach. New York: Plenum Press, 1995, pp. 495–524.
170. Moore A, McCarthy L, Mills KHG. The adjuvant combination monophosphoryl lipid A and QS21, switches T cell responses induced with a soluble recombinant HIV protein from Th2, to Th1. Vaccine 1999;17:2517–2527.

171. Salkowski CA. Lipopolysaccharide and monophosphoryl lipid A differentially regulate interleukin-12, gamma interferon, and interleukin-10, mRNA production in murine macrophages. Infect Immun 1997;65:3239–3247.
172. Baldridge JR, Yorgensen Y, Ward JR, Ulrich JT. Monophosphoryl lipid A enhances mucosal and systemic immunity to vaccine antigens following intranasal administration. Vaccine 2000;18:2416–2425.
173. Childers NK. Adjuvant activity of monophosphoryl lipid A for nasal and oral immunization with soluble or liposome-associated antigen. Infect Immun 2000; 68: 5509–5516.
174. Mikloska Z, Ruckholdt M, Ghadiminejad I, Dunckley H, Denis M, Cunningham AL. Monophosphoryl lipid A and QS21, increase CD8, T lymphocyte cytotoxicity to herpes simplex virus-2, infected cell proteins 4, and 27, through IFN-g and IL-12, production. Immunol J 2000;164:5167–5176.
175. Peteers CCAM, Lagerman PR, De Weers O, et al. Polysaccharide-conjugate vaccines. In: Robinson A, Farrar GH, Wiblin CH, eds. Vaccine Protocols. Totowa, NJ: Humana Press, 1996, pp. 111–134.
176. Lagos R, Valenzuela MT, Levine OS, et al. Economisation of vaccination against Haemophilus influenzae type b: a randomised trial of immunogenicity of fractional-dose and two-dose regimens. Lancet 1998;351:1472–1476.
177. Michetti P, Kreiss C, Kotloff KL, et al. Oral immunization with urease and Escherichia coli heat-labile enterotoxin is safe and immunogenic in Helicobacter pylori-infected adults. Gastroenterology 1999;116:804–812.
178. Gluck U, Gebbers JO, Gluck R. Phase 1 evaluation of intranasal virosomal influenza vaccine with and without Escherichia coli heat-labile toxin in adult volunteers. J Virol 1999;73:7780–7786
179. Gluck R, Mischler R, Durrer P, et al. Safety and immunogenicity of intranasally administered inactivated trivalent virosome-formulated influenza vaccine containing Escherichia coli heat-labile toxin as a mucosal adjuvant. J Infect Dis 2000; 181:1129–1132.
180. Mutsch M, Zhou W, Rhodes P, et al. Use of the inactivated intranasal influenza vaccine and the risk of Bell's palsy in Switzerland. N Engl J Med 2004;350:896–903.
181. van Ginkel FW, Jackson RJ, Yuki Y, McGhee JR. Cutting edge: the mucosal adjuvant cholera toxin redirects vaccine proteins into olfactory tissues. J Immunol 2000;165:4778–4782.
182. Cohen D, Orr N, Haim M, et al. Safety and immunogenicity of two different lots of the oral, killed enterotoxigenic Escherichia coli-cholera toxin B subunit vaccine in Israeli young adults. Infect Immun 2000;68:4492–4497.
183. Taylor DN, Cardenas V, Sanchez JL, et al. Two-year study of the protective efficacy of the oral whole cell plus recombinant B subunit cholera vaccine in Peru. J InFect Dis 2000;181:1667–1673.
184. Holmgren J, Svennerholm AM, Jertborn M, et al. An oral subunit B, whole cell vaccine against cholera. Vaccine 1992;10:911–914.
185. Bergquist C, Johansson, E-L, Lagergard T, Holmgren J, Rudin A. Intranasal vaccination of humans with recombinant cholera toxin B subunit induces systemic and local antibody responses in the upper respiratory tract and the vagina. Infect Immun 1997;65:2676-2684.

186. Hashigucci K, Ogawa H, Ishidate T, et al. Antibody responses in volunteers induced by nasal influenza vaccine combined with Escherichia coli heat-labile enterotoxin B subunit containing a trace amount of the holotoxin. Vaccine 1996; 14:113–119.
187. Stoute JA, Kester KE, Krzych U, et al. Long-term efficacy and immune responses following immunization with the RTSS malaria vaccine. J Infect Dis 1998;178: 1139–1144.
188. McCormack S, Tilzey A, Carmichael A, et al. A phase I trial in HIV negative healthy volunteers evaluating the effect of potent adjuvant on immunogenicity of a recombinant gp120W61D derived from dual tropic R5X4, HIV-1ACH320. Vaccine 2000;18:1166–1177.
189. Miller DL, Ross EM, Alderslade R, Bellman MH, Rawson NS. Pertussis immunisation and serious acute neurological illness in children. BMJ 1981;282:1595–1599.
190. Donnelly S, Loscher C, Lynch, Mills KHG. Whole cell but not acellular pertussis vaccines induce convulsive activity in mice: evidence of a role for toxin-induced IL-1β in a new murine model for analysis of neuronal side effects of vaccination. Infect Immun 2001;69:4217–4223.
191. Loscher CE, Donnelly S, McBennett S, Lynch MA, Mills KHG. Pro-inflammatory cytokines in the adverse systemic and neurologic effects associated with parenteral injection of a whole cell pertussis vaccine. Ann Acad NY Sci 1998;856: 274–277.
192. Loscher CL, Donnelly S, Mills KHG, Lynch MA. Interlukin-1b-dependent changes in the hippocampus following parenteral immunization with a whole cell pertussis vaccine. J Neuroimmunol 2000;111:68–76.
193. Yuhas Y, Shulman L, Weizman A, Kaminsky E, Vanichkin A, Ashkenazi S. Involvement of tumour necrosis factor alpha and interleukin-1β in enhancement of pentylenetetrazole-induced seizures caused by Shigella dysenteriae. Infect Immun 1999;67:1455–1460.
194. Armstrong ME, Lavelle EC, Loscher CE, Lynch MA, Mills KHG. Induction of proinflammatory responses in the murine hypothalamus following intranasal delivery of cholera toxin: implications for the use of AB toxins as adjuvants in nasal vaccines. J Infect Dis 2005 (in press).
195. Rennels MB, Deloria MA, Pichichero ME, et al. Extensive swelling after booster doses of acellular pertussis-tetanus-diphtheria vaccines. Pediatrics 2000;105:e12.
196. Ryan EJ, Nilsson L, Kjellman N-IM, Gothefors L, Mills KHG. Booster immunization of children with an acellular pertussis vaccine enhances Th2, cytokine production and serum IgE against pertussis toxin but not against common allergens. Clin Exp Immunol 2000;121:193–200.
197. Marinaro M, Di Tommaso A, Uzzau S, Fasano A, De Magistris MT. Zonula Occludens toxin is a powerful mucosal adjuvant for intranasally delivered antigens. Infect Immun 1999;67:1287–1291.
198. Mu H-H, Sewell WA. Enhancement of interleukin-4, production by pertussis toxin. Infect Immun 1993;61:2834–2840.

# 8

# Glycosylphosphatidylinositol Anchors As Natural Immunological Adjuvants Derived From Protozoan Parasites

## Ricardo T. Gazzinelli, Catherine Ropert, Igor C. Almeida, João S. Silva, and Marco A. Campos

## INTRODUCTION

Parasitism involves an intimate association between two different organisms. The host provides food and shelter for the parasite, and may or may not be injured by the parasite. As well elaborated in the book *Living Together* by William Trager *(1)*, it is not in the best interest of the parasite to destroy the host. In the case of intracellular protozoan parasites that proliferate inside the vertebrate host cells, the immune system has a crucial role in controlling parasite replication and maintaining a balanced interaction between the parasite and the host, until the parasite encounters the transmitting vector or is shed to the environment to propagate its life cycle.

At first view it seems paradoxical that a pathogen aiming to establish a chronic infection will elicit a strong effective protective immunity. However, it is clear from many studies that protozoan parasites have learned different strategies during evolution to stimulate the effector immunological mechanisms so that their hosts will survive and they can maintain persistent parasitism. On the other hand, the evasion of host immunological effector mechanisms appears to be essential for the protozoan parasites to establish persistent parasitism in the vertebrate hosts. For instance, residing inside the host cells will shelter the parasite against various immunological mechanisms for destruction of the intracellular parasites. Taking this in consideration, one would assume that a successful parasitism would emerge from parasites that manage to balance their mechanisms of evasion and activation of the immune system, so they can establish parasitism, but at the same time limit their replication, to avoid excessive tissue damage to host lethality.

From: *Vaccine Adjuvants: Immunological and Clinical Principles*
Edited by: C. J. Hackett and D. A. Harn, Jr. © Humana Press Inc., Totowa, NJ

Cell-mediated immunity (CMI) is the main compartment of the immune system involved in resistance of vertebrate host against intracellular protozoan parasites *(2)*. In the last decade a great deal has been learned regarding the ability of intracellular protozoan parasites to stimulate and sustain a parasite specific CMI. The activation of the immune system observed during early stages of infection relies on the ability of protozoan parasites to promote the synthesis of the proinflammatory cytokine interleukin (IL)-12. The parasite elicits IL-12 synthesis by cells of the innate immune system (i.e., cells from monocytic lineage to granulocytes), which will in turn initiate the synthesis of high levels of interferon (IFN)$\gamma$ by natural killer (NK) cells. IFN$\gamma$ is the central cytokine for activating macrophages and nonprofessional phagocytic cells to display effector mechanisms involved in the control of parasite replication and pathogenesis, before the establishment of the acquired immunity. This early production of IL-12 and IFN$\gamma$ is also essential for promoting protective acquired immunity, characterized by the development of T helper (Th)1 lymphocytes and progression of infection to a chronic stage. Thus, in many cases infection with intracellular protozoan parasites will result on the induction of a strong CMI, characterized by a highly polarized Th1 response, production of high levels of IFN$\gamma$, a dominance of murine immunoglobin (Ig)G2a or human IgG1 antibody isotypes, and establishment of a population of parasite specific CD8$^+$ T cells. This type I immune response induced by the protozoan parasites is highly effective in controlling tissue parasitism and parasitemia, and in most cases infection will evolve for a chronic and asymptomatic stage *(3)*.

Although the IL-12/IFN$\gamma$ axis appears to be crucial for host resistance to infection with different protozoan parasites (e.g., *Leishmania sp.*, *Plasmodium sp.*, *Toxoplasma gondii*, and *Trypanosoma cruzi*) *(3–7)*, the balance between evasion and activation of host innate immunity appears to vary, when comparing different species and genus of protozoan parasites. For instance, in the case of *Leishmania* species, which are slow-growing parasites and obligatory macrophage residents, evasion must prevail over activation of innate immunity, so the parasitism is established. Thus, during its early stages, infection with *Leishmania* parasites evolves in a quite silent way and induction of IL-12 and IFN$\gamma$ synthesis to CMI will occur only several weeks after infection, when an intense parasitism has been accumulated in the vertebrate host tissues *(8)*.

In contrast, in the case of more virulent protozoan parasites such as the *T. gondii* and *T. cruzi*, which infect and replicate inside any nucleated cell from the vertebrate host, strong stimulation of host innate immunity and high levels of proinflammatory cytokines (e.g., tumor necrosis factor [TNF]$\alpha$, IL-12, and IFN$\gamma$) are detected in the sera of mice in the first 2 weeks of infection *(9–11)*. This initial production of IL-12 and IFN$\gamma$ is so essential in the parasite–host interaction, that 100% of knockout (KO) mice lacking functional genes for such cytokines will die around 10 to 20 days postinfection with *T. gondii* or *T. cruzi*, as opposed to 100% survival in wild-type mice *(12–14)*. In many cases, this early activation of the immune system is so intense that some of the symptoms observed during acute infection with such protozoan parasites (e.g., *Plasmodium sp., T. gondii,* and *T. cruzi)* is thought to be dependent on immunological mediators, rather than tissue damage caused by excessive parasite replication *(10,11,15,16)*. In these cases, immunoregulatory mechanisms appear to have an important role in controlling excessive activation of the immune system, immunopathology, and lethality during acute infection with protozoan parasites.

As discussed above, many of the key cytokines and cell populations involved on innate resistance to protozoan infections have been defined. However, the molecular events involved on parasite interaction with host cells that will determine the degree of activation of host innate immunity are largely unknown. Studies at the cellular level performed by different groups are beginning to elucidate some important aspects related to the very initial steps of parasite interaction with host cells. Some of the interesting questions that are being pursued involve the route of parasite entry to the host cells, identification of parasite signaling molecules and their host counterpart receptors, to the involvement of host costimulatory molecules. These different aspects of parasite–host cell interaction may provide new information of how parasite activate or subvert specific signaling pathways and gene expression, affecting various host cell functions, including those involved on activation of the innate immunity, development of specific immunity, and ultimately determining the fate of parasitism in the vertebrate host (Fig. 1).

In many instances, the induction of a potent Th1 response is desired in various protocols aiming to induce protective immunity against intracellular pathogens, including various protozoan parasites. In this chapter, we review the studies performed in our laboratory and elsewhere, that try to dissect the molecular and cellular mechanisms involved on activation of the innate immunity by *T. cruzi* parasites, and lead to the induction of a highly polarized, but controlled type I immune response. We believe that the better understanding of how protozoan parasites elicit a polarized Th1 immune response may provide new insights to develop more efficient protocols for vaccination against intracellular pathogens.

## KEY STEPS INVOLVED IN ACTIVATION OF INNATE IMMUNITY AND EARLY RESISTANCE TO *T. CRUZI* PARASITES

As shown in Fig. 2, soon after the initial rounds of replications *T. cruzi* parasites initiate a cascade of events that will trigger cells from monocytic lineage (e.g., macrophages and dendritic cells [DCs]) to synthesize proinflammatory cytokines and express costimulatory molecules that will culminate in a strong

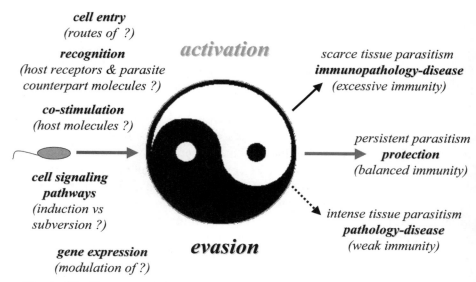

cell entry
(routes of ?)

recognition
(host receptors & parasite
counterpart molecules ?)

*activation*

scarce tissue parasitism
**immunopathology-disease**
(excessive immunity)

co-stimulation
(host molecules ?)

persistent parasitism
**protection**
(balanced immunity)

cell signaling
pathways
(induction vs
subversion ?)

intense tissue parasitism
**pathology-disease**
(weak immunity)

gene expression
(modulation of ?)

*evasion*

**Fig. 1.** Yin-Yang model for parasite activation/evasion of host innate immunity. The route of parasite entry to the host cells, the existence of parasite signaling molecules and their host counterpart receptors, to the involvement of host costimulatory molecules will define whether protozoan parasites activate or subvert specific signaling pathways and gene expression. These are important aspects of parasite–host cell interaction, which will ultimately determine the levels of activation of innate immunity, development of specific immunity and determining the fate of parasitism in the vertebrate host. Strong activation of host innate immunity, although efficiently controlling parasite replication, may lead to pathology because of excessive activation of immunological effector mechanisms. On the other hand if evasion of innate immunity prevails, excessive parasite replication may lead to intense tissue damage and pathology. Thus, a controlled activation of the cellular compartment of innate immunity may avoid intense host tissue injury, leading to induction of protective immunity and a balanced parasite–host interaction.

activation of cells from innate and acquired immune systems. This strong and systemic activation of the immune system is well illustrated at the peak of parasitemia, when one can detect increased serum levels of proinflammatory cytokines, such as IL-6, IL-12, IL-18, TNF-α, and IFNγ *(9,10)*, followed by an intense polyclonal activation of T and B lymphocytes to hypergammaglobulinemia *(17–19)*.

This early activation of the cellular compartment of the immune system, in particular the synthesis of IL-12 by cells from monocytic lineage is essential in initiating IFNγ synthesis by NK cells *(5,20)* and early resistance to *T. cruzi* infection. Whereas the IL-12 is indispensable, other cytokines such as TNF-α and IL-18 appear to play a role, potentiating the induction of IFNγ synthesis by

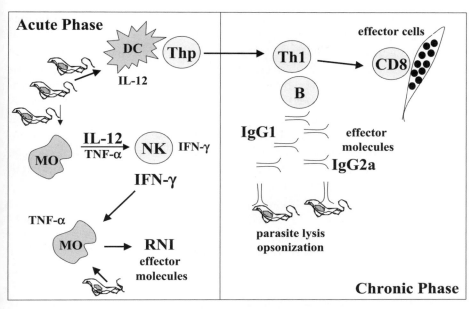

**Fig. 2.** After the initial rounds of replications *T. cruzi* initiates a cascade of events that will trigger cells from monocytic lineage (i.e., macrophages and dendritic cells) to synthesize interleukin (IL)-12 and express costimulatory molecules that culminates in a strong activation of cells from the innate and acquired immune system. This early activation of the innate cellular compartment of the immune system is essential in initiating interferon (IFN)γ synthesis by natural killer cells. IFNγ is a key cytokine that activate macrophages to kill *T. cruzi* parasites through the production of reactive nitrogen intermediates (RNI). Additionally, the early production of IL-12 and IFNγ also appears to be critical in directing differentiation of T Helper precursor (Thp) cells toward the Th1 phenotype. Once established the Th1 lymphocytes will be the basis for a very effective immunity that controls the parasite replication during the chronic stages of infection. High levels of IFNγ are produced by Th1 lymphocytes on antigen stimulation. Th1 lymphocytes will provide help for the development and activation of CD8⁺ T lymphocytes that are involved in the control of parasite replication by producing additional IFNγ to displaying cytotoxic activity. Furthermore, parasite specific Th1 lymphocytes will provide help for B lymphocytes to secrete high levels of parasite specific IgG2a antibodies that will promote parasite killing by complement-mediated lysis and favor opsonization, facilitating parasite uptake by macrophages.

IL-12 elicited during infection with *T. cruzi (21,22)*. Additionally, recent studies suggests that natural killer T (NKT) cells that produce high levels of IFNγ, in a IL-12 independent manner, may also be involved in the early control of *T. cruzi* infection *(23,24)*. However, the parasite molecules that stimulate the IFNγ production by NKT cell have not been defined and the protective effect of NKT cells against *T. cruzi* parasites appears to be parasite strain-dependent *(25)*.

Early studies showed that IFNγ is a key cytokine that activate macrophages to kill *T. cruzi* parasites *(26)*. Initial experiments suggested that the release of reactive oxygen intermediates *(27,28)* was the main mechanism involved in the microbicidal and/or microbiostatic effect against *T. cruzi* displayed by activated macrophages. However, other studies showed that IFNγ-activated macrophages deficient on respiratory burst and release of reactive oxygen intermediates were still able to control *T. cruzi* replication *(29,30)*. Thus, the production of reactive nitrogen intermediates (RNI) *(31)* was proposed as an alternative mechanism involved in killing of *T. cruzi* by activated macrophages with IFNγ. The RNI are products of arginine degradation by the inducible nitric oxide synthase (iNOS), which expression is induced in macrophages exposed to IFNγ. In fact, in the presence of specific inhibitors for iNOS, parasite replication is not controlled in murine macrophages activated with IFNγ *(32)*. Further, mice lacking functional iNOS gene are highly susceptible to acute infection with *T. cruzi* *(12)*. Because iNOS is mainly expressed by macrophages activated with IFNγ, these studies indicate a primary role for macrophages in early resistance to *T. cruzi* infection.

In addition to be involved in the control of parasite replication, this early production of IL-12 and IFNγ also appears to be critical in directing differentiation of Th precursor cells toward the Th1 phenotype (Fig. 2) *(5,33)*. Once established the Th1 lymphocytes will be the basis for a very effective immunity that controls the parasite replication during the chronic stages of infection. Interestingly, at later stages, after development of acquired immunity, iNOS and the RNI are no longer essential for the host to control parasite replication, and alternative mechanisms may be involved *(12,34)*. Thus, in addition to producing high levels of IFNγ on antigen stimulation the Th1 lymphocytes will provide help for the development and activation of CD8+ T lymphocytes that are involved in the control of parasite replication by producing additional IFNγ, to displaying cytotoxic activity *(35)*. Furthermore, parasite specific Th1 lymphocytes will provide help for B lymphocytes to secrete high levels of parasite specific IgG2a antibodies *(17,36)*, that will promote parasite killing by complement-mediated lysis to opsonization, facilitating parasite uptake by macrophage effector cells (Fig. 2).

## REGULATORY MECHANISMS AND EVASION FROM THE INNATE IMMUNITY DURING EARLY INFECTION WITH *T. CRUZI*

The activation of the immune system during acute infection with *T. cruzi* is so extreme that the host engages various immunoregulatory mechanisms to control excessive activation of the immune system and attenuate the deleterious effects of such a response. For instance, IL-10 appears to play a key role in modulating this early activation of the immune system by *T. cruzi* parasites. The experiments performed with IL-10 deficient mice infected with *T. cruzi* are very illustrative. On infection with *T. cruzi* IL-10 KO mice produce even higher levels of proinflammatory cytokines, including IL-12, TNF-α, and IFNγ. Yet they succumb at the acute phase of infection with *T. cruzi*. Importantly, the load of tissue parasitism and parasitemia are lower in IL-10 KO mice, as compared to wild-type animals, indicating that the effector mechanisms elicited by IFNγ are operative in mutant mice *(11)*. Thus, this study suggests that in absence of endogenous IL-10, mice will succumb because of an excessive production of proinflammatory cytokines and IFNγ-induced effector mechanisms, rather than parasite replication. These findings are supported by in vitro experiments showing the essential role of IL-10 in controlling IL-12 synthesis by macrophages exposed to *T. cruzi* glycolipids.

On the other hand, the production of high levels of RNI by macrophages has a potent inhibitory effect on the proliferation of T cells activated during infection with *T. cruzi (37)*. Additionally, a large proportion of T cells activated during *T. cruzi* undergo programmed cell death *(38)*. In fact, apoptosis should also be considered as an important regulatory mechanism during acute phase of experimental Chagas disease, and when it is combined with the RNI acts to minimize the deleterious effects of polyclonal lymphocyte activation. Interestingly, when ingested by macrophages the apoptotic cells induce production of high levels of TGF-β, which in turn inhibit the production of proinflammatory cytokines and RNI *(39)*, minimizing the activation of the host immune system. Importantly, in this model the blockade of apoptosis in mice infected with *T. cruzi* results in lower parasitemia and enhanced resistance to *T. cruzi* infection in mice.

In conclusion, to counteract the uncontrolled stimulation of host immunological effector functions, consequent tissue damage and lethality, the host engages various immunoregulatory mechanisms during the infection with *T. cruzi*. However, these mechanisms, involved in the control of the early activation of the immune system, may be used in the benefit of the parasite as evasion strategies for establishment and maintenance of persistent parasitism.

## INITIAL EVENTS AND CELL SIGNALING REQUIRED FOR ACTIVATION OF INNATE IMMUNITY *T. CRUZI* PARASITES

Different studies have shown that *T. cruzi* trypomastigotes directly signal both nonprofessional phagocytic and professional phagocytic cells. However, the signaling pathways, the genes modulated and cellular functions studied vary from cell to cell, and sometimes according to the parasite strain employed in each experimental set. Studies performed by Andrews and colleagues, show that fibroblast signaling through G protein promotes the process of exocytosis, favoring active entrance of the parasite via lysosomes *(40)*. This process involves an oligopeptidase from the parasite, possibly responsible for cleavage of another parasite molecule that releases the actual agonist of a yet undefined host counterpart receptor coupled to G protein *(41)*. Studies performed with human endothelial cells also showed that another protease, the cruzipain, a thiolprotease from the parasite, is able to process kininogen-releasing bradykinin that will activate a G protein-coupled serpentine receptor, also leading to the enhancement of the levels of cell invasion by *T. cruzi* parasites *(42)*. Consistently, β-chemokines that are agonists of G protein-coupled serpentine receptors were also shown to enhance parasite uptake by macrophages *(43)*. Notably, the enhanced parasite uptake in macrophage primed with β-chemokines resulted in an enhanced production of TNF-α and RNI *(43)*. Different protein kinases, such as the mitogen-activated protein kinases (MAPKs) *(44)*, protein kinase C *(45)*, those involved on NF-κB activation *(46)* to the TGF-β *(47)* signaling pathways have been shown to interfere with parasite entry and persistence within host cells.

Different studies also show the ability of *T. cruzi* parasites to modulate numerous genes and various cellular functions in macrophages, fibroblasts, endothelial cells and cardiomyocytes *(48–55)*. These studies suggest that the activation of host cells and expression of various genes are directly induced by parasite molecules or by immunologically active molecules previously elicited by *T. cruzi* parasites *(48–55)*. Among the cellular functions elicited by *T. cruzi* infection are the production of proinflammatory, chemoattractant, and adhesion molecules to molecules that control the extravascular extravasations, all thought to be important in the process of leukocyte activation and recruitment to the site of inflammation, and potentially in the immunological adjuvant activity observed during *T. cruzi* infection in the vertebrate host.

The ability of trypomastigotes to modulate gene expression on host macrophages appear to rely on parasite molecules that trigger signaling pathways involved on the activation of genes encoding molecules with proinflammatory activity. Among the molecules described to possess such proinflammatory activity, we can list the glycosylphosphatidylinositol (GPI)-linked mucin like glycoproteins (GPI-mucins) *(48,56)*, *trans*-sialidase *(57)*, Tc52 *(58)*, gp83 *(44)*, and deoxyribonucleic acid (DNA) *(59)*. In fact, our current studies show that the ability of trypomastigotes to induce the synthesis of proinflammatory cytokines and chemokines by macrophages is mimicked by both in vivo and in vitro stimulation with highly purified GPI anchors derived from GPI-mucins *(48–51,56, 60)*. In the next section, we review the structural analysis and functional studies that indicate the activity of GPI anchors derived from *T. cruzi* as potential immunological adjuvants.

## STRUCTURAL AND FUNCTIONAL ANALYSIS
## OF THE PROINFLAMMATORY ACTIVITY OF GPI
## ANCHORS DERIVED FROM *T. CRUZI*

The term pathogen-associated molecular patterns (PAMPs), has been coined to describe the molecular targets of the innate immune response *(61)*. Three main features characterize PAMPs: (a) they are usually expressed by microbes and not by host cells, (b) they show little variation among microorganisms of a given class, and (c) their expression is essential for the survival of the microbe. Whereas the first two characteristics allow class recognition of microbes and not of host cells, the latter prevents the development of mutants, which escape from recognition by the host immune system.

Different studies have documented the immunostimulatory and regulatory activities of GPI anchors derived from membrane of parasitic protozoa, such as *P. falciparum, T. brucei, and T. cruzi (48,56,63–66)*. The findings that protozoan-derived GPI anchors possess proinflammatory activity lead to the question regarding why mammalian GPI anchors do not ordinarily induce unrestrained autoimmunity. To answer that, first, mammalian cells typically express $10^5$ copies of GPI anchors per cell, whereas protozoan parasites express up to 1 to 10 million copies of GPI anchors per cell *(62)*. Second, there are subtle but significant structural differences between mammalian and protozoan GPIs. The existence of extra carbohydrate residues in the conserved GPI core, and/or an unsaturated fatty acid in the glycerolipid moiety, or a ceramide moiety in *T. cruzi* GPI anchors appears to confer their potency/ability to activate murine macrophages and B lymphocytes. Thus, we assume that both the amount and the fine structure of GPI anchors/GIPLs derived from protozoan parasites are critical for the activation of the vertebrate host innate immunity.

The most fundamental function of the GPI anchor is to allow a stable association of proteins to the cell surface plasma membrane *(62)*. The GPI anchors, which are also found in the surface of protozoan parasites on its free form, i.e., not attached to any surface protein, are named glycoinositolphospholipid (GIPL). The basic GPI structure consists of a hydrophilic core with a conserved domain of Manα1-2Manα1-6Manα1-4GlcNα1-6*myo*-inositol-1-HPO$_4$. Variant related structures can arise from this conserved domain as a result of phosphorylated substituents (e.g., ethanolamine phosphate or 2-aminoethylphosphonate) and extra carbohydrate residues. The ethanolamine phosphate or 2-aminoethylphosphonate will serve as the point of attachment to the GPI for the parasite surface proteins. The other extremity of the conserved hydrophilic domain contains a *myo*-inositol ring followed by a phosphate that is covalently linked to the hydrophobic moiety of the GPI anchor. In the case of *T. cruzi,* the hydrophobic moiety of the GPI anchors consist, in most cases, of alkylacylglycerol or ceramide lipid (Fig. 3) *(62,63)*.

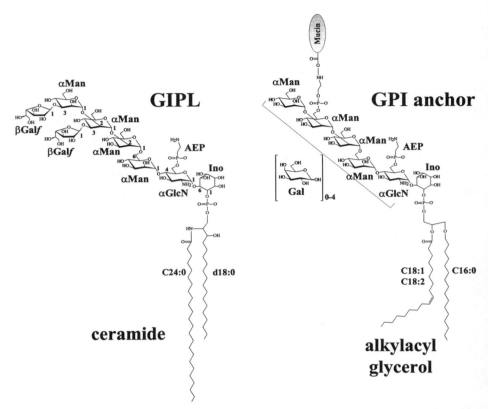

**Fig. 3.** The glycosylphosphatidylinositol (GPI) structure consists of a conserved domain of Manα1-2Manα1-6Manα1-4GlcNα1-6*myo*-inositol-1-HPO$_4$, which may have extra carbohydrate residues. The ethanolaminephosphate will serve as the point of attachment for the parasite surface proteins. The other extremity of the conserved hydrophilic domain contains a *myo*-inositol ring followed by a phosphate that is covalently linked to the hydrophobic moiety of the GPI anchor. GPI anchors derived from trypomastigotes derived GPI-mucins possess a potent proinflammatory activity and contain a PI moiety that is composed mainly by unsaturated (C18:1 or C18:2) fatty acids in the *sn*-2 position of the glycerol residue of the alkylacylglycerolipid. This feature together with the presence of extra galactose residues in the conserved glycan core seem to contribute to the proinflammatory activity of this glycolipid. Ceramide containing GPI anchor from *T. cruzi* will also activate IFNγ-primed macrophages triggering apoptosis and stimulate B lymphocytes enhancing antibody production, both in vitro and in vivo.

In our recent studies, we defined the structure of various GPI anchors and GIPLs from *T. cruzi* parasites by gas chromatography-mass spectrometry and electrospray ionization-mass spectrometry, aiming to establish a correlation between structure and bioactivity of GPI anchors, that is their ability to elicit the synthesis of proinflammatory cytokines by macrophages *(56,63)*. We observed that GPI anchors derived from the trypomastigote developmental stage of *T. cruzi* were highly active in inducing TNF-α, IL-12, and nitric oxide by IFNγ-primed murine macrophages. Highly purified GPI anchors activated macrophages in the concentration range of 1 to 10 nM. When the GPI-mucins, the source of purified GPI anchors, were treated with proteinase K, the specific activity on macrophages was maintained, indicating that the active moiety of the GPI-mucin was indeed located at the GPI anchor. However, after deamination of purified GPI anchors, it was observed that neither the phosphatidylinositol (PI) moiety nor the glycan core were able to activate macrophages *(48,56)*. Then, we conclude that an intact GPI anchor is necessary for the maximal biological activity on macrophages. Other important observations from these studies were that the PI moiety from the highly active GPI anchors contains mainly unsaturated fatty acids in the *sn*-2 position of the glycerol residue of the alkylacylglycerolipid, and extra galactose residues in the glycan. The absence of such components in less active GPI anchors, suggests that they may be responsible for the extreme potency of GPI anchors derived from *T. cruzi* trypomastigotes in eliciting the synthesis of proinflammatory cytokines by macrophages.

Studies performed elsewhere, show that ceramide containing GIPLs purified from *T. cruzi* parasites, although at higher concentrations (i.e., low μM range) also activate macrophages triggering apoptosis in cells primed with IFNγ *(67)*. Furthermore, the ceramide-containing GIPLs were also shown to activate T and B lymphocytes to enhance antibody production, both in vitro and in vivo *(68–72)*. Hence, they maybe pointed as parasite molecules potentially involved on the polyclonal lymphocyte activation to hypergammaglobulinemia observed during acute phase of infection with *T. cruzi*. For more details on the structural analysis and proinflammatory activity of GPI anchors from protozoan parasites, please refer to review by Almeida and Gazzinelli *(63)*.

## SIGNALING PATHWAYS TRIGGERED BY THE GPI ANCHORS FROM *T. CRUZI* TRYPOMASTIGOTES

MAPKs are components of signaling pathways that amplify and integrate signals from several extracellular stimuli, guiding cellular maturation, inducing inflammation and apoptosis *(73)*. The main components of the MAPKs family include the extracellular signal-regulated kinases (ERKs), c-jun NH2-terminal kinases (JNKs), and p38 MAPK cascades, which are partially involved on the ability of lipopolysaccharide (LPS) from *E. coli* to induce the synthesis of proinflammatory cytokines by macrophages *(74,75)*. The abilities of GPI-mucins (or purified GPI) and bacterial LPS to trigger MAPKs pathways were compared by Ropert and associates *(76)*. In experiments using murine macrophages, it was shown that the kinetics of ERKs, JNKs, and p38 phosphorylation triggered by LPS and GPI-mucins were similar. Furthermore, it was demonstrated the importance of these different signaling pathway induced GPI-mucin or tGPI in the cytokine production in macrophages. It was also shown that GPI-mucins activate the NF-κB transcription factor through the phosphorylation of the IκB. The use of SN50 peptide, an inhibitor of NF-κB nuclear translocation, resulted in 85% inhibition of TNF-α synthesis, in macrophages exposed to GPI-mucins. Therefore, very similar pathways of the MAPKs and NF-κB nuclear translocation in C57BL/6 murine macrophages were triggered after stimulation with LPS, purified GPI anchors or GPI-mucins *(76)*.

## ACTIVATION OF TOLL-LIKE RECEPTORS BY HIGHLY PURIFIED GPI ANCHORS FROM *T. CRUZI*

Innate immunity can discriminate between pathogens and self through the recognition of PAMPs by pattern recognition receptors. The recently discovered germline-encoded receptors of the Toll-like family (TLRs) are signal transducers responsible for the dendritic cells/macrophage activation and induction of the synthesis of proinflammatory cytokines, including IL-12 and TNF-α *(61, 77–80)*. PAMPs recognized through TLRs by IFN-exposed phagocytic leukocytes are also responsible for the rapid induction of a variety of immunological effector functions, including the synthesis of reactive oxygen and nitrogen intermediates *(81,82)*.

It is now well established that a member of the Toll family, TLR4, mediates the cellular activation of LPS *(77)*. The C3H/HeJ mice contain a point mutation in the TLR4 gene, causing a modified cytoplasmatic domain of the protein, which results in a hyporesponse from macrophages to LPS *(83)*. Accordingly, Ropert and associates *(76)* observed that LPS did not induce any MAPKs or IκB, whereas GPI-mucins still trigger the phosphorylation of IκB, ERK, JNK, and p38 MAPKs in C3H/HeJ macrophages. Then, we can conclude that, although LPS and GPI/GPI-mucins possess similar proinflammatory activity, their receptors are not physically the same.

Although we knew that GPI anchors were responsible for the induction of cytokine production and for effector functions in macrophages, not much was known about the functional receptors from macrophage that recognized the protozoan-derived GPI anchors. Because LPS was identified as the responsible molecule that induces the innate immune response through TLR4/CD14 in murine macrophages, and because LPS, GPI, and GPI-mucins trigger the same MAPKs pathways to IκB phosphorylation in mice macrophages, our group evaluated the ability of GPI anchors and GIPLs from *T. cruzi* to trigger TLR2 and TLR4, in chinese hamster ovary (CHO) cells transfected with TLRs and in macrophages from KO mice deficient on specific TLRs *(84)*. This was possible using

CHO cells stably transfected with a gene reporter (CD25) plus CD14, or CD14 and TLR2 or CD14 and TLR4, and then exposing these cells to diverse stimuli of interest, with the posterior evaluation of the CD25 expression by flow cytometry. This gene reporter (CD25) is under the control of the human E-selectin promoter, which contains a NFκB binding site and then the expression of CD25 is totally dependent on the transport of NFκB to the nucleus *(78)*. The synthesis of cytokines and nitric oxide (NO) were studied in inflammatory/bone marrow macrophages derived from TLR2 or TLR4 KO mice exposed to different stimuli. We showed that live *T. cruzi* trypomastigotes and GPI or GPI-mucins purified from trypomastigotes were able to activate cells through TLR2/CD14, but not through TLR4/CD14, and that this activation was dependent on the parasite-to-cell ratio. Then, we showed that whereas highly active trypomastigote-derived GPI-mucins (or its purified GPI) trigger TLR2 at picomolar to low nanomolar concentration range, epimastigote-derived ceramide-containing GIPLs only trigger TLR2 above 100 nM. Neither the PI nor the glycan part from GPI anchors was able to activate cells transfected with TLRs. We also evaluated the functionality of the *T. cruzi*-derived GPI anchors and found that TLR2 could not mediate cell activation without CD14. Finally, we showed, through the induction of cytokines (IL-12 and TNF-α) and NO, that inflammatory or bone marrow macrophages from TLR2 KO mice didn't respond to GPI-mucins or to GPI anchors purified from *T. cruzi* parasites *(84)*.

## *T. CRUZI*-DERIVED GPI ANCHORS AS POTENTIAL IMMUNOLOGICAL ADJUVANTS

Actually the only adjuvants for human vaccine approved by the US Food & Drug Administration are the alum (salts based on aluminum) and MF59 (emulsion water/squalene oil) *(85)*. These adjuvants do not trigger the immune response through TLRs, and tend to induce responses that differentiate to Th2 *(85,86)*. In 1942, complete Freund's adjuvant was used with success for the first time *(87)*. But for a long time, nobody knew the molecular mechanism by which this adjuvant works. Now, with the discovery of TLRs and its functions, we know that bacterial adjuvants work through TLRs. For this reason TLRs were already defined as the "general adjuvant receptors in the body" *(88)*. In addition to macrophages, dendritic cells bear TLRs on their surface *(61,88,89)*. On activation via TLRs, the maturation of antigen-presenting cell will occur, followed by their migration to the lymph nodes, in which they will activate naïve T cells and initiate adaptive immunity. To obtain an efficient clonal T-cell expansion, an upregulation of expression of the major histocompatability complex molecules and CD80/CD86 costimulatory molecules are necessary *(88)*. In fact, both these phenomena occur associated with the production of various proinflammatory cytokines, including IL-12, after the activation of DCs via TLRs, which creates an environment that favors the differentiation of Th precursor cells into Th1 phenotype.

Returning to our yin-yang model shown in Fig. 1, there are normally two major opposite problems in the use of adjuvants: (a) the adjuvant may be not strong enough, leading to weak immune response and incomplete protection on vaccination; and (b) the adjuvant may stimulate a strong immune response, but leads to undesirable side effects because of an excessive stimulation of the cellular compartment of the innate immune system. Again, the ideal adjuvant would be the one that induces the aimed immune response, without showing the undesirable side effects. In fact, distinct TLRs may induce cellular functions with different intensities. Thus, recent reports suggest that TLR-dependent inflammatory responses are not identical. TLR2 signaling resulted in both quantitatively and qualitatively different responses compared with TLR4 signaling *(90)*. Another group, using DCs, confirmed that TLR4 agonists promote a stronger production of IL-12 and development of a more polarized Th1 response, although TLR2 stimulation produces conditions that are predicted to favor a Th2 response *(91)*. However, all TLRs for which an agonist has been identified appear to activate similar signaling pathways including MAPKs and NF-κB *(61,89)*. Thus, further dissecting and identifying signaling pathways triggered by specific TLRs may be immediately applicable as one might define new classes of adjuvants aiming to stimulate a specific type of inflammatory reaction/immune response desired to establish acquired host resistance to infectious diseases.

As previously discussed in this chapter, the GPI anchors derived from *T. cruzi* trypomastigotes is one of the most powerful stimulant of TLR2 *(63,84)* and induce macrophages to produce high levels of proinflammatory cytokines, leading to IFNγ production by NK cells. Because the DCs express TLR2 *(61,89)*, *T. cruzi*-derived GPI anchors may potentially work for stimulating maturation of DCs. Consistent with the studies mentioned above, the ability of *T. cruzi*-derived GPI anchors to stimulate IL-12 and the chemokine monocyte chemoattractant protein (MCP)-1 production is highly dependent on macrophage priming with IFNγ *(48,60)*. These results are in contrast with those using LPS, which does not require IFNγ to stimulate IL-12 and MCP-1 synthesis by macrophages and/or DCs. Thus, one would predict that using *T. cruzi*-derived GPI anchors as adjuvant would lead to a less polarized Th1 response as compared to LPS. However, the ability to induce a polarized Th1 response could be overcome if *T. cruzi*-derived GPI anchors are used in association with other adjuvant molecules, such as the α-galactosylceramide *(86)*, which induces the production of IFNγ response by NK cells in a IL-12-independent manner.

To date we have defined the precise molecular structure of GPI anchors with the ability to stimulate cytokine synthesis to antibody responses by macrophages and B-lymphocytes, respectively. By comparing the structure of various GPI anchors, we defined part of the molecules that may be critical for these immunological activities. For example, we know that the unsaturated fatty acid at the *sn*-2 position of the glycerol residue in the alkylacylglycerolipid, and the terminal galactose residues from these GPI anchors are likely to confer their potent proinflammatory activity. However, the main impediments for using *T. cruzi*-derived GPI anchors as immunological adjuvants are the methodological difficulties to obtain large quantities of synthetic glycolipids. Producing complex oligosaccharides containing defined carbohydrate sequences is a rather laborious and time-consuming process. Once we overcome these methodological barriers, one could produce in the laboratory different structural changes in the protozoan-derived GPI anchors, and test how it alters its proinflammatory properties, aiming to eliminate undesirable side effects, and favor the desirable immunological activities. Regardless, these are early but exciting days that are now allowing the rational development of new adjuvants based on the knowledge acquired from TLR functionality and structure of TLR agonists.

## ACKNOWLEDGMENTS

We wish to express our gratitude to all undergraduate and graduate students, as well as many collaborators, particularly Profs. Michael A.J. Ferguson and Luiz R. Travassos, from different institutions that have contributed to the studies reviewed here. We would also like to acknowledge the financial support of FAPEMIG (EDT 24000/01), WHO/TDR/World Bank (AA0047 and 990942), CNPq, CNPq/PADCT, and FAPESP (No.98 /10495-5).

## REFERENCES

1. Trager W. Living Together. The biology of animal parasitism. New York, NY: Plenum Press, 1986, pp. 1–467.
2. Pearce E, Scott PA, Sher A. Immune regulation in parasitic diseases. In: Paul W, ed. Fundamental of Immunology, 4th ed. Philadelphia: Lippincott-Raven, 1999, pp. 1271–1295.
3. Biron C, Gazzinelli RT. IL-12 effects on immune responses tomicrobial infections: a key mediator in regulating disease outcome. Curr Opin Immunol 1995;7: 485–496.
4. Gazzinelli RT, Wysocka M, Hayashi S, Denkers E, Hieny S, Caspar P, Trinchieri G, Sher A. Parasite Induced IL-12 stimulates early IFN-g synthesis and resistance during acute infection with *Toxoplasma gondii*. J Immunol 1994;153:2533–2543.
5. Aliberti JCS, Cardoso MAG, Martins GA, Gazzinelli RT, Vieira LQ, Silva JS. IL-12 mediates resistance to *Trypanosoma cruzi* infection in mice and is produced by normal murine macrophages in response to live trypomastigote. Infect Immunol 1996;64:1961–1967.
6. Mattner F, Magram J, Ferrante J, et al. Genetically resistant mice lacking interleukin-12 are susceptible to infection with Leishmania major and mount a polarized Th2 cell response. Eur J Immunol 1996;26:1553–1559.

7. Su Z, Stevenson MM. IL-12 is required for antibody-mediated protective immunity against blood-stage Plasmodium chabaudi AS malaria infection in mice. J Immunol 2002;168:1348–1355.

8. Belkaid Y, Mendez S, Lira R, Kadambi N, Milon G, Sacks D. A natural model of Leishmania major infection reveals a prolonged "silent" phase of parasite amplification in the skin before the onset of lesion formation and immunity. J Immunol 2000;165:969–977.

9. Roggero E, Perez A, Tamae-Kakasu M, et al. Differential susceptibility to acute *Trypanosoma cruzi* infection in BALB/c and C57BL/6 mice is not associated with a distinct parasite load but cytokine abnormalities. Clin Exp Immunol 2002;128: 421–428.

10. Gazzinelli RT, Hieny S, Wysocka M, et al. In the absence of endogenous IL-10 mice acutely infected with *Toxoplasma gondii* succumb to a lethal CD41 T cell response associated with Type 1 cytokine synthesis. J Immunol 1996;157:798–805.

11. Hunter CA, Ellis-Neyes LA, Slifer T, et al. IL-10 is required to prevent immune hyperactivity during infection with *Trypanosoma cruzi*. J Immunol 1997;158: 3311–3316.

12. Michailowsky V, Silva NM, Rocha CD, Vieira LQ, Lannes-Vieira J, Gazzinelli RT. Pivotal role of interleukin-12 and interferon-γ axis in controlling tissue parasitism and inflammation in the heart and central nervous system during *Trypanosoma cruzi* infection. Am J Pathol 2001;159:1723–1733.

13. Scharton-Kersten T, Wynn TA, Denkers EY, et al. In absence of endogenous IFN-γ mice develop unimpaired IL-12 responses to *Toxoplasma gondii* while failing to control acute infection. J Immunol 1996;157:4045–4054.

14. Yap G, Pesin M, Sher A. Cutting edge: IL-12 is required for the maintenance of IFN-gamma production in T cells mediating chronic resistance to the intracellular pathogen, Toxoplasma gondii. J Immunol 2000;165:628–631.

15. Clark IA, Schofield L. Pathogenesis of malaria. Parasitol Today 2000;16:451–454.

16. Linke A, Kuhn R, Muller W, Honarvar N, Li C, Langhorne J. Plasmodium chabaudi chabaudi: differential susceptibility of gene-targeted mice deficient in IL-10 to an erythrocytic-stage infection. Exp Parasitol 1996;84:253–263.

17. d'Imperio Lima MR, Eisen H, Minoprio P, Joskowicz, Coutinho A. Persistence of polyclonal B cell activation with undetectable parasitemia in late stages of experimental Chagas' disease. J Immunol 1986;137:353–356.

18. Minoprio PM, Eisen H, Forni L, et al. Polyclonal lymphocyte responses to murine *Trypanosoma cruzi* infection. I. Quantitation of both T- and B-cell responses. Scand J Immunol 1986;24:661–668.

19. Minoprio P, Eisen H, Joskowicz M, Pereira P, Coutinho A. Suppression of polyclonal antibody production in *Trypanosoma cruzi*-infected mice by treatment with anti-L3T4 antibodies. J Immunol 1987;139:545–550.

20. Cardillo F, Voltarelli JC, Reed SG, Silva JS. Regulation of Trypanosoma cruzi infection in mice by gamma interferon and interleukin 10: role of NK cells. Infect Immun 1996;64:128–134.

21. Une C, Andersson J, Eloranta ML, Sunnemark D, Harris RA, Orn A. Enhancement of natural killer (NK) cell cytotoxicity and induction of NK cell-derived interferon-gamma (IFN-gamma) display different kinetics during experimental infection with *Trypanosoma cruzi*. Clin Exp Immunol 2000;121:499–505.

22. Hunter CA, Slifer T, Araujo F. Interleukin-12-mediated resistance to *Trypanosoma cruzi* is dependent on tumor necrosis factor alpha and gamma interferon. Infect Immun 1996;64:2381–2386.
23. Muller U, Kohler G, Mossmann H, et al. IL-12-independent IFN-gamma production by T cells in experimental Chagas' disease is mediated by IL-18. J Immunol 2001;167:3346–3353.
24. Duthie MS, Wleklinski-Lee M, Nakayama T, Taniguchi M, Kahn SJ. During *Trypanosoma cruzi* infection CD1d-restricted NK T cells limit parasitemia and augment the antibody response to a glycophosphoinositol-modified surface protein. Infect Immun 2002;70:36–48.
25. Duthie MS, Kahn SJ. Treatment with alpha-galactosylceramide before Trypanosoma cruzi infection provides protection or induces failure to thrive. J Immunol 2002;168:5778–5785.
26. Procópio DO, Almeida IC, et al. Glycosylphosphatidylinositol-Anchored Mucin-Like Glycoproteins from *Trypanosoma cruzi* bind to CD1d but do not elicit dominant innate or adaptive immune responses via the CD1d/NKT cell pathway. J Immunol 2002;169:3929–3933.
27. James SL, Kipnis TL, Sher A, Hoff R. Enhanced resistance to acute infection with *Trypanosoma cruzi* in mice treated with an interferon inducer. Infect Immun 1982; 35:588–593.
28. Nathan C, Nogueira N, Juangbhanich, Ellis J, Cohn Z. Activation of macrophages in vivo and in vitro. Correlation between hydrogen peroxide release and killing of *Trypanosoma cruzi*. J Exp Med 1979;149:1056–1068.
29. Tanaka Y, Kiyotaki C, Tanowitz H, Bloom BR. Reconstitution of a variant macrophage cell line defective in oxygen metabolism with a $H_2O_2$-generating system. Proc Natl Acad Sci USA 1982;79:2584–2588.
30. McCabe RE, Mullins BT. Failure of *Trypanosoma cruzi* to trigger the respiratory burst of activated macrophages. Mechanism for immune evasion and importance of oxygen-independent killing. J Immunol 1990;144:2384–2388.
31. Gazzinelli RT, Oswald IP, Hieny S, James SL, Sher A. The microbicidal activity of interferon-gamma-treated macrophages against Trypanosoma cruzi involves an L-arginine-dependent, nitrogen oxide-mediated mechanism inhibitable by interleukin-10 and transforming growth factor-beta. Eur J Immunol 1992;22:2501–2506.
32. Vespa GN, Cunha FQ, Silva JS. Nitric oxide is involved in control of *Trypanosoma cruzi*-induced parasitemia and directly kills the parasite in vitro. Infect Immun 1994;62:5177–5182.
33. Seder RA, Gazzinelli RT, Sher A, Paul WE. IL-12 acts directly on CD4+ T cells to enhance priming for IFN-γ production and diminishes IL-4 inhibition of such priming. Proc Natl Acad Sci USA 1993;90:10188–10192.
34. Saeftel M, Fleischer B, Hoerauf A. Stage-dependent role of nitric oxide in control of *Trypanosoma cruzi* infection. Infect Immun 2001;69:2252–2259.
35. Tarleton RL, Koller BH, Latour A, Postan M. Susceptibility of beta 2-microglobulin-deficient mice to *Trypanosoma cruzi* infection. Nature 1992; 356:338–340.
36. Brodskyn CI, da Silva AM, Takehara HA, Mota I. Characterization of antibody isotype responsible for immune clearance in mice infected with *Trypanosoma cruzi*. Immunol Lett 1988;18:255–258.

172 *Gazzinelli et al.*

37. Abrahamsohn I, Coffman RL. Cytokine and nitric oxide regulation of the immunosuppression in *Trypanosoma cruzi* infection. J Immunol 1995;155:3955–3963.
38. Lopes MF, da Veiga VF, Santos AR, Fonseca ME, dosReis GA. Activation-induced CD4+ T cell death by apoptosis in experimental Chagas' disease. J Immunol 1995; 154:744–752.
39. Freire-de-Lima CG, Nascimento DO, Soares MB, et al. Uptake of apoptotic cells drives the growth of a pathogenic trypanosome in macrophages. Nature 2000;403: 199–203.
40. Tardieux I, Webster P, Ravesltoot J, et al. Lysosome recruitment and fusion are early events required for trypanosome invasion of mammalian cells. Cell 1992;71: 1117–1130.
41. Burleigh BA, Caler EV, Webster P, Andrews NW. A cytosolic serine endopeptidase from Trypanosoma cruzi is required for the generation of Ca2+ signaling in mammalian cells. J Cell Biol 1997;136:609–620.
42. Scharfstein J, Schmitz V, Morandi V, et al. Host cell invasion by *Trypanosoma cruzi* is potentiated by activation of bradykinin B (2) receptors. J Exp Med 2000; 192:1289–1300.
43. Aliberti JCS, Machado FS, Souto JT, et al. β-chemokines enhance parasite uptake and promote nitric oxide-dependent microbiostatic activity in murine inflammatory macrophages infected with *Trypanosoma cruzi*. Infect Immun 1999;67:4819–4826.
44. Villalta F, Zhang Y, Bibb KE, Burns JM Jr, Lima M. Signal transduction in human macrophages by gp83 ligand of *Trypanosoma cruzi*: trypomastigote gp83 ligand up-regulates trypanosome entry through the MAP kinase pathway. Biochem Biophys Res Commun 1998;249:247–252.
45. Villalta F, Zhang Y, Bibb KE, Pratap S, Burns JM Jr, Lima MF. Signal transduction in human macrophages by gp83 ligand of Trypanosoma cruzi: trypomastigote gp83 ligand up-regulates trypanosome entry through protein kinase C activation. Mol Cell Biol Res Commun 1999;2:64–70.
46. Hall BS, Tam W, Sem R, Pereira ME. Cell-specific activation of nuclear factor-kappaB by the parasite Trypanosoma cruzi promotes resistance to intracellular infection. Mol Biol Cell 2000;11:153–160.
47. Ming M, Ewen ME, Pereira ME. Trypanosome invasion of mammalian cells requires activation of the TGF beta signaling pathway. Cell 1995;82:287–296.
48. Camargo MM, Almeida IC, Pereira MES, Ferguson MAJ, Travassos LR, Gazzinelli RT. Glycosylphosphatidylinositol anchored mucin-like glycoproteins isolated from *Trypanosma cruzi* trypomastigotes initiate the synthesis of proinflammatory cytokines by macrophages. J Immunol 1997;158:5980–5991.
49. Camargo MM, Andrade AC, Almeida IC, Travassos LR, Gazzinelli RT. Glycoconjugates isolated from *Trypanosoma cruzi* but not from *Leishmania sp.* membranes trigger nitric oxide synthesis as well as microbicidal activity in IFN-γ primed macrophages. J Immunol 1997;159:6131–6139.
50. Ferreira LRP, Silva AM, Michailowsky V, Reis LFL, Gazzinelli RT. Expression of serum amyloid A3 mRNA by inflammatory macrophages exposed to membrane glycoconjugates from *Trypanosoma cruzi*. J Leuk Biol 1999;66:593–600.

51. Talvani A, Ribeiro CS, Aliberti JCS, et al. Kinetics of cytokine genes expression in experimental chagasic cardiomyopathy: tissue parasitism and IFN-γ as important determinants of chemokine mRNAs expression during infection with *Trypanosoma cruzi*. Microb Infect 2000; 2:851–866.

52. Huang H, Calderon TM, Berman JW, et al. Infection of endothelial cells with *Trypanosoma cruzi* activates NF-kappaB and induces vascular adhesion molecule expression. Infect Immun 1999; 67:5434–5440.

53. Huang H, Petkova SB, Pestell RG, et al. *Trypanosoma cruzi* infection (Chagas' disease) of mice causes activation of the mitogen-activated protein kinase cascade and expression of endothelin-1 in the myocardium. J Cardiovasc Pharmacol 2000; 36(Suppl 1):S148–S150.

54. Machado FS, Martins GA, Aliberti JC, Mestriner FL, Cunha FQ, Silva JS. *Trypanosoma cruzi*-infected cardiomyocytes produce chemokines and cytokines that trigger potent nitric oxide-dependent trypanocidal activity. Circulation 2000;102: 3003–3008.

55. de Avalos SV, Blader IJ, Fisher M, Boothroyd JC, Burleigh BA. Immediate/early response to *Trypanosoma cruzi* infection involves minimal modulation of host cell transcription. J Biol Chem 2002;277:639–644.

56. Almeida IC, Camargo MM, Procopio DO, et al. Highly-purified glycosylphosphatidylinositols from Trypanosoma cruzi are potent proinflammatory agents. EMBO J 2000;19:1476–1485.

57. Saavedra E, Herrera M, Gao W, Uemura H, Pereira MA. The *Trypanosoma cruzi* trans-sialidase, through its COOH-terminal tandem repeat, upregulates interleukin 6 secretion in normal human intestinal microvascular endothelial cells and peripheral blood mononuclear cells. J Exp Med 1999;190:1825–1836.

58. Ouaissi A, Guilvard E, Delneste Y, et al. The *Trypanosoma cruzi* Tc52-released protein induces human dendritic cell maturation, signals via Toll-like receptor 2, and confers protection against lethal infection. J Immunol 2002;168:6366–6374.

59. Norimine J, Suarez CE, McElwain TF, Florin-Christensen M, Brown WC. Immunodominant epitopes in Babesia bovis rhoptry-associated protein 1 that elicit memory CD4(+)-T-lymphocyte responses in *B. bovis*-immune individuals are located in the amino-terminal domain. Infect Immun 2002;70:2039–2048.

60. Coelho SC, Klein A, Talvani A, et al. Glycosylphosphatidylinositol-anchored mucin-like glycoproteins isolated from *Trypanosoma cruzi* trypomastigotes induce in vivo leuckocyte recruitment dependent on MCP-1 production by IFN-γ-primed macrophages. J Leuk Biol 2002;71:837–844.

61. Janeway CA Jr, Medzhitov R. Innate immune recognition. Annu Rev Immunol 2002;20:197–216.

62. Ferguson MAJ. The structure, biosynthesis and functions of glycosylphosphatidylinositol anchors, and the contributions of *Trypanosome* research. J Cell Sci 1999; 112:2799–2809.

63. Almeida IC, Gazzinelli RT. Proinflammatory activity of glycosylphosphatidylinositol anchors derived from *Trypanosoma cruzi*: structural and functional analyses. J Leuk Biol 2001;70:467–477.

64. Schofield L, Hackett F. Signal transduction in host cells by a glycosylphosphatidylinositol toxin of malaria parasites. J Exp Med 1993;177:145–153.

65. Naik RS, Branch OLH, Wood AS, et al. Glycosylphosphatidylinositol anchors of *Plasmodium falciparum*: molecular characterization and naturally elicited antibody response that may provide immunity to malaria pathogenesis. J Exp Med 2000;192:1563–1575.

66. Magez S, Stijlemans B, Radwanska M, Pays E, Ferguson MAJ, Debestlier P. The glycosyl-inositol-phosphate and dimyristoylglycerol moieties of the glycosylphosphatidylinositol anchor of the *Trypanosoma* variant-specific surface glycoprotein are distinct macrophage activating factors. J Immunol 1998;160:1949–1956.

67. Freire-de-Lima CG, Nunes MP, Corte-Real S, et al. Proapoptotic activity of a *Trypanosoma cruzi* ceramide-containing glycolipid turned on in host macrophages by IFN-γ. J Immunol 1998; 161:4909–4916.

68. Bellio M, Oliveira ACSC, Mermelstein CS, et al. Costimulatory action of glycoinositolphospholipids from *Trypanosome cruzi*: increased interleukin 2 secretion and induction of nuclear translocation of the nuclear factor of activated T cells 1. FASEB J 1999;13:1627–1635.

69. Bento CA, Melo MB, Previato JO, Mendonça-Previato L, Peçanha LM. Glycoinositolphospholipids purified from *Trypanosoma cruzi* stimulate Ig production in vitro. J Immunol 1996;157:4996–5001.

70. De Arruda Hinds LB, Previato LM, et al. Modulation of B-lymphocyte and NK cell activities by glycoinositolphospholipid purified from *Trypanosoma cruzi*. Infect Immun 1999;67:6177–6180.

71. Bilate AM, Previato JO, Medonça-Previato L, Peçanha LM. Glycoinositolphospholipids from *Trypanosoma cruzi* induce B cell hyper-responsiveness in vivo. Glycoconj J 2000;17:727–734.

72. De Arruda Hindas LB, Alexandre-Moreira MS, Decote-Ricardo D, Nunes MP, Peçanha LM. Increased immunoglobulin secretion by B lymphocytes from Trypanosoma cruzi infected mice after B lymphocytes-natural killer cell interaction. Parasite Immunol 2001;23:581–586.

73. Weston CR, Lambright DG, Davis RJ. MAP kinase signaling specificity. Science 2002;296:2345–2347.

74. Bhat NR, Zhang P, Lee JC, Hogan EL. Extracellular signal-regulated kinase and SAPK-2/p38 subgroups of mitogen-activated protein kinases regulate inducible nitric oxide synthase and tumor necrosis factor-α gene expression in endotoxin-stimulated primary glial cultures. J Neurosci 1998;18:1633–1641.

75. Kyriakis JM, Avruch J. Sounding the alarm: protein kinase cascades activated by stress and inflammation. J Biol Chem 1996;271:24313.

76. Ropert C, Almeida IC, Closel M, et al. Requirement of MAP kinases and IκB phosphorylation for induction of proinflammatory cytokines synthesis by macrophages indicates functional similarity of receptors triggered by glycosylphosphatidylinositol anchors from parasitic protozoa and bacterial LPS. J Immunol 2001; 166:3423–3431.

77. Medzhitov R, Preston-Hurlburt P, Janeway CA. A human homologue of the *Drosophila* Toll protein signals activation of adaptive immunity. Nature 1997;388: 394–397.

78. Lien E, Sellati TJ, Yoshimura A, et al. Toll-like receptor-2 functions as a pattern recognition receptor fro diverse bacterial products. J Biol Chem 1999;274:33419–33425.

79. Hemmi H, Takeuchi O, Kawai T, et al. A Toll-like receptor recognizes bacterial DNA. Nature 2000;408:740–745.
80. Alexopoulou L, Holt AC, Medzhitov R, Flavell RA. Recognition of double-stranded RNA and activation of NF-kappaB by Toll-like receptor 3. Nature 2001;413:732–738.
81. Shiloh MU, MacMicking JD, Nicholson S, et al. Phenotype of mice and macrophages deficient in both phagocyte oxidase and inducible nitric oxide synthase. Immunity 1999;10:29–38.
82. Brightbill HD, Libraty HD, Krutzick SR, et al. Host defense mechanisms triggered by microbial lipoproteins through Toll-like receptors. Science 1999;285:732–736.
83. Poltorak A, He X, Smirnova I, et al. Defective LPS signaling in C3H/HeJ and C57BL/10ScCr mice: mutations in Tlr4 gene. Science 1998;282:2085–2088.
84. Campos MAS, Almeida IC, Takeuchi O, et al. Activation of Toll-like receptor-2 by glycosylphosphatidylinositol anchors from a protozoan parasite. J Immunol 2001; 167:416–423.
85. Singh M, O'Hagan D. Advances in vaccine adjuvants. Nat Biotech 1999;17:1075–1081.
86. Bendelac A, Medzhitov R. Adjuvants of immunity: Harnessing innate immunity to promote adaptive immunity. J Exp Med 2002;195:F19–F23.
87. Freund J, McDermottt K. Sensitization to horse serum by means of adjuvants. Proc Soc Exp Biol Med 1942;49:548–553.
88. Kaisho T, Akira S. Toll-like receptors as adjuvant receptors. Biochem Biophys Acta 2002;1589:1–13.
89. Akira S, Takeda K, Kaisho T. Toll-like receptors: critical proteins linking innate and acquired immunity. Nat Immunol 2001;2:675–680.
90. Hirschfeld M, Weis JJ, Toshchakov V, et al. Signaling by toll-like receptor 2 and 4 agonists results in differential gene expression in murine macrophages. Infect Immun 2001;69:1477–1482.
91. Re F, Strominger JL. Toll-like receptor 2 (TLR2) and TLR4 differentially activate human dendritic cells. J Biol Chem 2001;276:37692–37699.

# 9

# The Immunomodulatory Glycan LNFPIII/Lewis X Functions As a Potent Adjuvant for Protein Antigens

## Mitsuhiro Okano, Kazunori Nishizaki, Akram Da'dara, Paul Thomas, Michele Carter, and Donald A. Harn, Jr.

## INTRODUCTION

There has been tremendous effort aimed at developing adjuvants that promote proinflammatory and/or strong cell-mediated immunity; many are discussed in this book. Interestingly, little effort is being placed on development of adjuvants that promote T helper (Th)2-type antibody responses. In part, this may be because alum has proven to be a safe, well-tolerated adjuvant that does bias the immune response in vaccine recipients toward Th2-type responses (1,2). Additionally, it may because of the perception that Th2-biased immune responses will not provide protection, or that they will not elicit strong cell-mediated responses to vaccine antigens, which is generally true for viral vaccines. However, there are disease situations in which driving Th2 responses is warranted, in particular for helminth infections, many of which require Th2-type responses for immune elimination of parasites (3–5). The second major category would be for preventive and/or therapeutic vaccines for proinflammatory-based autoimmune diseases. This category of diseases is increasing dramatically in humans and their pets. Clearly the use of adjuvants, which drive Th2-biased and/or anti-inflammatory responses, would be beneficial here. In fact, the tremendous increase in proinflammatory autoimmune diseases suggests that it is prudent to limit exposure to strong proinflammatory driving adjuvants and vaccines that promote Th1-type responses.

In regards to driving Th2-type responses numerous studies have demonstrated that infection with helminth parasites, or injection of extracts from helminths, drives polarized Th2-type immune responses in patients and animals (6–10). Using various biochemical methods, the immune responses of helminth-infected individuals or animals were shown to be largely directed at helminth-expressed carbohydrates. A number of glycan structures from helminths

From: *Vaccine Adjuvants: Immunological and Clinical Principles*
Edited by: C. J. Hackett and D. A. Harn, Jr. © Humana Press Inc., Totowa, NJ

have been identified and Lewis X and other fucosylated sugars are prominent Lewis X, originally identified from *Schistosoma mansoni* has now been shown to be common among many helminths. Lewis X and Lewis X containing gly-can structures have been shown to drive Th2-biasing and immunomodulatory properties in vivo and in vitro. In this chapter we cover the history leading up to the use of Lewis X glycoconjugates in vivo and in vitro to demonstrate that this molecule functions as a Th2-driver. Further, that Lewis X functions as a Th2-driving adjuvant for irrelevant, third-party protein antigens. This chapter closes with a discussion of putative mechanisms that Lewis X containing gly-cans activate antigen presenting cells to drive Th2-type immune responses.

## HELMINTH PARASITES DRIVE TH2-TYPE AND ANTI-INFLAMMATORY IMMUNE RESPONSES

The immune response to most bacterial and viral pathogens is generally proinflammatory coincident with production of interleukin (IL)-12, interferon (IFN)$\gamma$, tumor necrosis factor (TNF)-$\alpha$, IL-18, and other mediators associated with driving maturation of CD4$^+$ Th1-type effector cells that produce IFN$\gamma$ *(11,12)*. In contrast to the proinflammatory responses driven by the majority of microbial pathogens, helminth infection drives immune responses dominated by a Th2-type CD4$^+$ T-cell response characterized by production of IL-4, IL-5 IL-10, IL-13, and often, large amounts of immunoglobin (Ig)E antibodies. This polarized Th2 CD4$^+$ T-cell response to helminth infection is seen in both experimental infections and in helminth infected patients *(6–10)*. In addition to driving polarized Th2 responses, helminth infection also induces production of the immunoregulatory cytokine IL-10, which downregulates IFN$\gamma$ and can induce immune anergy by reducing expression of major histocompatibility complex (MHC) and costimulatory molecules on antigen-presenting cells (APCs) *(13–16)*. To better understand the nature of Th biasing in helminth infection, early studies on experimental schistosome infection in mice examined the nature of the CD4$^+$ Th responses at varying times postinfection. Pearce and associates *(17)* and later Gryzch and associates *(18)* demonstrated that there was a measurable shift from IFN$\gamma$ production and Th1 responses to predominant production of IL-4 and Th2 responses in spleens of infected mice coincident with the onset of egg deposition. These same groups and numerous others subsequently demonstrated that simple injection of schistosome eggs or a soluble extract of schistosome eggs was capable of inducing this polarized Th2 CD4$^+$ T-cell response *(13,14,19)*. Importantly, these studies occurred simultaneous with the discovery of the Lewis X glycan in extracts of schistosome eggs *(20–24)* leading to studies on the role of the biologically interesting Lewis X molecule in driving Th2 responses in experimental infections and in patients infected with schistosomes *(16,25–29)*.

## LNFPII

$$Gal\beta 1— 4G\underset{3}{l}cNAc\beta 1 — 3Gal\ \beta 1 — 3Glc$$

$$|$$

$$Fuc\ \alpha 1$$

## LNnT

$$Gal\beta 1— 4GlcNAc\beta 1 — 3Gal\ \beta 1 — 3Glc$$

**Fig. 1.** Structures of LNFPIII and LNnT.

## HELMINTH GLYCANS AS IMMUNOMODULATORS

Using antischistosome egg monoclonal antibodies, the structures of two car-bohydrates were identified. One of the carbohydrates recognized was Lewis X *(20)*. The human milk sugar Lacto-*N*-Fucopentaose III (LNFPIII) contains the Lewis X trisaccharide. Using synthetically produced LNFPIII polyvalently linked to a backbone/carrier molecule, we demonstrated that this carbohydrate alone could produce some of the immunological effects associated with the Th2-response in schistosome infected mice, including B-cell proliferation, IL-10 and prostaglandin $E_2$ production *(28)*. The second study to directly link Lewis X to schistosome immunomodulation involved studies of chronically infected schistosomiasis patients *(16)*. These patients have a profound IL-10-induced anergy and show decreased proliferation of their peripheral blood mononuclear cells to stimulation with schistosome antigen. Interestingly, proliferation could be restored and IL-10 levels reduced if the peripheral blood mononuclear cells were first pretreated with free monovalent LNFPIII. We concluded that although polyvalent LNFPIII activates cells to produce IL-10 among other activities, monovalent LNFPIII might actually work to block those same activities by interfering with the interaction between polyvalent LNFPIII and a receptor com-plex. Monovalent LNFPIII on its own has not been shown to have any signifi-cant activities. Figure 1 shows the structures of LNFPIII and lacto-*N*-neotetra-ose (LNnT), and Fig. 2 provides a representation of the sugar-conjugates that were produced and used to show biologic activity in vitro and in vivo.

## FUCOSYLATED SUGARS INDUCE PRODUCTION
## OF ANTIBODIES DURING SCHISTOSOME INFECTION

Interestingly, the majority of monoclonal antibodies produced in schistosome infected mice or mice immunized with schistosome extracts bound to carbohy-

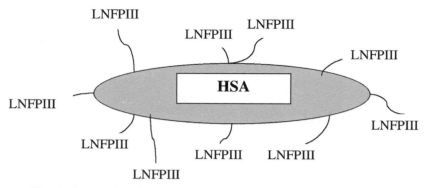

**Fig. 2.** Structures of LNFPIII conjugated to human serum albumin.

drate epitopes, including Lewis X containing structures *(20–24,30)*. Following the study by Ko and associates *(20)*, several groups used patient sera or sera from experimentally infected or immunized animals as probes to identify other glycan structures on schistosomes including LacDiNac (GalNAc$\beta$1->4GlcNAc-R) and LDNF ($\alpha$1,3-fucosylated lacdiNAc) *(21,31,32)*. Whether antibodies to these sugars have a protective effect, are neutral, or actually inhibit protective immune mechanisms of the host is controversial. The monoclonal antibodies that were initially used to detect Lewis X and poly-Lewis X were able to passively transfer protection to challenge infection in mice *(33)*. Similarly, highly protective sera from mice or chimpanzees immunized with radiation attenuated cercariae also contain antibodies to Lewis X, LacdiNAC and fucosylated LacdiNAC *(34)*. Thus, schistosome infection leads to production of antibodies to Lewis X and other schistosome fucosylated sugars.

## SCHISTOSOME EGG CARBOHYDRATES ARE LARGELY RESPONSIBLE FOR INDUCTION OF TH2 RESPONSES AND HAVE ADJUVANT ACTIVITY

Following the observations on the Th2 and anti-inflammatory driving properties of LNFPIII-human serum albumin (HSA) conjugates, we asked if carbohydrates were the major drivers of Th2 responses in schistosome eggs. We examined cellular and humoral immune responses in mice immunized with schistosome egg antigen (SEA), or SEA treated with 10 mM sodium meta-periodate. Sodium meta-periodate treatment opens up the glycan structures but does not remove them *(25)*. Comparison of the responses of these mice showed that as expected, SEA drives elevated IgE production, recruitment of nasal eosinophils and elevated levels of IL-4, IL-5, and IL-10. By comparison, mice sensitized with periodate-treated SEA had significantly lower levels of total and SEA-specific IgE, no nasal recruitment of eosinophils and no production of Th2-associated cytokines. These results clearly demonstrated that on schistosome eggs or egg extracts it is the carbohydrate structures that are necessary for driving Th2-type responses, including the high levels of total and antigen-specific IgE that are a hallmark in schistosomiasis and most other helminth infections. Importantly, although carbohydrates were required to drive these responses, this same study showed that they were not targets of the IgE response, suggesting that they were functioning as adjuvants to promote enhanced IgE production. This early observation was followed by a larger study that examined the role of helminth carbohydrates in driving Th2-type responses in parasitic and free-living helminths. They concluded that carbohydrates were essential for driving Th2 type responses in all helminths (35). Both of these studies supported the hypothesis that LNFPIII/Lewis X would function as an adjuvant for unrelated, third-party antigens, to enhance Th2-type antibody responses.

## LNFPIII/LEWIS X FUNCTIONS AS AN ADJUVANT FOR THIRD-PARTY ANTIGENS

For these studies we utilized HSA (or bovine serum albumin as our third-party antigens. Mice were immunized with HSA alone, HSA-LNFPIII conjugate, HSA-LNnT conjugate, and HSA-Lacto-$N$-fucopentaose I (LNFPI) conjugate. We utilized HSA-LNnT conjugate and HSA-LNFPI conjugate to determine how important Lewis X was in driving these responses (26). Further, immunization with HSA-LNFPI conjugate would allow us to determine if the fucose residue alone was critical for adjuvant activity in mice, as unlike the Lewis X $\alpha(1-3)$ linked fucose, LNFPI has the same tetrasaccharide backbone as LNnT and LNFPIII but has the fucose linkage as $\alpha(1-2)$. The level of substitution of LNFPIII, LNnT, and LNFPI was 10 to 12 molecules per molecule of HSA (Fig. 2).

For the majority of experiments mice were primed and boosted by intranasal instillation of HSA or the various sugar conjugates mixed in phosphate buffered saline. Additional experiments were done in which mice were immunized with saline, HSA in saline, HSA in alum, HSA-LNFPIII in saline, and HSA-LNFPIII in alum by intraperitoneal or subcutaneous injection. Mice were bled after the prime, boost, and final boost and sera tested by ELISA for levels of total IgG HSA-specific antibodies and for IgM, IgA, IgE, and isotypes of IgG HSA-specific antibodies.

From intranasally immunized mice we obtained dramatic results showing that mice immunized with HSA alone produced very low levels of anti-HSA total IgG in which mice immunized with HSA-LNFPIII had endpoint titers of 5000, 80,000, and 700,000 after the primary, first, and second boosts respectively (Table 1). The elevated levels of anti-HSA antibodies detected in the HSA-LNFPIII group were specific to the adjuvant activity of LNFPIII as sera from mice vaccinated with HSA-LNnT did not have detectable levels of anti-HSA IgGs

**Table 1**
**Endpoint Titers of Anti-HSA IgG in Immunized Mice**

|   | Saline | HSA | HSA-LNFPIII | HSA-LNnT |
|---|--------|-----|-------------|----------|
| 1 | 100 | 200 | 5000 | 100 |
| 2 | 100 | 180 | 80,000 | 100 |
| 3 | 100 | 100 | 700,000 | 200 |

Balb/c mice were primed and boosted intranasally with saline HSA, HSA-LNFPIII, or HSA-LNnT as described. Sera was collected after the primary (1), first (2), and second (3) boosts, then analyzed for endpoint titers of anti-HSA total IgGs by ELISA.

**Table 2**
**Endpoint Titers of Anti-HSA Antibody Classes and IgG Isotypes in Immunized Mice**

|   | IgM | IgA | IgG1 | IgG2a | IgG2b | IgG3 |
|---|-----|-----|------|-------|-------|------|
| 1 | 100 | 100 | 5000 | 100 | 100 | 100 |
| 2 | 100 | 100 | 500,000 | 900 | 2000 | 500 |
| 3 | 100 | 100 | 1,000,000 | 6000 | 25,000 | 200 |

Balb/c mice were primed and boosted intranasally with HSA-LNFPIII as described. Sera was collected after the primary (1), first (2), and second (3) boosts, then analyzed for endpoint titers of anti-HSA IgM, IgA, and isotypes of IgG by ELISA.

(Table 1). Vaccination of mice with HSA-LNFPIII increased the levels of HSA-specific IgG and IgE antibodies, but not IgM or IgA anti-HSA antibodies (Tables 1–3). We next examined the anti-HSA specific antibody response by class of antibody and IgG isotypes. For saline, HSA and HSA-LNnT, we were unable to detect any IgM, IgA, or isotypes of IgG anti-HSA specific antibodies (not shown). Similarly, as shown in Table 2, we were unable to detect significant levels of IgM or IgA antibodies to HSA following intranasal immunization with HSA-LNFPIII. However, immunization with HSA-LNFPIII did induce production of large amounts of anti-HSA specific IgGs, notably the endpoint titers of the Th2 associated IgG1 isotype were 5000, 500,000, and 1 million following the prime and second and third boosts respectively (Table 2).

Immunization with HSA-LNFPIII also induced significant levels of anti-HSA specific IgG2a and IgG2b antibodies were nominally 400-fold lower than the IgG1 antibody endpoints (Table 2). Interestingly, we were able to detect an increase in the endpoint titers of anti-HSA IgE in HSA-LNFPIII immunized mice; however, the overall levels were far lower than the IgG levels with IgE endpoints of 6000 and 3000 following first and second boosts (Table 3). Thus, LNFPIII/Lewis X functions as an adjuvant for a third party antigen when administered intranasally, and further, the adjuvant activity of LNFPIII/Lewis X is

**Table 3**
**Endpoint Titers of IgE Anti-HSA Antibodies in Immunized Mice**

|   | Saline | HSA | HSA-LNFPIII | HSA-LNnT |
|---|--------|-----|-------------|----------|
| 1 | 100 | 100 | 100 | 100 |
| 2 | 100 | 100 | 6000 | 100 |
| 3 | 100 | 100 | 3000 | 100 |

Values were determined by ELISA. Sera was collected after the primary (1), first (2), and second (3) boosts then analyzed for IgE anti-HSA end point titers by ELISA.

specific to LNFPIII/Lewis X as mice immunized with either HSA-LNnT or HSA-LNFPI did not produce a significant anti-HSA response of any antibody class or IgG isotype.

We wanted to test the general applicability of LNFPIII as an adjuvant. Therefore we performed similar vaccination trials in mice only we changed the route of vaccination to intraperitoneal and subcutaneous. For these experiments we also compared levels of IgG and IgE obtained when HSA or HSA-LNFPIII were formulated with alum. Endpoint titer for IgG or capture assay for HSA-specific IgE analysis showed that in mice immunized intraperitoneally or subcutaneously, levels of total anti-HSA IgG and IgE were equivalent from HSA-alum and HSA-LNFPIII immunized mice with endpoint titers of approx 600,000 for IgG compared to undetectable titers of HSA-specific IgG for saline or HSA immunized mice. For IgE we detected an optical density (O.D.) value of 0.5 for IgE as compared to undetectable O.D.s for saline or HSA immunized mice (data not shown). Similar results were obtained with subcutaneously immunized mice although the endpoint titers and IgE O.D. values were lower, at 100,000 and 0.1 values, respectively. Interestingly mice immunized with the combination of HSA-LNFPIII in alum had increased IgG endpoint titers and IgE O.D. value using both immunization routes. For IgG levels in intraperitoneally immunized mice, the endpoint titers increased from approx 600,000 to 5 million or about ninefold. The increase in HSA-specific IgG was 10-fold in mice immunized subcutaneously, rising from 100,000 for HSA-LNFPIII or HSA-alum to 1 million for HSA-LNFPIII-alum. This important finding shows that there is a synergistic effect of LNFPIII on alum. Thus, although LNFPIII is not more potent than alum, the standard criterion Th2-adjuvant, it does act synergistically with alum increasing IgG-HSA specific antibody titers from 9- to 10-fold over that seen when either adjuvant is used alone.

The adjuvant activity was specific for LNFPIII/Lewis X as mice immunized with LNnT-HSA or LNFPI-HSA did not have an increase in HSA-specific antibody titers over that of mice immunized with HSA alone. This experiment also demonstrated that the adjuvant effect of LNFPIII was not solely because of the

**Table 4**
**Levels of Cytokines Produced by Nasal Lymphocytes Postimmunization**

|        | Saline | HSA | HSA-LNFPIII |
|--------|--------|-----|-------------|
| IL-4   | 0      | <5  | 25          |
| IL-5   | 12     | 45  | 110         |
| IL-10  | 200    | 250 | 800         |

Nasal lymphocytes were harvested as described and restimulated in vitro with 10 μg/mL HSA or 10 μg/mL HSA-LNFPIII for 48 hours. Culture supernatants were collected and levels of cytokines (pg/mL) determined by ELISA.

fucose residue, but was related to the structural linkage of the fucose, apparently requiring an $\alpha(1\text{-}3)$ linkage suggesting that the adjuvant effect was specific for the Lewis X portion of LNFPIII. The adjuvant effect was shown to be requiring conjugation of LNFPIII to HSA. In experiments in which LNFPIII was simply mixed with HSA there was no increase in anti-HSA antibody titers. Conversely, if we added free, nonconjugated sugar to HSA or HSA-LNFPIII, this had no effect on either increasing the anti-HSA-specific antibody titer, or in lowering it.

Examination of the proliferative and cytokine responses of nasal lymphocytes from mice restimulated with HSA in vitro showed that mice immunized with HSA-LNFPIII also had an upregulation of Th2-associated cytokines (IL-4, IL-5, IL-10) compared to mice immunized with HSA alone (Table 4). IL-4 levels were low at 25 pg/mL, IL-5 levels were 110 pg/mL compared to 45 pg/mL in HSA immunized mice and IL-10 levels were 800, 250, and 200 pg/mL for HSA-LNFPIII, HSA, and saline immunized mice respectively (Table 4). This study also tested the adjuvant effect of an analogue of LNFPIII, LNnT, which is identical to LNFPIII except that it does not contain a fucose residue. This analogue had no effect on cytokine production supporting the antibody data, and indicating that the adjuvant effect in these experiments was dependent of the presence of the fucose residue. The requirement of the fucose certainly reflects the specificity of the cell surface receptor for LNFPIII/Lewis X.

## POTENTIAL MECHANISMS OF ADJUVANT ACTIVITY AND/OR IMMUNE BIASING BY LNFPIII/LEWIS X

Whether the adaptive CD4[+] Th response is directed toward Th1 or Th2 type is dependent on the events that occur during the interaction of naïve CD41 T cells with activated APCs. Activated APCs present pathogen peptide bound to MHC II to T-cell receptor (TCR) on CD4[+] Th cells simultaneous with ligation of costimulatory molecules (*11,12,36,37*). Among APCs, dendritic cells (DCs) are arguably the most powerful antigen sampling and presenting cells driving

T-cell adaptive immune responses to pathogens *(38–44)*. In 1989, Charles Janeway proposed that the innate immune system had evolved to recognize conserved molecular patterns across multiple pathogens and that the innate response of DCs and macrophages (Macs) to these conserved molecular patterns would determine the direction that the adaptive immune response would take *(45)*. The receptors for these conserved molecular patterns were named pattern recognition receptors, and the conserved molecular patterns are now called pathogen-associated molecular patterns (PAMPs). Examples of conserved PAMPs include mannans, zymosan, lipopolysaccharide (LPS), lipoteichoic acids, peptidoglycans, and unmethylated deoxyribonucleic acid (DNA) or CpG motifs, each of which are not expressed on mammalian cells *(40)*.

Cell surface C-type lectin receptors that have single or multiple carbohydrate recognition domains are most often associated with endocytosis of pathogens and not directly involved in cell-surface signaling leading to APC activation *(46–50)*. By comparison, the ligation of Toll-like receptors (TLRs) on DCs and Macs leads to immediate signaling and activation events (40). Currently, 10 different TLRs have been described (51). PAMP activation of DCs through the Toll receptors is generally described as inducing type-1, proinflammatory responses *(40)*, although there have been some reports of TLR ligands inducing IL-4 or anti-inflammatory responses *(15,52)*. DCs activated and responding via type 1 mediators have been termed DC1s, which promote the maturation of Th1-type CD4$^+$ T cells whereas DCs that promote Th2-type responses are defined as DC2s. A large body of literature describes PAMP binding to TLR4, TLR2, and TLR9 activating immature DCs toward proinflammatory responses and giving rise to DC1s *(40)*. By contrast, comparatively little is known regarding the generation of Th2-type responses via PAMP activation of DCs, and less is known about defined molecules that function as Th2 PAMPs *(15,52)*. This chapter focuses on how infection with, or exposure to helminths/helminth molecules drives dominant and polarized Th2-type and anti-inflammatory CD4$^+$ T-cells responses, the molecular nature of a few defined helminth glycans, and how they are able to activate various types of APCs leading to Th2-type immune responses.

## LNFPIII/LEWIS X ACTIVATES APCs IN A TLR4-DEPENDENT MECHANISM THAT LEADS TO INDUCTION OF TH2 RESPONSES

As mentioned earlier, Pearce and associates *(17)* and Gryzch and associates *(18)* demonstrated that schistosome eggs drive polarized Th1 to Th2 shifts. One glycan is the pentasaccharide LNFPIII, also known as stage-specific embryonic antigen 1 and the second is the nonfucosylated homolog, LNnT. In addition to schistosome parasites LNFPIII is found in human milk and in the urine of pregnant women *(53–55)*. LNFPIII also contains the asialo, asulfo-Lewis X trisaccharide, which is a ubiquitous structure on SEA.

These observations on the immunomodulatory properties of LNFPIII conjugates have important implications for potential drug design in the future based on schistosome carbohydrates, in that it suggests that multiple fucosylations on a carbohydrate may produce a more potent Th2-driver in host tissue. These findings are also important in light of the fact that several fucose containing glycans with varying structures have been identified in schistosomes (which contain their own fucosyltransferase) *(56)*. These include several variations of repeating difucosylated GlcNAc structures *(30)* and several asparagine-linked and mannosylated structures *(57)*. None of these have been rigorously examined from the point of view of immunoregulation and might produce interesting differences in terms of the degree and quality of response that they effect.

## LNFPIII/LEWIS X DRIVES TH2-TYPE
## RESPONSES AND FUNCTIONS AS A TH2 PAMP

How alum drives Th2 responses is not clearly understood. On contrast, the mechanisms of multiple Th1-associated adjuvants have been identified including LPS (lipid A), peptidoglycan, and CpG motifs. These all function by activating APCs through TLRs, TLR4, TLR2, and TLR9 respectively *(38,40)*. Signaling through the respective TLRs for each of these adjuvants eventually leads to production of proinflammatory mediators and a Th1-biased CD4[+] Th response. However, until recently, few Th2 PAMPs have been identified. SEA has been useful in these studies as a known Th2-promoter and two studies showed that SEA could indeed act as a DC2 maturation agent in both human and mouse DCs *(58–60)*. These papers also demonstrated that DC2 cells have a very different phenotype than DC1 cells, in that they do not upregulate many immunological markers associated with strong DC maturation. However, when incubated with T cells, they do promote strong Th2 responses.

We initiated studies on LNFPIII-Lewis X conjugate activation on murine DCs to determine if this was a potential mechanism behind the adjuvant activity of LNFPIII/Lewis X. We were able to demonstrate that LNFPIII, when used as a multivalent conjugate, is capable of activating immature bone marrow-derived DCs and inducing their maturation to DC2s *(61)*. Similar to what we reported for adjuvant activity, the ability to mature DCs was dependent on the fucose-moiety, as LNnT was unable to activate either immature bone marrow-derived DCs (BMDCs) or murine Macs. To determine if, like CpGs or peptidoglycans or even LPS, adjuvant activity of LNFPIII/Lewis X is associated with this molecule activating DCs in a TLR-dependent mechanism, we initiated studies in mice using either antibodies that block TLR4-MD2 activation, or performing experiments in mice with a functional mutation in TLR4. Surprisingly we found that the ability of LNFPIII/Lewis X to activate DCs was dependent on TLR4, a TLR-associated with driving proinflammatory responses in cells stimulated with LPS.

In contrast to LPS stimulation via TLR4, the Th2 driving adjuvant LNFPIII/ Lewis X drives alternative activation of mitogen-activated protein kinases, activating predominantly extracellular receptor kinase and not c-Jun NH2-terminal kinase or p38 as LPS stimulation does. Additionally, LNFPIII/Lewis X-stimulated cells have only transient activation of NF$\kappa$B compared to persistent and long-lasting activation of NF$\kappa$B seen in LPS-stimulated cells. Another difference between LPS and LNFPIII/Lewis X activation of DCs is that although LPS drives production of nitric oxide, LNFPIII/Lewis X does not. How then, can both of these PAMPs signal via TLR4 but drive such disparate pathways? This is currently a major area of research in our lab. We do know from the excellent study of Kaisho and associates *(62)* that even LPS stimulation of Macs can lead to a Th2-biased immune response in cells that are deficient in the TIR adaptor protein MyD88. Thus, our hypothesis is that LNFPIII/Lewis X activates cells via TLR4, inducing a MyD88-independent signaling pathway that gives rise to a DC2 maturational pathway. How LNFPIII/Lewis X is able to differentially signal through TLR4 as compared to LPS is another area of research ongoing in our lab. We believe that it depends on the nature of the cell receptors for LNFPIII/ Lewis X that eventually bring this signalosome complex including TLR4, together. One obvious candidate is DC-specific intercellular cell adhesion molecule-3-grabbing nonintegrin, as several laboratories have shown this cell surface molecule to bind Lewis X *(63)*. Thus, LNFPIII/Lewis X appears to be the first molecularly defined Th2-PAMP and one of the more molecularly defined PAMPs of either type, with specificity being fucose dependent. As more Th2-driving helminth glycans are defined, similar to LNFPIII/Lewis X, they should prove to be useful reagents for studying the immune response to helminth parasites but also as a means to understand how immature dendritic cells and other APCs can be specifically activated to drive Th2-type and anti-inflammatory responses, which may have use as adjuvants for vaccines, and for development of novel anti-inflammatory therapeutics that could be used to treat Th1-mediated autoimmune diseases.

## CONCLUSION

The use of small oligosaccharides as adjuvants, and/or Th2-drivers in general is still very young. The findings of these studies clearly show that LNFPIII/ Lewis X represents a novel, potent, Th2-driving adjuvant that functions equivalent to the criterion standard Th2 adjuvant alum in driving IgG and IgE antigen specific responses. Importantly, this study demonstrated an amazing synergistic effect when LNFPIII-conjugated antigen was mixed with alum, driving increases in IgG endpoints from 9- to 10-fold higher than the levels seen in mice immunized with HSA-LNFPIII or HSA-alum alone. The synergy in antibody responses suggests that this combination of adjuvants could safely be employed for antigens that are poorly immunogenic, although caution should be used when testing such a combination because of the small increase in IgE antibodies. In addition to the use of small oligosaccharides such as LNFPIII/Lewis X as adjuvants we believe that the study of immunomodulatory glycans from helminth parasites represents an area of research that will provide tremendous findings in the area of innate immunity, particularly in defining how Th2 PAMPs activate and drive DC2 maturation. We also believe that these helminth glycans likely have many other as yet undescribed immunomodulatory properties and that taken together, will provide much insight into understanding the evolution and maintenance of polarized Th2 responses in chronic infections or other disease states. The fact that LNFPIII/Lewis X functions to drive Th2-responses and activate DC2 maturation programs suggests that this molecule can be used as a therapy or perhaps a preventative treatment for proinflammatory mediated autoimmune diseases such as diabetes and colitis. We are currently testing this interesting possibility.

## REFERENCES

1. Lindblad EB. Aluminium compounds for use in vaccines. Immunol Cell Biol 2004; 82:497.
2. Lindblad EB. Aluminium adjuvants—in retrospect and prospect. Vaccine 2004; 22:3658.
3. Bancroft AJ, Artis D, Donaldson DD, Sypek JP, Grencis RK. Gastrointestinal nematode expulsion in IL-4 knockout mice is IL-13 dependent. Eur J Immunol 2000;30:2083.
4. Madden KB, Urban JF Jr, Ziltener HJ, et al. Antibodies to IL-3 and IL-4 suppress helminth-induced intestinal mastocytosis. J Immunol 1991;147:1387.
5. Urban JF Jr, Maliszewski CR, Madden KB, Katona IM, Finkelman FD. IL-4 treatment can cure established gastrointestinal nematode infections in immunocompetent and immunodeficient mice. J Immunol 1995;154:4675.
6. Finkelman FD, Urban JF Jr. The other side of the coin: the protective role of the TH2 cytokines. J Allergy Clin Immunol 2001;107:772.
7. Rogerie F, Gallissot MC, et al. Sex-dependent neutralizing humoral response to Schistosoma mansoni 28GST antigen in infected human populations. J Infect Dis 2000;181:1855.
8. Urban JF Jr, Fayer R, Sullivan C, et al. Local TH1 and TH2 responses to parasitic infection in the intestine: regulation by IFN-gamma and IL-4. Vet Immunol Immunopathol 1996;54:337.
9. Urban JF Jr, Schopf L, Morris SC, et al. Stat6 signaling promotes protective immunity against Trichinella spiralis through a mast cell- and T cell-dependent mechanism. J Immunol 2000;164:2046.
10. Fallon PG, Fookes RE, Wharton GA. Temporal differences in praziquantel- and oxamniquine-induced tegumental damage to adult Schistosoma mansoni: implications for drug-antibody synergy. Parasitology 112 1996(Pt 1):47.

11. Jankovic D, Sher A, Yap G. Th1/Th2 effector choice in parasitic infection: decision making by committee. Curr Opin Immunol 2001;13:403.
12. O'Garra A. Cytokines induce the development of functionally heterogeneous T helper cell subsets. Immunity 1998;8:275.
13. Vella AT, Pearce EJ. CD4+ Th2 response induced by Schistosoma mansoni eggs develops rapidly, through an early, transient, Th0-like stage. J Immunol 1992;148: 2283.
14. Cook GA, Metwali A, Blum A, Mathew R, Weinstock JV. Lymphokine expression in granulomas of Schistosoma mansoni-infected mice. Cell Immunol 1993; 152:49.
15. van der Kleij D, Latz E, Brouwers JF, et al. A novel host-parasite lipid cross-talk. Schistosomal lyso-phosphatidylserine activates toll-like receptor 2 and affects immune polarization. J Biol Chem 2002;277:48122.
16. Velupillai P, dos Reis EA, dos Reis MG, Harn DA. Lewis(x)-containing oligosaccharide attenuates schistosome egg antigen-induced immune depression in human schistosomiasis. Hum Immunol 2000;61:225.
17. Pearce EJ, Caspar P, Grzych JM, Lewis FA, Sher A. Downregulation of Th1 cytokine production accompanies induction of Th2 responses by a parasitic helminth, Schistosoma mansoni. J Exp Med 1991;173:159.
18. Grzych JM, Pearce E, Cheever A, et al. Egg deposition is the major stimulus for the production of Th2 cytokines in murine schistosomiasis mansoni. J Immunol 1991;146:1322.
19. Henderson GS, Conary JT, Summar M, McCurley TL, Colley DG. In vivo molecular analysis of lymphokines involved in the murine immune response during Schistosoma mansoni infection. I. IL-4 mRNA, not IL-2 mRNA, is abundant in the granulomatous livers, mesenteric lymph nodes, and spleens of infected mice. J Immunol 1991;147:992.
20. Ko AI, Drager UC, Harn DA. A Schistosoma mansoni epitope recognized by a protective monoclonal antibody is identical to the stage-specific embryonic antigen 1. Proc Natl Acad Sci USA 1990;87:4159.
21. Eberl M, Langermans JA, Vervenne RA, et al. Antibodies to glycans dominate the host response to schistosome larvae and eggs: is their role protective or subversive? J Infect Dis 2001;183:1238.
22. Van Roon AM, Van de Vijver KK, Jacobs W, et al. Discrimination between the anti-monomeric and the anti-multimeric Lewis X response in murine schistosomiasis. Microbes Infect 2004;6:1125.
23. Robijn ML, Wuhrer M, Kornelis D, et al. Mapping fucosylated epitopes on glycoproteins and glycolipids of Schistosoma mansoni cercariae, adult worms and eggs. Parasitology 2005;130:67.
24. Remoortere A, Hokke CH, van Dam GJ, et al. Various stages of schistosoma express Lewis(x), LacdiNAc, GalNAcbeta1-4 (Fucalpha1-3G) lcNAc and GalNAc beta1-4(Fucalpha1-2Fucalpha1-3G) lcNAc carbohydrate epitopes: detection with monoclonal antibodies that are characterized by enzymatically synthesized neoglycoproteins. Glycobiology 2000;10:601.
25. Okano M, Satoskar AR, Nishizaki K, Abe M, Harn DA Jr. Induction of Th2 responses and IgE is largely due to carbohydrates functioning as adjuvants on Schistosoma mansoni egg antigens. J Immunol 1999;163:6712.

26. Okano M, Satoskar AR, Nishizaki K, Harn DA Jr. Lacto-N-fucopentaose III found on Schistosoma mansoni egg antigens functions as adjuvant for proteins by inducing Th2-type response. J Immunol 2001;167:442.

27. Palanivel V, Posey C, Horauf AM, et al. B-cell outgrowth and ligand-specific production of IL-10 correlate with Th2 dominance in certain parasitic diseases. Exp Parasitol 1996;84:168.

28. Velupillai P, Harn DA. Oligosaccharide-specific induction of interleukin 10 production by B220+ cells from schistosome-infected mice: a mechanism for regulation of CD4+ T-cell subsets. Proc Natl Acad Sci USA 1994;91:18.

29. Velupillai P, Secor WE, Horauf AM, Harn DA. B-1 cell (CD5+B220+) outgrowth in murine schistosomiasis is genetically restricted and is largely due to activation by polylactosamine sugars. J Immunol 1997;158:338.

30. Levery SB, Weiss JB, Salyan ME, et al. Characterization of a series of novel fucose-containing glycosphingolipid immunogens from eggs of Schistosoma mansoni. J Biol Chem 1992;267:5542.

31. Nyame AK, Leppanen AM, Bogitsh BJ, Cummings RD. Antibody responses to the fucosylated LacdiNAc glycan antigen in Schistosoma mansoni-infected mice and expression of the glycan among schistosomes. Exp Parasitol 2000;96:202.

32. Van der Kleij D, Van Remoortere A, Schuitemaker JH, et al. Triggering of innate immune responses by schistosome egg glycolipids and their carbohydrate epitope GalNAc beta 1-4(Fuc alpha 1-2Fuc alpha 1-3G) lcNAc. J Infect Dis 2002;185:531.

33. Harn DA, Mitsuyama M, David JR. Schistosoma mansoni. Anti-egg monoclonal antibodies protect against cercarial challenge in vivo. J Exp Med 1984;159:1371.

34. Richter D, Incani RN, Harn DA. Lacto-N-fucopentaose III (Lewis x), a target of the antibody response in mice vaccinated with irradiated cercariae of Schistosoma mansoni. Infect Immun 1996;64:1826.

35. Tawill S, Le Goff L, Ali F, Blaxter M, Allen JE. Both free-living and parasitic nematodes induce a characteristic Th2 response that is dependent on the presence of intact glycans. Infect Immun 2004;72:398.

36. Mosmann TR, Coffman RL. TH1 and TH2 cells: different patterns of lymphokine secretion lead to different functional properties. Annu Rev Immunol 1989;7:145.

37. Mosmann TR, Sad S. The expanding universe of T-cell subsets: Th1, Th2 and more. Immunol Today 1996;17:138.

38. Barton GM, Medzhitov R. Control of adaptive immune responses by Toll-like receptors. Curr Opin Immunol 2002;14:380.

39. Shortman K, Wu L. Parentage and heritage of dendritic cells. Blood 2001;97:3325.

40. Medzhitov R. Toll-like receptors and innate immunity. Nat Rev Immunol 2001;1:135.

41. Banchereau J, Briere F, Caux C, et al. Immunobiology of dendritic cells. Annu Rev Immunol 2000;18:767.

42. Banchereau J, Steinman RM. Dendritic cells and the control of immunity. Nature 1998;392:245.

43. Lane PJ, Brocker T. Developmental regulation of dendritic cell function. Curr Opin Immunol 1999;11:308.

44. Moser M, Murphy KM. Dendritic cell regulation of TH1-TH2 development. Nat Immunol 2000;1:199.

45. Janeway CA Jr. Approaching the asymptote? Evolution and revolution in immunology. Cold Spring Harb Symp Quant Biol 1989;54 Pt 1:1.
46. Stahl PD, Ezekowitz RA. The mannose receptor is a pattern recognition receptor involved in host defense. Curr Opin Immunol 1998;10:50.
47. Hoyle GW, Hill RL. Molecular cloning and sequencing of a cDNA for a carbohydrate binding receptor unique to rat Kupffer cells. J Biol Chem 1988;263:7487.
48. Geijtenbeek TB, Engering A, Van Kooyk Y. DC-SIGN, a C-type lectin on dendritic cells that unveils many aspects of dendritic cell biology. J Leukoc Biol 2002; 71:921.
49. Figdor CG, van Kooyk Y, Adema GJ. C-type lectin receptors on dendritic cells and Langerhans cells. Nat Rev Immunol 2002;2:77.
50. Shepherd VL, Konish MG, Stahl P. Dexamethasone increases expression of mannose receptors and decreases extracellular lysosomal enzyme accumulation in macrophages. J Biol Chem 1985;260:160.
51. Reis e Sousa C. Dendritic cells as sensors of infection. Immunity 2001;14:495.
52. Pulendran B, Kumar P, Cutler CW, et al. Lipopolysaccharides from distinct pathogens induce different classes of immune responses in vivo. J Immunol 2001;167: 5067.
53. Pfenninger A, Karas M, Finke B, Stahl B, Sawatzki G. Mass spectrometric investigations of human milk oligosaccharides. Adv Exp Med Biol 2001;501:279.
54. Erney R, Hilty M, Pickering L, Ruiz-Palacios G, Prieto P. Human milk oligosaccharides: a novel method provides insight into human genetics. Adv Exp Med Biol 2001;501:285.
55. Kelder B, Erney R, Kopchick J, Cummings R, Prieto P. Glycoconjugates in human and transgenic animal milk. Adv Exp Med Biol 2001;501:269.
56. DeBose-Boyd R, Nyame AK, Cummings RD. Schistosoma mansoni: characterization of an alpha 1-3 fucosyltransferase in adult parasites. Exp Parasitol 1996;82:1.
57. Srivatsan J, Smith DF, Cummings RD. Schistosoma mansoni synthesizes novel biantennary Asn-linked oligosaccharides containing terminal beta-linked N-acetylgalactosamine. Glycobiology 1992;2:445.
58. de Jong EC, Vieira PL, Kalinski P, et al. Microbial compounds selectively induce Th1 cell-promoting or Th2 cell-promoting dendritic cells in vitro with diverse th cell-polarizing signals. J Immunol 2002;168:1704.
59. MacDonald AS, Straw AD, Bauman B, Pearce EJ. CD8-dendritic cell activation status plays an integral role in influencing Th2 response development. J Immunol 2001;167:1982.
60. MacDonald AS, Straw AD, Dalton NM, Pearce EJ. Cutting edge: Th2 response induction by dendritic cells: a role for CD40. J Immunol 2002;168:537.
61. Thomas PG, Carter MR, Atochina O, et al. Maturation of dendritic cell 2 phenotype by a helminth glycan uses a Toll-like receptor 4-dependent mechanism. J Immunol 2003;171:5837.
62. Kaisho T, Hoshino K, Iwabe T, et al. Endotoxin can induce MyD88-deficient dendritic cells to support Th)(2 cell differentiation. Int Immunol 2002;14:695.
63. van Die I, van Vliet SJ, Nyame AK, et al. The dendritic cell-specific C-type lectin DC-SIGN is a receptor for Schistosoma mansoni egg antigens and recognizes the glycan antigen Lewis x. Glycobiology 2003;13:471.

# 10

# Immune and Antiviral Effects of the Synthetic Immunomodulator Murabutide

## *Molecular Basis and Clinical Potential*

### George M. Bahr

## INTRODUCTION

The field of immunomodulation started with the concept of vaccination to protect against infectious diseases, an approach successfully employed by Edward Jenner over 200 years ago. From this initial concept and based on the progress in understanding the functions of the immune system, it became evident that several immune pathways could be regulated, either positively or negatively, to restore the disrupted immune homeostasis in a wide array of human diseases. Today, therapeutic approaches aimed at modulating immune mechanisms extend from interventions in cancer and organ transplantation to reach infectious, autoimmune, immunodeficiency, and neurological diseases.

Early studies have focussed on the use of live, attenuated, or killed microbial organisms to modulate immune responses and to generate protective vaccines. Heat-killed mycobacterial cells suspended in mineral oil, a formulation referred to as Freund complete adjuvant (FCA), was known since 1956 to be the most potent immunoadjuvant for the induction of cell-mediated immunity and antibody formation *(1)*. Later studies clearly demonstrated that the cell wall skeleton fraction was the important adjuvant-active component of the cells of mycobacteria and related bacteria *(2)*. Then, Ellouz and associates in 1974 *(3)* reported that the minimal adjuvant-active subunit of bacterial cell-wall skeleton was $N$-acetylmuramyl-L-alanyl-D-isoglutamine, called muramyl dipeptide (MDP) (Fig. 1). This molecule was synthesized and its biological activities were studied by several laboratories. Besides a classical adjuvant effect and a capacity to replace whole mycobacterial cells in FCA, MDP was found to exert numerous immunomodulatory activities. However, the administration of MDP

From: *Vaccine Adjuvants: Immunological and Clinical Principles*
Edited by: C. J. Hackett and D. A. Harn, Jr. © Humana Press Inc., Totowa, NJ

into different hosts was always associated with serious toxicity that hampered its use in man *(4)*. Therefore, in an effort to generate MDP analogs with reduced toxicity and enhanced biological activities, several hundred derivatives were synthesized by chemical modification of the parent molecule. Evaluation of the activity to toxicity ratio was carried out on most of these derivatives and has led to the selection of few molecules that were projected for clinical development. In this chapter, a brief overview on muramyl peptides (MPs) is presented followed by a detailed analysis of the biological activities, the molecular mechanism of action, and the clinical applications of a selected safe derivative named Murabutide (Fig. 1). Starting from a single biological effect and absence of associated toxicity, we will present the exciting scientific efforts that lead to the identification of various immunomodulatory and antiviral activities of Murabutide. Moreover, the recent clinical data obtained with the use of this synthetic derivative in the field of chronic viral infections suggest that Murabutide could well represent a new generation of nonspecific immunotherapeutics.

## MURAMYL PEPTIDES:
## A FAMILY OF SYNTHETIC MOLECULES
## WITH MULTIPLE BIOLOGICAL ACTIVITIES

*Hydrophilic and Lipophilic Structural Derivatives*

Starting from the parent molecule MDP, few hundred derivatives were produced by chemical synthesis and modification or substitution of the sugar and/or the amino acid moieties. Two major classes of MPs were generated that could be classified into hydrophilic or lipophilic analogs. The hydrophilic derivatives were produced with the aim of reducing the frequently observed MDP toxicities including pyrogenicity, transient leukopenia, sensitization to endotoxin, and induction of arthritis, granuloma, and uveitis *(5,6)*. On the other hand, lipophilic analogs were prepared to reproduce the antitumor activity of bacterial cell walls, which have a high lipid content, and to increase the limited adjuvant activity of MDP when administered as an aqueous solution in vivo, because of its rapid excretion into urine. Detailed analysis of the biological and pharmacological effects of different MPs revealed that certain structural modifications were associated with reduced toxicity and enhanced efficacy whereas others rendered analogs totally inactive *(7–10)*. Moreover, although the biological activities of MDP derivatives were mostly observed following parenteral administration, few analogs presented effects when given by the oral route *(10,11)*. The activities of hydrophilic and lipophilic MPs were also reported to be significantly enhanced by polymerization, conjugation with an appropriate carrier, or incorporation into liposomes *(12,13)*. These approaches are believed to enhance the uptake, by the reticuloendothelial system, and the bioavailability of the

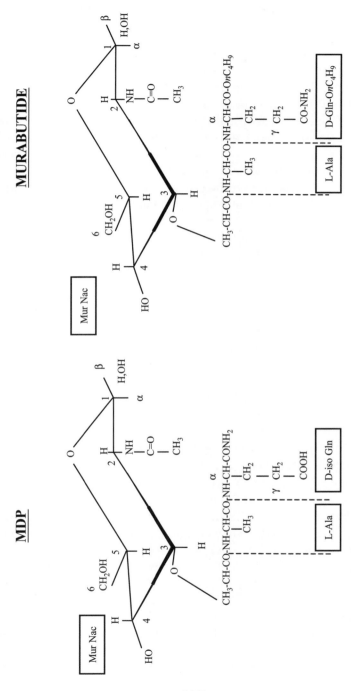

**Fig. 1.** Chemical structure of muramyl dipeptide (MDP) and of Murabutide. Mur Nac, *N*-acetyl-muramyl.

195

immunostimulants. Taken together, the studies which were spread over a period of two decades lead to the selection of few derivatives and the extensive profiling of their immunopharmacological activities. Among the hydrophilic derivatives that eventually reached a clinical stage of development are Murabutide (*N*-acetyl-muramyl-L-alanyl-D-glutaminyl-*N*-butyl ester), Temurtide (threonyl-MDP), Nor-MDP (*N*-acetyl-glucosamin-3-yl-acetyl-L-alanyl-D-isoglutamine), and GMDP (*N*-acetyl-D-glucosaminyl-$\beta$(1-4)-*N*-acetyl-muramyl-L-alanyl-D-isoglutamine). On the other hand, Romurtide (MDP-Lys[18]$N^2$-acetylmuramoyl]-L-alanyl-D-isoglutaminyl-$N^6$-stearoyl-L-Lysine) and MTP-PE (muramyl-tripeptide phosphatidylethanolamine), and Immther (*N*-acetyl-glucosaminyl-*N*-acetylmuramyl-L-alanyl-glyceryl dipalmitate) were the three major lipophilic derivatives to be developed by pharmaceutical industries *(5,8–10)*. Importantly, the biological effects of MPs were found to extend far beyond the initially described adjuvant activity, and to target cells of the immune, hematopoietic, and central nervous system (CNS). The multiple activities of key MPs have been the subject of extensive reviews *(4,5,9,10,14)* and are only summarized in the next section.

## Biological Effects Targeting the Immune System

Synthetic MPs are generally believed to exert direct effects on monocytes/macrophages, granulocytes, and B lymphocytes, but to affect indirectly the functions of T lymphocytes and natural killer cells *(14–16)*. The immunological activities of MDP and several of its derivatives are mediated by multiple effector mechanisms including macrophage activation, regulation of cell-surface receptor expression, and induction of cytokine release *(5,10,15,17)*. These mechanisms translate into different biological activities that have found a potential therapeutic value in different immune-based strategies. For instance, MPs administered in saline together with an antigen result in enhanced antibody responses to the antigen in question, an effect classically known as the adjuvant effect. However, potentiation of cell-mediated immunity by MPs was mostly achieved when the antigen and the adjuvant were administered as a water-in-oil emulsion *(4,14)*. Interestingly, MDP and only few other derivatives were found to exert an adjuvant effect when given orally, even if the antigen was administered by a different route *(18)*. It is relevant to mention that although few MPs have presented adjuvant effects in man *(5,9)*, no commercial vaccine has yet been developed incorporating a MP as the adjuvant-active ingredient.

A second well-studied immunological activity of MPs is their capacity to enhance the host's nonspecific resistance against bacterial, viral, fungal, and parasitic infections. Thus, treatment with MDP or analogs has been shown to enhance resistance in mice to a variety of pathogens, and this activity could be observed in immunocompromised or in malnourished and aged animals *(4)*. By studying several derivatives with defined and selective effects, it has been shown that neither adjuvanticity nor pyrogenicity was a prerequisite for eliciting increased resistance to infections. The mechanisms implicated in this latter activity were further differentiated from those mediating the adjuvant effect by the findings that repeated injections of large doses of MDP, which resulted in inhibiting specific antibody responses and abrogating the adjuvant activity, did not impair the capacity of the molecule to protect against infections. Recently, the MDP-induced resistance to bacterial infections has been linked with its capacity to trigger the secretion of microbicidal α-defensins by intestinal Paneth cells in response to bacteria *(19)*. Moreover, in different models of infection-induced mortality, increased host survival in MP-treated animals was correlated with a better containment of the organisms, restricted dissemination of the infection, efficacious activation of tissue macrophages, and increased cytokine release *(10,13,20,21)*. These effector mechanisms were also found to attribute to MPs the capacity of enhancing non-specific immunity against tumors *(4)*. In this respect, the lipophilic derivative MTP-PE, encapsulated in liposomes, has demonstrated an important potential for cancer therapy and has been evaluated in several clinical studies *(22)*.

Besides the immune potentiating and proinflammatory effects of MPs, selected derivatives were found, when administered by the oral route, to inhibit ongoing, anamnestic, isotype-specific immunoglobin (Ig)E responses *(5)*. This activity was associated with a local effect on Peyer's patches, and with a selective down-regulation of interleukin (IL)-4 expression in gut-associated lymphoid tissues and mesenteric lymph nodes *(23)*. These findings suggest a potential application of immunomodulators of this type in the therapeutic management of IgE-mediated diseases such as allergic rhinitis and asthma. Finally, the potential application of lipophilic muramyl peptides as anti-inflammatory molecules has been provided by the findings that topical application of certain derivatives could suppress ear swelling in mouse models of phorbol ester- and oxazolone-induced ear inflammation. This effect was linked to a selective capacity of inhibiting the release of inflammatory cytokines by activated macrophages *(24)*.

## Biological Effects Targeting the Hematopoietic System

Nearly two decades ago, several MPs including MDP and Murabutide were reported to induce, in vitro and in vivo, the release of factors with colony-stimulating activity. Additionally, increased serum levels of macrophage-colony-stimulating factor (M-CSF), increased proliferation of multipotential stem cells in the bone marrow, and expansion of granulocyte-macrophage progenitors in the spleen were observed following parenteral administration of some adjuvant-active molecules into mice *(25)*. These effects were reproduced by lipophilic glyceryl dipalmitate-MDP (MDP-GDP) derivatives, were associated with analogs presenting either anti-infectious or adjuvant activity, and constituted the basis for the clinical development and eventual marketing of Romurtide. This drug is currently used for the restoration of leukopenia associated with cancer chemotherapy and/or radiotherapy *(26)*, and is believed to induce a battery of cytokines and growth factors that are essential for hematopoiesis and the increase of white blood cells and platelets *(27)*.

Using a mouse model of Azidothymidine (AZT)-induced bone marrow toxicity, the iv administration of MDP or MDP-GDP, before AZT, was found to protect bone marrow cellularity and the numbers of circulating leukocytes and erythrocytes *(28)*. Recently, we have employed a similar model to analyze the ability of a safe, hydrophilic, orally active analog Muradimetide (dimethyl ester of *N*-acetyl-muramyl-L-alanyl-D-glutamic acid) in the protection of AZT-immunocompromised mice against death induced by a challenge with an opportunistic infection namely *Mycobacterium fortuitum*. Besides the reported adjuvant activity and the ability of Muradimetide to enhance resistance against infections in normal mice *(7,8)*, this molecule presented a somewhat unique capacity of restoring the resistance against opportunistic infections in AZT-immunosuppressed mice and resulted in 60 to 100% protection against death. More interestingly, a daily oral administration of Muradimetide with AZT on 4 successive days induced the appearance of immature cells (myelocytes) in the peripheral blood. These stem cells were then observed to differentiate within few days into mature leukocytes, erythrocytes, and platelets (Table 1). This effect could not be observed by the administration of either drug alone, and the co-administration of Muradimetide with the nucleoside analogue totally protected mice against AZT-induced leukopenia and anemia (Table 1). These findings demonstrate the capacity of orally administered Muradimetide with AZT to mobilize stem cells from the bone marrow to peripheral blood, a phenomenon that was verified by observing a similar level of stem cell mobilization in splenectomized mice, and by the identification of cobblestone area forming cells and long-term culture initiating cells among the mobilized myelocyte population (Bahr et al., manuscript in preparation). Awaiting the demonstration of this activity in nonhuman primates, the combination of Muradimetide with AZT, even at low and nontoxic doses, could become the first generation of orally-active drugs to be employed in multiple indications necessitating bone marrow stem cell mobilization. It is of interest to note that among 12 different MPs tested in this model, 10 of them, including Murabutide, MTP-PE, and Romurtide, were totally inactive, and only MDP presented a weak activity, which was far below that observed with Muradimetide. This further emphasizes the structural requirements for a MP to exert a defined biological effect.

**Table 1**
**Effect of Orally Administrated AZT, Muradimetide, or Combination
of the Two Compounds on the Changes in the Number of Circulating
Leukocytes, Red Blood Cells, Platelets, and Immature Stem Cells** [a]

| Cell type studied | Day tested | Muradimetide (50 mg/kg) | AZT (50 mg/kg) | $p$ value [d] | AZT + Muradimetide (50 mg/kg + 50 mg/kg) |
|---|---|---|---|---|---|
| Leukocytes | 0 | $64 \pm 15$ [b] | $68 \pm 16$ | NS | $68 \pm 8$ |
| ($\times 10^5$/mL) | 2 | $68 \pm 10$ | $45 \pm 11$ [c] | $p < 0.05$ | $88 \pm 6$ [c] |
| | 4 | $65 \pm 12$ | $63 \pm 13$ | $p < 0.05$ | $120 \pm 10$ [c] |
| | 7 | $66 \pm 8$ | $66 \pm 14$ | $p < 0.05$ | $84 \pm 10$ [c] |
| | 9 | $68 \pm 12$ | $67 \pm 15$ | NS | $72 \pm 9$ |
| Red blood cells | 0 | $85 \pm 11$ | $91 \pm 5$ | NS | $86 \pm 10$ |
| ($\times 10^8$/mL) | 2 | $89 \pm 18$ | $71 \pm 6$ [c] | $p < 0.05$ | $97 \pm 11$ |
| | 4 | $88 \pm 8$ | $59 \pm 4$ [c] | $p < 0.05$ | $81 \pm 15$ |
| | 7 | $87 \pm 5$ | $71 \pm 2$ [c] | NS | $84 \pm 12$ |
| | 9 | $87 \pm 9$ | $86 \pm 5$ [c] | NS | $84 \pm 8$ |
| Platelets | 0 | $87 \pm 11$ | $84 \pm 6$ | NS | $93 \pm 10$ |
| ($\times 10^7$/mL) | 2 | $88 \pm 8$ | $95 \pm 12$ [c] | $p < 0.05$ | $135 \pm 20$ [c] |
| | 4 | $85 \pm 12$ | $104 \pm 10$ [c] | $p < 0.05$ | $155 \pm 26$ [c] |
| | 7 | $90 \pm 13$ | $106 \pm 18$ [c] | $p < 0.05$ | $155 \pm 28$ [c] |
| | 9 | $89 \pm 11$ | $99 \pm 10$ [c] | $p < 0.05$ | $114 \pm 14$ [c] |
| Immature cells | 0 | $7 \pm 7$ | $5 \pm 4$ | NS | $6 \pm 7$ |
| ($\times 10^4$/mL) | 2 | $5 \pm 5$ | $4 \pm 7$ | $p < 0.05$ | $166 \pm 41$ [c] |
| | 4 | $8 \pm 4$ | $3 \pm 5$ | $p < 0.05$ | $27 \pm 27$ [c] |
| | 7 | $9 \pm 6$ | $9 \pm 9$ | $p < 0.05$ | $70 \pm 25$ [c] |
| | 9 | $8 \pm 7$ | $5 \pm 6$ | NS | $12 \pm 13$ |

NS, not statistically significant; AZT, azidothymidine.

[a] Groups of female BALB/C mice (five per group) were administered orally the indicated doses of the compounds, once a day and on 4 consecutive days (day 0–3). Different blood cell types were enumerated before treatment (day 0) and up to 9 days after the start of treatment. Leukocytes, platelets, and red blood cells were counted using Unopette kits from Beckton Dickinson. Differential counts were performed on smear preparations stained with May-Grunwald/Giemsa to enable the morphological identification of immature cells of the promyelocyte, myelocyte, and neutophilic metamyelocyte populations.

[b] Mean ± standard deviation.

[c] Significantly different from the corresponding values on day 0 before treatment (Wilcoxon matched-pairs test).

[d] Mann-Whitney U Rank test.

# BASIS FOR THE SELECTION OF MURABUTIDE: SAFETY AND ADJUVANT ACTIVITY

Following the synthesis of hundreds of MDP analogs, Murabutide was selected on the basis that it was water soluble, apyrogenic, and adjuvant active *(29)*. The immunomodulator was then subjected to a series of in vivo testing comparing its pharmacological, inflammatory, and toxic effects with those of the parent molecule MDP (Table 2). It was striking to observe that whereas the minimal pyrogenic dose of MDP could be defined at 30 μg/kg body weight, doses of Murabutide up to 10 mg/kg did not induce detectable elevation in rabbit body temperature. Similarly, injection of high doses of Murabutide into rabbits did not result in the release of endogenous pyrogen transferable in the serum. Furthermore, and in contrast to MDP, the administration of Murabutide into different hosts did not lead to the modification of plasma metal levels, increased prostaglandins in the brain, appearance of transient leukopenia, or enhancement of slow wave sleep (Table 2). It is of interest to note that the absence of Murabutide effects on the CNS, as judged by its apyrogenicity and lack of induction of slow wave sleep, were confirmed not only after iv administration, but also when the molecule was given by the intracerebroventricular route. On the other hand, administration of Murabutide into experimental animals did not increase the levels of serum amyloid A protein, and did not cause acute joint inflammation, edematous swelling of paws, vascular leakage, or uveitis *(6,30–34)*. All these inflammatory reactions were repeatedly observed with MDP and several other structural derivatives. Similarly, the toxic effects classically reported with MDP and other bacterial cell wall components such as distress syndrome in guinea pigs, autoimmune thyroiditis in the mouse, adjuvant polyarthritis in mice and rats, and toxic synergism with lipopolysaccharide (LPS) were all absent with Murabutide *(29, 35–37)*. Taken together, these studies clearly established the safety of Murabutide, the absence of undesirable effects on the CNS, and the lack of induction of inflammatory responses.

Regarding the adjuvant activity of Murabutide, it was clearly evident that this synthetic glycopeptide was able to present, when administered parenterally but not orally, adjuvant effects that were identical to those detected with the parent molecule MDP *(29)*. Enhancement of antibody responses to natural or to synthetic antigens could be reproducibly observed, in different animal species, when the antigen was administered mixed with Murabutide *(29,38)*. Moreover, the titers of total antibodies produced in the presence of Murabutide were equivalent to those detected using alum hydroxide as adjuvant. However, the levels of allergy-associated IgE antibodies were significantly lower in Murabutide-vaccinated animals *(38)*. Interestingly, the combination of alum-containing vaccine with Murabutide was found to induce higher titers of antibodies than the vaccine alone. Moreover, cell-mediated immunity against the antigenic component could be detected more efficiently in the Murabutide-supplemented vaccine recipients. Using synthetic hepatitis B antigen conjugated to a toxoid carrier and comparing the adjuvanticity of Murabutide, alum hydroxide, and FCA, it was revealed that high titered antibodies against the synthetic antigen could

**Table 2**
**Differences in Pharmacologic, Inflammatory, and Toxic Effects
Between MDP and Murabutide**

| Activity studied | Host tested | Route administered | Effect of compound studied MDP | Murabutide | Ref. |
|---|---|---|---|---|---|
| Pyrogenicity | Rabbit | IV | ++ | – | 29 |
| | | icv | +++ | – | 29 |
| Induction of transferable endogenous pyrogen | Rabbit | IV | ++ | – | 29 |
| Decrease in plasma iron levels | Rabbit | IV | ++ | – | 30 |
| Decrease in plasma copper level | Rabbit | IV | ++ | – | 30 |
| Increased prostaglandins in brain | Rat | IV | ++ | – | 30 |
| Induction of slow wave sleep | Rabbit | IV | ++ | – | 31 |
| | | ICV | +++ | – | 31 |
| Transient leukopenia | Rabbit | IV | ++ | – | 29 |
| Induction of serum amyloid A protein | Mouse | IP | ++ | – | 32 |
| Induction of acute joint inflammation | Mouse | IV | ++ | – | 33 |
| Induction of edematous swelling of paws | Rats | PO | ++ | – | 34 |
| | | SC | ++ | – | 34 |
| Induction of uveitis | Rabbit | IV | 11 | – | 6 |
| Induction of vascular leakage | Rabbit | IV | ++ | – | 6 |
| Induction of distress syndrome | Guinea pig | IV | ++ | – | 35 |
| Induction of auto immune thyroiditis | Mouse | IP | ++ | – | 36 |
| Induction of adjuvant polyarthritis | Mouse | IV | ++ | – | 37 |
| | Rat | IV | ++ | – | 37 |
| Toxic synergism with endotoxin | Mouse | IV | ++ | – | 29 |
| | Guinea pig | IV | ++ | – | 29 |

MDP, Muramyl dipeptide; IV, intravenous; ICV, intracerebroventricular; IP, intraperitoneal; SC, subcutaneous; PO, per os.

be generated with any of the three adjuvants. However, the use of Murabutide resulted in modulating the antibody specificity allowing a better recognition of the natural hepatitis antigen *(39)*. Based on these experimental studies and on a safe toxicological profile, Murabutide was evaluated as adjuvant to a natural streptococcal M protein vaccine in adults *(40)*, and to a weakly immunogenic, fluid-phase tetanus toxoid vaccine in children *(41)*. The ability of Murabutide to enhance the immunogenicity of vaccines could be demonstrated in both studies, although the optimal Murabutide dosage to include in vaccine preparation is yet to be determined. It is worthwhile to mention that single or repeated administrations of Murabutide, either alone or in combination with antigens, did not elicit detectable antibodies against its own structure. Thus, Murabutide is totally nonimmunogenic, and this evidently presents advantages for its use in the same subject on repeated occasions.

## TARGET CELLS, RECEPTORS, AND SIGNALING EVENTS

Similar to most other MPs, Murabutide has been known to regulate the functions of different cell types. Using highly purified cell populations or cell lines, Murabutide was found to interact directly with blood monocytes, tissue macrophages, astrocytes, dendritic cells, polymorphonuclear neutrophils, B lymphocytes, and endothelial cells *(5,15,42,43)*. However, the identification of receptors for this molecule has not yet been resolved. Cell-surface, intracellular, and nuclear receptors have been claimed for MPs, and conflicting data were frequently reported. For instance, although one study suggested that the major LPS receptor CD14 is involved in the recognition of MPs, another demonstrated that MDP was not recognized by CD14 *(42)*. On the other hand, recent developments in the identification of Toll-like receptors (TLRs) recognizing different bacterial cell wall components *(44)* suggested that TLR2, the peptidoglycan receptor in macrophages, may also be the receptor for MPs. However, using cell lines transfected with CD14 and TLR2 or CD14 and TLR4 (the receptor for LPS), no signal transduction by any of these receptors could be put into evidence following stimulation with MDP or with Murabutide *(42)*. These studies, and others reported from different laboratories *(45)*, indicate that MPs exhibit their activities in a CD14-, TLR2-, and TLR4-independent manner. Nevertheless, taking into consideration that there are already 10 different known TLRs *(44)*, it is reasonable to suggest that one of these receptors may potentially be implicated in Murabutide signaling. Moreover, the potential presence of multiple receptors capable of interacting with MPs cannot be ruled out in view of the large spectrum of biological effects induced by these molecules in different cell populations. It remains a challenging question for future studies to clone the receptor(s) of Murabutide, and to explain how minor modification of the molecule can render the derivative with extended, with restricted, or with no biological activity.

Another research area in the MP field that has been quite neglected is the understanding of the signaling events mediating the biological readout. Recently, an effort was made to analyze the profile of signaling molecules that are rapidly activated in antigen-presenting cells (APCs) following stimulation with Murabutide *(42,43)*. Using monocyte-derived macrophages in vitro, phosphorylation of the extracellular signal-regulated kinases 1 and 2 was noted as early as 20 minutes after stimulation with the synthetic immunomodulator. In contrast, other kinases including p38 mitogen-activated protein kinase and the Jun-N-terminal kinases 1 and 2 remained without detectable activation over a 3-hour testing period *(42)*. The profile of kinase activation by Murabutide was also different from that observed in LPS-treated macrophages in which all the tested kinases were found to become phosphorylated within 20 to 30 minutes. It was of interest to note the absence of p38 mitogen-activated protein kinase activation by Murabutide because this specific kinase has been highly implicated in the initiation of inflammatory responses. In contrast, when kinase activation was tested in Murabutide-treated monocyte-derived immature dendritic cells, the three classes of kinases were found to be rapidly phosphorylated *(43)*. This suggests that either the same Murabutide-specific receptor could induce different signaling events in different cell types or that the immunomodulator interacts with different receptors that are specific for each cell population. Future studies aimed at cloning and identifying the Murabutide receptor will help to explain these issues. On the other hand, besides the important role of kinases in the signaling events, different transcription factors and adaptor molecules are known to be key mediators in this process. Among these factors, the signal transducers and activators of transcription (STATs) were found to play a primordial role in transducing signals delivered by different exogenous or endogenous immunomodulators. In general, three members of the STAT family of molecules, namely STAT 1, STAT 3, and STAT 5, have been mostly implicated in macrophage signaling events, and the activation of these factors have been recently analyzed following stimulation with Murabutide. In contrast to LPS signaling, which highly activates the three STATs under study, Murabutide induced a potent activation of STAT 1, a weak activation of STAT 3, and no detectable activation of STAT 5 *(42)*. Additionally, whereas AP-1 and C/EBP-β were equally activated by Murabutide and by LPS, only a weak and transient activation of NF-κB was evident in Murabutide-stimulated macrophages. Once again, these studies reveal a selective activation of transcription factors by this synthetic immunomodulator, and the absence or weak activation of factors that are highly implicated in mediating inflammatory reactions. This could explain, in part, the good clinical tolerance of Murabutide and the lack of associated toxicities that have been frequently observed with inflammatory compounds such as MDP and LPS.

## IMMUNE-MEDIATED EFFECTS OF MURABUTIDE:
## A SPECTRUM OF IMMUNOMODULATORY ACTIVITIES

Extensive studies have characterized the responses of monocytes/macrophages to stimulation with Murabutide, and the consensus is that the immunomodulator, in vitro, induces the release of a battery of proinflammatory cytokines, which are identical to those induced by other MPs, including the toxic molecule MDP *(5)*. However, the administration of Murabutide into experimental animals or into healthy volunteers was associated with the release of anti-inflammatory cytokines and G-CSF without detectable levels of IL-1, IL-8, or TNF-$\alpha$ *(5)*. This paradox between the in vitro and the in vivo effects still awaits resolution or explanation. Because of this and in the interest of understanding relevant biological functions, we will focus the presentation of the immune-mediated effects of Murabutide to those that have been observed in vivo. As stated above, the initial and most frequently studied activity of Murabutide has been its adjuvant effect. However, this safe adjuvant was also found, in different bacterial or viral infection models, to present an important capacity of enhancing host's resistance against microbial infections, even in newborn or in splenectomized mice *(13,29)*. This was not surprising considering the fact that Murabutide could reproducibly activate macrophages and neutrophils to release several classes of antimicrobial mediators. Similarly, a limited capacity to enhance nonspecific resistance against tumors has also been reported for this molecule *(12)*. On the other hand, because Murabutide was found to induce the release of CSFs and other cytokines implicated in hematopoiesis, the administration of this compound into mice was closely associated with induced differentiation and proliferation of bone marrow progenitor cells *(25)*.

In addition to the above mentioned immune-mediated effects of Murabutide, two additional activities need to be emphasized in view of the fact that one is not shared with many other adjuvant-active derivatives, and the second is the only known activity of Murabutide to be exerted following oral administration. In contrast to MDP or to many other active MPs, Murabutide has demonstrated anti-inflammatory effects in different mouse models. For instance, the administration of Murabutide into galactosamine-sensitized and LPS-challenged mice resulted in a significant protection against lethality induced by the inflammatory endotoxic shock *(5)*. Similarly, in a model of acute hepatitis induced by the administration of the mitogen concanavalin-A, prophylactic or therapeutic treatment of mice with Murabutide resulted in 40 to 65% inhibition of the elevation in serum transaminases levels. This activity correlated with inhibition, in the liver, of the expression of the interferon (IFN)$\gamma$, responsible for the mitogen-induced hepatotoxicity *(46)*. Under a completely different set-up and using a model to analyze the regulation of IgE production, it was demonstrated that the administration of Murabutide by gavage, but not parenterally, resulted in an isotype-specific suppression of IgE synthesis as evaluated by measuring either IgE serum levels or the number of IgE antibody-forming cells in the spleen and gut-associated lymphoid tissues *(47)*. This potential anti-allergic activity is the only known effect of Murabutide to be manifested following oral administration of the compound. An overall presentation of the immune-mediated effects of Murabutide and the corresponding mechanism of action are shown in Table 3.

## SYNERGISTIC EFFECTS BETWEEN MURABUTIDE AND SELECTED THERAPEUTIC CYTOKINES

Many in vitro studies have analyzed the potential synergistic effects between a cytokine and a MP with the aim of potentiating the tumoricidal activity of macrophages. Moreover, it was hoped that such costimulatory signals could also induce a better activation of B lymphocytes, and a selective increase in the release of protective cytokines under defined conditions *(5)*. Similar studies were performed with Murabutide in which stimulation of human blood with IFNα and the immunomodulator resulted in selective upregulation of anti-inflammatory cytokines *(5)*. On the other hand, when human peripheral blood mononuclear cells (PBMCs) were costimulated with IL-2 and Murabutide, a different set of cytokines appeared to be synergistically induced comprising T-helper 1 cytokines (IFNγ and IL-12) and CSFs *(48)*. These studies, paved the way for the evaluation, in vivo, of whether a combination therapy between Murabutide and a cytokine could potentiate the therapeutic efficacy of the latter. Thus, using the meth A fibrosarcoma tumor model, it was demonstrated that treatment of tumor-bearing mice with Murabutide and IFNα or with Murabutide and IL-2 result in synergistic potentiation of the antitumor activity of either cytokine *(47,48)*. The combination therapy over a period of 2 weeks resulted in 60 to 70% of tumor-free mice, an effect which could not be achieved even by 10-fold higher doses of either Murabutide or the cytokine separately. Moreover, the anti-inflammatory and antiviral activities of IFNα in different mouse models were found to be significantly potentiated when the cytokine was administered with Murabutide *(46,49)*. On the other hand, using the inflammatory model of endotoxic shock in galactosamine-sensitized mice, the prophylactic co-administration of Murabutide with IFNα attributed new biological effects to the cytokine resulting in 70% protection against mortality. In this model, the use of the cytokine alone presented no efficacy whatsoever *(5)*. Taken together, these studies strongly suggested that the combination of a safe exogenous immunomodulator with a therapeutic cytokine could present several advantages in the management of difficult diseases in which the existing treatment is far from being satisfactory. Moreover, it was evident that such a combination therapy might allow the reduction of the cytokine dosage needed to achieve a therapeutic effect, thereby reducing the toxicity which is frequently associated with high-dose

**Table 3**
**Immune-Medicated Effects of Murabutide, In Vivo, and the Proven or Probable Mechanism of Activity**

| Activity observed | Route of administration | Target cells or tissues | Proven or probable mechanism of action |
|---|---|---|---|
| Adjuvant effect | IV, IP, SC | Macrophages/dendritic cells/ B lymphocytes | Release of cytokines with adjuvant activity<br>Enhanced antigen-presentation to T-helper lymphocytes<br>Enhanced B-cell differentiation and Ig secretion |
| Enhancement of nonspecific resistance against infections | IV, IP | Macrophages/neutrophils/ NK cells | Release of cytokines with anti-infectious activity<br>Containment of infection within restricted sites<br>Enhanced phagocytosis and release of antimicrobial mediators<br>Enhanced NK cell activity |
| Enhancement of nonspecific resistance against tumors | IV, IP | Macrophages/dendritic cells/ NK cells | Enhanced macrophage tumoricidal activity and cytokine release<br>Enhanced dendritic cells tumorostatic activity and cytokine release<br>Enhanced NK cell cytotoxicity |
| Hematopoietic effect | IV, IP | Endothelical cells/macrophages/ bone marrow/stromal cells | Release of colony-stimulating factors and other cytokines affecting hematopoiesis |
| Anti-inflammatory effect | IV, IP | Hepatocytes/macrophages | Downregulation of inflammatory cytokines in tissues<br>Downregulation of multiple cellular factors implicated in inflammation |
| Anti-allergic effect | PO | Peyer's patches/mesenteric lymph nodes | Downregulation of IL-4 expression leading to suppression of IgE synthesis |

IV, intravenous; IP, intraperitoneal; SC, subcutaneous; PO, per os; NK, natural killer; Ig, immunoglobulin; IL-4, interleukin-4.

administration of cytokines. Based on these preclinical models, the safety and efficacy of the co-administration of Murabutide and IFNα in man has been evaluated and will be described in the section titled Use of Murabutide in the Treatment of Chronic Hepatitis C.

## MURABUTIDE-MEDIATED SUPPRESSION OF HIV-1 REPLICATION

In the last few years, the use of highly-active antiretroviral therapy (HAART) for the management of human immunodeficiency virus (HIV)-1 infection has led to substantial advances in the control of viral replication. However, this therapeutic strategy is now believed to be insufficient for eliminating the pool of latently infected cells and for bringing about normalization of immune functions. Therefore, immune-based strategies are being sought to correct the considerable dysfunction caused by HIV infection in cells implicated in innate and acquired immunity. One such strategy involves the use of nonspecific immunomodulators to restore the capacity of APCs in orchestrating an efficacious and protective response against the virus. Based on the ability of Murabutide to regulate the function of cells of the innate immune system, we have evaluated its effects on HIV-infected macrophages and dendritic cells. Surprisingly, stimulation of acutely infected cells with Murabutide lead to a dramatic inhibition of viral replication and to the release of HIV-suppressive β-chemokines. However, the two phenomena were not directly linked because neutralization of the released chemokines by polyclonal antibodies had no measurable effect on the observed viral inhibition *(50)*. On the other hand, experiments aimed at defining the steps in the virus life cycle that are blocked or inhibited by Murabutide revealed that the immunomodulator significantly interfered with the nuclear transport of viral pre-integration complexes and with virus transcription. These effects did not target the virus directly but appeared to correlate with the regulation of different cellular factors needed at critical steps of the viral replication process. These factors will be presented and discussed in the following section on the molecular basis of Murabutide activity.

Recently we have addressed the question of whether stimulation of infected cells with Murabutide could potentiate the efficacy of antiretrovirals (ARVs). Thus, macrophages were infected with the macrophage-tropic HIV-1 Bal, and were then cultured for 2 weeks in the absence or presence of Murabutide (1 μg/mL) and various concentrations ($0.1-10^3$ n$M$) of the protease inhibitor saquinavir. The dose of Murabutide used was verified to be ineffective on its own in inducing a significant inhibition of HIV replication. Supernatants were collected at the end of the culture period and were assessed for the levels of virus reverse transcriptase *(50)*. The concentration of Saquinavir needed to exert 50, 70, or 90% inhibition of HIV replication, when used alone or in association

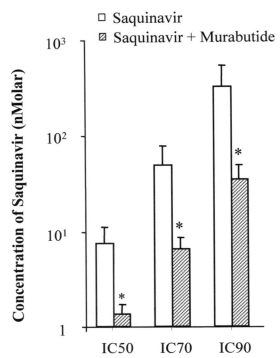

**Fig. 2.** Murabutide potentiates human immunodeficiency virus (HIV) suppression by the protease inhibitor Saquinavir. Monocyte-derived macrophages from seven separate donors were infected with HIV-1 Bal and were cultured in the absence or presence of various concentrations of Saquinavir or/and 1 μg/mL of Murabutide. Supernatants were collected 14 days postinfection and were evaluated for virus reverse transcriptase activity. The inhibitory concentration (IC) of Saquinavir necessary for inducing 50, 70, or 90% virus suppression was calculated from constructed curves. Bars represent the mean ± standard error of the mean from seven independent experiments. The asterisks indicate statistically significant reduction ($p < 0.05$ by Wilcoxon matched-pairs test) in the ICs of Saquinavir when used in combination with Murabutide. The use of 1 μg/mL of Murabutide, on its own, did not induce any significant inhibition (<10%) of viral replication.

with Murabutide, was calculated following construction of standard curves. Results from seven independent experiments shown in Fig. 2 clearly demonstrate that the combination of Murabutide with the protease inhibitor significantly enhanced the efficacy of the ARV drug. This was evident by the fact that the concentrations of Saquinavir needed to induce 50, 70, or even 90% virus suppression (IC50, IC70, or IC90) were dramatically reduced in cultures costimulated with Murabutide. Similar results were also observed when the immunomodulator was combined with the reverse transcriptase inhibitor AZT.

These encouraging results on HIV suppression by Murabutide in APCs led us to investigate the activity of this immunomodulator in endogenously infected lymphocytes obtained from HIV-1 patients. Thus, following depletion of CD8 cells and activation of the remaining PBMCs (mostly CD4 lymphocytes) with phytohemagglutinins to induce viral replication, cells were cultured in the presence of IL-2 and without or with Murabutide. These studies, which were recently published *(51)*, demonstrated a highly potent capacity of Murabutide to induce HIV suppression, and this effect was equally evident in cells harboring macrophage-tropic, dual-tropic, or T-tropic virus strains. Additionally, the immunomodulator presented a similar capacity to inhibit HIV replication in lymphocytes originating from asymptomatic, symptomatic, or acquired immune deficiency syndrome patients. The antiviral activity of Murabutide targeted HIV transcription and correlated with the regulation of the expression of cellular factors. More importantly, Murabutide also exhibited a capacity to suppress viral loads in severe combined immunodeficiency mice repopulated with human PBMCs and infected with HIV-1 *(51)*. Taken together, these studies provide the evidence on the capacity of Murabutide to regulate the expression of multiple cellular factors thereby rendering infected cells nonpermissive for viral replication. This strategy of targeting host cells may prove to be complementary to the use of ARVs and could lead to highly efficient, long-term control of the virus.

## MOLECULAR BASIS OF THE IMMUNE AND ANTIVIRAL EFFECTS OF MURABUTIDE

The progress achieved in technologies aimed at profiling changes in gene expression has allowed us to address, at the molecular level, the mechanisms implicated in the Murabutide-induced cell activation process. Because macrophage have been reproducibly observed as the major target cells mediating several of the immunomodulatory effects of Murabutide, we first analyzed the profile of regulated genes in this cell population following a 6-hour stimulation with Murabutide. Employing microarrays technology to evaluate changes in the expression of 1081 genes, stimulation with Murabutide induced or enhanced the expression of 40 genes, and inhibited that of 16 others *(52)*. The Murabutide-regulated genes belonged to different families of immune mediators or their receptors, transcription factors and kinases, matrix proteins and their inhibitors, ion channels and transporters, and proteins involved in cell metabolic pathways. In addition to the upregulation of cytokines and chemokines which may contribute to the adjuvant activity of Murabutide, the microarray analysis revealed a strong induction of heat shock protein 70, a factor known to be endowed with potent adjuvant effect. Furthermore, the identification of several other genes that were regulated by Murabutide has considerably contributed to the understanding of some of the described biological effects of this immunomodulator *(52)*. More interesting was the identification of two sets of Murabutide-upregulated genes that had never been reported in previous studies. One set included transcripts encoding proteins involved in bone formation such as insulin-like growth factor-binding protein 5 and bone morphogenetic protein 8. The second cluster consisted of genes involved in functions of the nervous system, including *ninj-1* and the neural cell adhesion molecule L1, and could potentially be of relevance to the mechanisms leading to nerve regeneration *(52)*. This approach has clearly shed light on the mode of action of Murabutide and also suggested new therapeutic indications for this compound. Future efforts to determine the potential application of Murabutide in these new areas could carry the field of immunomodulation far beyond the current conception.

To understand the molecular events mediating the described activity of Murabutide in HIV-infected lymphocytes, we opted for the technology of differential display-reverse transcription-polymerase chain reaction (DD-RT-PCR) to identify genes that are implicated in the virus-suppressive effects of the immunomodulator *(53)*. This approach has the advantage of identifying regulated genes with known and with unknown sequences or/and functions. The DD-RT-PCR analysis has revealed the upregulation of 15 known genes and the downregulation of another 8 in Murabutide-treated CD8 depleted lymphocytes from HIV-1-infected subject. As shown in Table 4, the Murabutide-regulated genes in this cell type were totally different from those identified in macrophages *(52)*, and clustered into genes implicated in signal transduction, transcription, splicing, translation, protein translocation, and proteolysis. Additionally, six partial complementary deoxyribonucleic acid (cDNA) sequences with unmatched sequence identity in the data banks were found to be induced by Murabutide whereas four others were observed to be inhibited. We then undertook the task of full-length cloning two of the four unknown and inhibited genes by Murabutide. The first one, named *SS56*, turned out to be a new member of the Sjogren syndrome family of autoantigens and was found to be a target of autoantibody responses in patients with Sjogren syndrome and systemic lupus erythematosus *(53)*. The second Murabutide-inhibited gene was named *RH116* and it revealed to be a new member of the DExH family of ribonucleic acid (RNA) helicases. Recently, *RH116* has been shown to play a major role in driving HIV-1 replication *(54)*. Bringing together the collected information so far on the Murabutide-regulated genes in HIV-infected cells, one can define 2 sets of cellular factors that could potentially mediate the virus-suppressive effects of the compound (Table 5). Thus, Murabutide is able, on one hand, to enhance the expression of factors that are known to down-regulate HIV replication and, on the other hand, to inhibit other factors used by the virus for cell entry, nuclear translocation, and transcription.

**Table 4**
**List of Known Genes Regulated by Murabutide in CD8-depleted PBMCs From HIV-1-Infected Subject**

| Murabutide-induced genes | Function | Murabutide-inhibited genes | Function |
|---|---|---|---|
| Transcription elongation factor B | Transcription elongation | Replication factor C large subunit | DNA Replication |
| SLAM-associated protein | Signal transduction | RNA polymerase II transcription cofactor 4 | Transcription coactivator |
| Formin-binding protein 21 | Splicing | | |
| Spliceosomal-associated protein 155 | Splicing | Eurokaryotic initiation factor p66 | Initiation of Translation |
| SRp25 nuclear protein | Splicing | Raf | Signal transduction |
| Ribosomal protein S17 | Translation | Calcium-activated neutral protease | Proteolysis |
| Ribosomal protein S23 | Translation | Proteasome subunit Z | Proteolysis |
| Ribosomal protein L26 | Translation | ATPase subunit 6 | ATPase |
| Translocation protein-1 | Protein translocation | | |
| Nascent-polypeptide-associated complex | | | |
| Alpha polypeptide | Protein translocation | | |
| Cell differentiation cycle 2 | Cell cycle regulation | | |
| BRCA1-associated RING protein | Tumor suppression | | |
| Guanylate-binding protein isoform II | GTPase activity | | |
| Stromal derived-factor 2 | Chemotaxis | | |

PBMCs, peripheral blood mononuclear cells; HIV-1, human immunodeficiency virus type 1.

**Table 5**
**Murabutide-Regulated Cellular Factors, Identified by Different Gene Expression Assays, With Potential Implication in Mediating the HIV-Suppressive Activity of the Immunomodulator**

| Target cell studied | Identified cellular factor | Known function | Regulated expression by Murabutide | Established role in HIV replication |
|---|---|---|---|---|
| T lymphocyte | c-Myc | Oncogene | Inhibited | Essential for nuclear transport of viral preintegration complexes |
| | RH116 | RNA Helicase | Inhibited | Increase HIV transcription |
| | RNA pol II | Transcription factor | Inhibited | Increase RNA polymerase II-dependent virus transcription |
| | Cofactor | | | |
| Macrophages | MIP-Iβ | Chemokine | Enhanced | Inhibition of cell binding and entry of macrophage-tropic HIV |
| | α-1 acid glycoprotein | Acute phase protein | Enhanced | Binding to HIV envelop protein and inhibiting virus entry |
| | P100 NFκB | Transcription factor | Enhanced | Inhibition of tat-transactivation of HIV long terminal repeat |
| | CCR5 | Chemokine receptor | Inhibited | Coreceptor for cell entry of macrophage-tropic HIV strains |
| | CXCR4 | Chemokine receptor | Inhibited | Coreceptor for cell entry of T-tropic HIV strains |
| | NF90 | Nuclear receptor | Inhibited | Increase viral replication at post-transcriptional level |

HIV, human immunodeficiency virus.

## CLINICAL DEVELOPMENT OF MURABUTIDE

Following the selection of Murabutide on the basis of its safe pharmacological profile and its adjuvant activity in different animal models, the molecule was subjected to acute, subacute and chronic toxicity studies in two or three animal species. These studies, and mutagenicity and embryo/fetal toxicity analyses, revealed the absolute safety of Murabutide at doses which are 10- to 100-fold the expected human dose (0.1–0.2 mg/kg body weight). The immunomodulator then received investigational new drug approval in the 80s and was aimed to be used as adjuvant in vaccines. Based on results obtained in few clinical studies *(40,41)*, which did not meet the high expectations of finding a more efficacious alternative to the only approved adjuvant (alum hydroxide) in man, the development of Murabutide as vaccine adjuvant was halted.

### Use of Murabutide in the Treatment of Chronic Hepatitis C

The clinical development of Murabutide took a different route after the discovery of its synergistic effects with human therapeutic cytokines. Because Murabutide was found to improve the efficacy of IFNα in different inflammatory, tumor, and viral models *(5,46,48,49)*, phase I and IIa studies were initiated in healthy volunteers to determine the safety and surrogate markers of activity of the simultaneous administration of Murabutide with human IFNα. Three studies were performed, using different dosages of Murabutide and of IFNα, which solidly established the absence of synergistic or even additive toxicity between the two molecules *(5,55)*. In contrast, these two immunomodulators, when co-administered simultaneously, were found to exhibit synergistic induction of the anti-inflammatory cytokine IL-1 receptor antagonist and of the HIV-suppressive chemokine macrophage inflammatory protein (MIP)-1β. Serum levels achieving 70 ng/mL of the former cytokine and 1.2 ng/mL of the latter one were detected in volunteers administered simultaneously 0.1 mg/kg Murabutide and 6 MU IFNα *(55)*. These trials have established the safety and markers of synergy between Murabutide and IFNα, and allowed the evaluation of the two drugs in patients with chronic hepatitis C virus (HCV) infection. Recently, two phase I studies were performed in HCV patients who had been nonresponders to prior treatment with IFNα and ribavirin. A Murabutide dosage of 0.1 mg/kg and 3 MU of IFNα, administered subcutaneously three times a week and for a period of 12 weeks, were found to produce no prohibiting toxicity. In contrast, serious grade IV toxicity was noted when the frequency of administration of Murabutide was increased to 5 consecutive days per week. The evaluation of Murabutide as a component of triple therapy, together with pegylated IFNα and ribavirin, is currently undergoing in two separate studies targeting HCV-infected patients naïve to treatment and HIV/HCV co-infected patients who failed to respond to prior treatment with classical IFNα and ribavirin. The results of these trials will soon determine the future development of Murabutide in the management of patients with HCV.

## Use of Murabutide in the Treatment of HIV-1 Infection

The ability of Murabutide to regulate the functions of APCs, together with its capacity to inhibit HIV-1 replication in different cell populations, have prompted its evaluation in the management of HIV disease. The aim of this development is not to place the immunomodulator in competition with potent ARVs but, on the contrary, to introduce a non-specific immune-based therapy as adjunct to HAART. It is hoped that the co-administration of Murabutide will help in correcting deficits in innate immunity, in restoring immune homeostasis, and in providing additional control of viral replication. Recently, the results of two phase I/IIa studies employing single and repeated administrations of Murabutide in 30 HIV-1 patients under HAART, have been published *(56)*. These studies clearly indicated the excellent clinical tolerance of Murabutide in HIV patients, and have provided further evidence on the capacity of Murabutide to induce the release of HIV-suppressive β-chemokines without any detrimental effect on viral loads and CD4 counts. A third study in 18 HIV-1-infected individuals, naïve to ARV therapy, addressed the safety and the biological effects of a 6-week cycle of immunotherapy with Murabutide, administered for 5 consecutive days per week and at a dosage of 7 mg (generally corresponding to 0.1 mg/kg). This clinical trial provided a clear cut evidence on the safety of long-term administration of Murabutide in patients who are not receiving any ARV therapy and, more importantly, on the efficacy of nonspecific immunotherapy to potentiate immune responses including those directed against the virus *(57)*. Additional trials addressing the efficacy of the combination of Murabutide immunotherapy with HAART are currently ongoing. Finally, the future development of Murabutide together with IFNα or with IL-2, as novel immunotherapeutic approaches in the management of HIV infection, are being seriously envisaged.

## CONCLUSIONS AND FUTURE PROSPECTS

Among several hundreds of MP derivatives, Murabutide presented a highly safe toxicological profile accompanied with desirable immunomodulatory effects. Although the initial activities of the molecule had targeted the adjuvant field or the nonspecific enhancement of resistance against infections, its development under these indications has been hampered by limited efficacy and a lack of understanding of its mechanism of action. A revived interest in this molecule came about following an extensive scientific program demonstrating its synergistic activity with human therapeutic cytokines, and the capacity to induce selective cell activation leading to HIV suppression. Moreover, recent studies aimed at profiling the molecular mechanism of action of Murabutide revealed the immunomodulatory nature of the molecule and its ability to regulate multiple cellular factors, thereby giving a credible explanation for some of the observed biological effects. These studies also projected several potential and new therapeutic indications for Murabutide. Today, this synthetic immunomodulator is being developed within the context of nonspecific immune-based therapies and targeting chronic viral diseases. Its use as a component of triple therapy for hepatitis C, together with pegylated IFNα and ribavirin, may soon provide the proof of concept that correction of defective and nonspecific elements of the immune system is a critical factor in achieving efficacious treatment. Furthermore, ongoing clinical studies in HIV patients may further substantiate the need for nonspecific immunotherapy, together with HAART, to restore immune homeostasis and protective responses against the virus. Nevertheless, future fundamental research should address the identification of the receptor(s) of Murabutide, the dissection of signal transduction pathways, and the development of experimental models to evaluate the potential therapeutic effects of Murabutide in conditions necessitating rapid bone formation and nerve regeneration. Finally, based on the reported T-helper 1-inducing and anti-tumor activities of Murabutide when associated with IFNα or with IL-2, it will be a high priority to undertake the clinical evaluation of such combination therapies in certain cancer indications. These could easily include melanoma and renal cell carcinoma in which the use of the cytokine alone had shown very limited and unsatisfying therapeutic value.

## REFERENCES

1. Freund J. The mode of action of immunologic adjuvants. Adv Tuberc Res 1956;7: 130–148.
2. Azuma I, Kishimoto S, Yamamura Y, Petit J-F. Adjuvanticity of mycobacterial cell wall. Jpn J Microbiol 1971;15:193–197.
3. Ellouz F, Adam A, Ciorbaru R, Lederer E. Minimal structural requirements for adjuvant activity of bacterial peptidoglycan derivatives. Biochem Biophys Res Commun 1974;59:1317–1325.
4. Lederer E. Natural and synthetic immunomodulators derived from the mycobacterial cell wall. In: Bizzini B, Bonmassar E, eds. Advances in Immunomodulation. Roma: Pythagora Press, 1988, pp. 9–36.
5. Bahr GM, Darcissac E, Bevec D, Dukor P, Chedid L. Immunopharmacological activities and clinical development of muramyl peptides with particular emphasis on murabutide. Int J Immunopharmacol 1995;17:117–131.
6. Waters RV, Terrell TG, Jones GH. Uveitis induction in the rabbit by muramyl dipeptides. Infect Immun 1986;51:816–825.
7. Chedid L, Audibert F, Lefrancier P, Choay J, Lederer E. Modulation of the immune response by a synthetic adjuvant and analogs. Proc Natl Acad Sci USA 1976;73: 2472–2475.

8. Lefrancier P, Derrien M, Jamet X, et al. Apyrogenic, adjuvant-active N-acetyl-muramyl-dipeptides. J Med Chem 1982;25:87–90.
9. Werner GH, Jolles P. Immunostimulating agents: what next? A review of their present and potential medical applications. Eur J Biochem 1996;242:1–19.
10. Azuma I, Otani T. Potentiation of host defense mechanism against infection by a cytokine inducer, an acyl-MDP derivative, MDP-Lys(L18) (romurtide) in mice and humans. Med Res Rev 1994;14:401–414.
11. Chedid L, Parant M, Parant F, Lefrancher P, Choay J, Lederer E. Enhancement of nonspecific immunity to *Klebsiella pneumoniae* infection by a synthetic immuno-adjuvant (N-acetylmuramyl-L-alanyl-D-isoglutamine) and several analogs. Proc Natl Acad Sci USA 1977;74:2089–2093.
12. Phillips NC, Chedid L. Muramyl peptides and liposomes. In: Gregoriadis GE, ed. Liposomes as Drug Carriers. Chichester: John Wiley and Sons Ltd, 1988, pp. 243–259.
13. Parant M. Muramyl peptides as enhancers of host resistance to bacterial infections. In: Majde JA, ed. Immunopharmacology of Infectious Diseases: Vaccine Adjuvants and Modulators of Non-Specific Resistance. New-York: Alan R. Liss, Inc., 1987, pp. 235–244.
14. Parant M, Chedid L. Muramyl dipeptides. In: Bray MA, Morley J, eds. Handbook of Experimental Pharmacology, vol. 85. Berlin: Springer-Verlag, 1988, pp. 503–516.
15. Bahr GM, Chedid L. Immunological activities of muramyl peptides. Fed Proc 1986; 45:2541–2544.
16. Souvannavong V, Brown S, Adam A. The synthetic immunomodulator muramyl dipeptide (MDP) can stimulate activated B cells. Mol Immunol 1988;25:385–391.
17. Heinzelmann M, Mercer-Jones MA, Gardner SA, Wilson MA, Polk HC. Bacterial cell wall products increase monocyte HLA-DR and ICAM-1 without affecting lymphocyte CD18 expression. Cell Immunol 1997;176:127–134.
18. Warren HS, Chedid LA. Future prospects for vaccine adjuvants. Crit Rev Immunol 1988;8:83–101.
19. Ayabe T, Satchell DP, Wilson CL, Parks WC, Selsted ME, Ouellette AJ. Secretion of microbicidal alpha-defensins by intestinal Paneth cells in response to bacteria. Nat Immunol 2000;1:113–118.
20. Polk HC Jr, Lamont PM, Galland RB. Containment as a mechanism of nonspecific enhancement of defenses against bacterial infection. Infect Immun 1990;58: 1807–1811.
21. O'Reilly T, Zak O. Enhancement of the effectiveness of antimicrobial therapy by muramyl peptide immunomodulators. Clin Infect Dis 1992;14:1100–1109.
22. Asano T, Kleinerman ES. Liposome-encapsulated MTP-PE: a novel biologic agent for cancer therapy. J Immunother 1993;14:286–292.
23. Kricek F, Zunic M, Ruf C, De Jong G, Dukor P, Bahr GM. Suppression of in vivo IgE and tissue IL-4 mRNA induction by SDZ 280.636, a synthetic muramyl dipeptide derivative. Immunopharmacology 1997;36:27–39.
24. Zunic M, Bahr GM, Mudde GC, Meingassner JG, Lam C. MDP(Lysyl)GDP, a nontoxic muramyl dipeptide derivative, inhibits cytokine production by activated macrophages and protects mice from phorbol ester- and oxazolone-induced inflammation. J Invest Dermatol 1998;111:77–82.

25. Galelli A, Chedid L. Modulation of myelopoiesis in vivo by synthetic adjuvant-active muramyl peptides: induction of colony-stimulating activity and stimulation of stem cell proliferation. Infect Immun 1983;42:1081–1085.
26. Azuma I. Development of the cytokine inducer romurtide: experimental studies and clinical application. Trends Pharmacol Sci 1992;13:425–428.
27. Namba K, Nitanai H, Otani T, Azuma I. Romurtide, a synthetic muramyl dipeptide derivative, accelerates peripheral platelet recovery in nonhuman primate chemotherapy model. Vaccine 1996;14:1322–1326.
28. Phillips NC, Tsoukas C, Chedid L. Abrogation of azidothymidine-induced bone marrow toxicity by free and liposomal muramyl dipeptide. In: Masihi KN, Lange W, eds. Immunotherapeutic Prospects of Infectious Diseases. Berlin: Springer-Verlag, 1990, pp. 135–139.
29. Chedid LA, Parant MA, Audibert FM, et al. Biological activity of a new synthetic muramyl peptide adjuvant devoid of pyrogenicity. Infect Immun 1982;35:417–424.
30. Riveau GJ, Chedid L. Comparison of the immuno- and neuropharmacological activities of MDP and murabutide. In: Majde JA, ed. Immunopharmacology of Infectious Diseases: Vaccine Adjuvants and Modulators of Non-Specific Resistance. New-York: Alan R Liss, Inc, 1987, pp. 213–222.
31. Krueger JM, Walter J, Karnovsky ML, et al. Muramyl peptides. Variation of somnogenic activity with structure. J Exp Med 1984;159:68–76.
32. McAdam KP, Foss NT, Garcia C, et al. Amyloidosis and the serum amyloid A protein response to muramyl dipeptide analogs and different mycobacterial species. Infect Immun 1983;39:1147–1154.
33. Koga T, Kakimoto K, Hirofuji T, Kotani S, Sumiyoshi A, Saisho K. Muramyl dipeptide induces acute joint inflammation in the mouse. Microbiol Immunol 1986;30:717–723.
34. Zidek Z. Differences in proinflammatory activity of several immunomodulatory derivatives of muramyl dipeptide (MDP) with special reference to the mechanism of the MDP effects. Agents Actions 1992;36:136–145.
35. Byars NE. Two adjuvant-active muramyl dipeptide analogs induce differential production of lymphocyte-activating factor and a factor causing distress in guinea pigs. Infect Immun 1984;44:344–350.
36. Kong YC, Audibert F, Giraldo AA, Rose NR, Chedid L. Effects of natural or synthetic microbial adjuvants on induction of autoimmune thyroiditis. Infect Immun 1985;49:40–45.
37. Chang YH, Pearson CM, Chedid L. Adjuvant polyarthritis. V. Induction by N-acetylmuramyl-L-alanyl-D- isoglutamine, the smallest peptide subunit of bacterial peptidoglycan. J Exp Med 1981;153:1021–1026.
38. Audibert FM, Przewlocki G, Leclerc CD, et al. Enhancement by murabutide of the immune response to natural and synthetic hepatitis B surface antigens. Infect Immun 1984;45:261–266.
39. Przewlocki G, Audibert F, Jolivet M, Chedid L, Kent SB, Neurath AR. Production of antibodies recognizing a hepatitis B virus (HBV) surface antigen by administration of murabutide associated to a synthetic pre-S HBV peptide conjugated to a toxoid carrier. Biochem Biophys Res Commun 1986;140:557–564.

*Bahr*

40. Olberling F, Morin A, Duclos B, Lang JM, Berchey EH, Chedid L. Enhancement of antibody response to a natural fragment of streptococcal M protein by Murabutide administered to healthy volunteers. Int J Immunol 1983;7:398.
41. Telzak E, Wolff SM, Dinarello CA, et al. Clinical evaluation of the immunoadjuvant murabutide, a derivative of MDP, administered with a tetanus toxoid vaccine. J Infect Dis 1986;153:628–633.
42. Vidal VF, Casteran N, Riendeau CJ, et al. Macrophage stimulation with Murabutide, an HIV-suppressive muramyl peptide derivative, selectively activates extracellular signal-regulated kinases 1 and 2, C/EBP-β and STAT1: role of CD14 and Toll- like receptors 2 and 4. Eur J Immunol 2001;31:1962–1971.
43. Vidal V, Dewulf J, Bahr GM. Enhanced maturation and functional capacity of monocyte-derived immature dendritic cells by the synthetic immunomodulator Murabutide. Immunology 2001;103:479–487.
44. Medzhitov R. Toll-like receptors and innate immunity. Nature Rev Immunol 2001; 1:135–145.
45. Yang S, Tamai R, Akashi S, et al. Synergistic effect of muramyldipeptide with lipopolysaccharide or lipoteichoic acid to induce inflammatory cytokines in human monocytic cells in culture. Infect Immun 2001;69:2045–2053.
46. Bahr GM, Pouillart PR, Chedid LA. Enhancement in vivo of the antiinflammatory and antitumor activities of type I interferon by association with the synthetic immunomodulator murabutide. J Interferon Cytokine Res 1996;16:297–306.
47. Auci DL, Carucci JA, Chice SM, Smith MC, Dukor P, Durkin HG. Control of IgE responses. 4. Isotype-specific suppression of peak BPO- specific IgE antibody-forming cell responses and of BPO-specific IgE in serum by muramyldipeptide or murabutide after administration to mice by gavage. Int Arch Allergy Immunol 1993; 101:167–176.
48. Bahr GM, Darcissac E, Pouillart PR, Chedid LA. Synergistic effects between recombinant interleukin-2 and the synthetic immunomodulator murabutide: selective enhancement of cytokine release and potentiation of antitumor activity. J Interferon Cytokine Res 1996;16:169–178.
49. Pouillart PR, Audibert FM, Chedid LA, Lefrancier PL, Bahr GM. Enhancement by muramyl peptides of the protective response of interferon-alpha/beta against encephalomyocarditis virus infection. Int J Immunopharmacol 1996;18:183–192.
50. Darcissac EC, Truong MJ, Dewulf J, Mouton Y, Capron A, Bahr GM. The synthetic immunomodulator murabutide controls human immunodeficiency virus type 1 replication at multiple levels in macrophages and dendritic cells. J Virol 2000; 74:7794–7802.
51. Bahr GM, Darcissac EC, Casteran N, et al. Selective regulation of human immunodeficiency virus-infected CD4+ lymphocytes by a synthetic immunomodulator leads to potent virus suppression in vitro and in hu-PBL-SCID mice. J Virol 2001;75: 6941–6952.
52. Goasduff T, Darcissac ECA, Vidal V, Capron A, Bahr GM. The transcriptional response of human macrophages to murabutide reflects a spectrum of biological effects for the synthetic immunomodulator. Clin Exp Immunol 2002;128:474–482.
53. Billaut-Mulot O, Cocude C, Kolesnitchenko V, et al. SS-56, a novel cellular target of autoantibody responses in Sjogren syndrome and systemic lupus erythematosus. J Clin Invest 2001;108:861–869.

54. Cocude C, Truong MJ, Billaut-Mulot O, et al. A novel cellular RNA helicase, RH116, differentially regulates cell growth, programmed cell death and human immunodeficiency virus type 1 replication. J Virol 2003;84:3215–3225.
55. Darcissac EC, Vidal V, Guillaume M, Thebault JJ, Bahr GM. Clinical tolerance and profile of cytokine induction in healthy volunteers following the simultaneous administration of ifn-alpha and the synthetic immunomodulator murabutide. J Interferon Cytokine Res 2001;21:655–661.
56. Amiel C, de la Tribonniere X, Vidal V, Darcissac E, Mouton Y, Bahr GM. Clinical tolerance and immunologic effects after single or repeated administrations of the synthetic immunomodulator Murabutide in HIV-1-Infected Patients. JAIDS 2002;30:294–305.
57. De la Tribonniere X, Mouton Y, Vidal V, et al. A phase I study of a six-week cycle of immunotherapy with Murabutide in HIV-1 patients naive to antiretrovirals. Med Sci Monit 2003;9:143–150.

# 11
# Effects of QS-21 on Innate and Adaptive Immune Responses

## Charlotte Read Kensil, Gui Liu, Christine Anderson, and James Storey

## INTRODUCTION

Immunological adjuvants typically fall within two classifications: (a) "vehicle" adjuvants that transport antigen from injection sites to lymphoid tissues (generally particulate adjuvants such as emulsions, liposomes, or mineral salts) and (b) "immunomodulators" that act on antigen-presenting cells (APCs) or other cells to induce a cytokine response that influences the immune response to a co-adminstered antigen *(1)*. Most immunomodulators are derived from bacterial sources *(2)*. These include lipopolysaccharides and derivatives such as lipid A or unmethylated deoxyribonucleic acid (DNA) or oligonucleotide sequences, such as CpG enriched sequences from bacteria. However, natural products from other sources can also act as immunomodulators. One such product is the plant saponin QS-21.

### Source

QS-21 is a purified natural product derived from the bark of *Quillaja saponaria* Molina, a tree native to Chile and Argentina. QS-21 is from the class of compounds known as "saponins," plant glycosides in which an oligosaccharide or oligosaccharides are linked to an aglycone consisting of a triterpene or steroid *(3)*. Saponins from the bark of *Quillaja* are triterpene glycosides. Saponins constitute up to 10% of the bark of this tree *(3)*.

*Quillaja* saponins have been long known to have significant adjuvant activity *(4,5)*. There are estimated to be close to 50 unique saponins from *Quillaja* saponaria *(6)*. Most have the same triterpene base, quillaic acid, and are acylated 3,28 bisdesmonosides (with oligosaccharide linked to the 3- and 28-carbons of quillaic acid). Differences between unique saponins are primarily found in the glycosylation pattern or acylation pattern. These structural differences affect their biological activity, for example adjuvant function, effects on cell membranes,

From: *Vaccine Adjuvants: Immunological and Clinical Principles*
Edited by: C. J. Hackett and D. A. Harn, Jr. © Humana Press Inc., Totowa, NJ

and toxicity. QS-21 was noted to have strong adjuvant activity compared to other saponins, but with minimal toxicity *(7)*. This saponin was purified by reversed-phase high performance liquid chromatography and has been extensively evaluated as a vaccine adjuvant in both preclinical and clinical studies.

## QS-21 ADJUVANT EFFECTS

### Influence of QS-21 on Adaptive Immune Responses

Studies in various species show significant effect on various measures of adaptive immunity. This includes humoral and cell-mediated immune responses.

QS-21 has been shown to have a strong adjuvant effect for antibody responses with a number of different antigens in preclinical and clinical studies. Additionally, QS-21 also stimulates cell-mediated immune responses, including CD8+ cytotoxic T-cell (CTL) responses in animal and clinical studies.

*Humoral Immune Response*

QS-21 has been shown to potentiate strong antibody responses to various antigens *(8–13)* in animal studies. The minimum effective dose is typically 5 to 10 µg in mice *(8)*. Surprisingly, not much more QS-21 is required for adjuvant responses in human clinical studies. Addition of a dose of 100 µg QS-21 to human immunodeficiency virus (HIV)-1 gp120 *(14)*, a malaria simplified by removing "NANP" peptide *(15)*, and to GM2-KLH *(16,17)* resulted in improved antibody responses in clinical studies. The adjuvant effect of QS-21 on antibody is sometimes more notable when low-dose antigen is used. The use of QS-21 reduced the minimum immunogenic dose of formalin-inactivated influenza virus vaccine in mice by a factor of approx 100 compared to a nonadjuvanted vaccine (assessed as virus-specific serum EIA titers) *(18)*. In a human clinical study of an experimental HIV-1 vaccine in healthy uninfected volunteers, QS-21 enabled the use of a 100-fold reduced gp120 antigen dose to yield comparable neutralizing antibody titers to an aluminum-hydroxide adjuvanted vaccine *(14)*.

The use of QS-21 in experimental vaccines in mice typically results in both strong immunoglobin (Ig)G1 and IgG2a responses *(7–9,19,20)*. The stimulation of IgG2a responses suggests that QS-21 stimulates T-helper (Th)1 cytokines, in contrast to the response provoked by standard adjuvants such as aluminum hydroxide, which is primarily limited to IgG1 response (associated with a Th2 cytokine pattern). However, it has been noted that QS-21 may produce a mixed Th1/Th2 cytokine response. Both IgG1 and IgG2a responses are elevated by QS-21. In a clinical evaluation of a QS-21 adjuvanted melanoma vaccine (GM2-KLH), the GM2-specific antibody consisted of IgM and IgG; the IgG subclasses consisted primarily of IgG1 and particularly, IgG3 *(17)*. In contrast, immunization of breast cancer patients with globo H-KLH resulted primarily in IgG1 responses with a few patients also generating IgG2, IgG3, and IgG4 responses *(21)*. Hence, there is no clear pattern of subclass response in humans receiving QS-21 adjuvanted vaccines.

In addition to standard parenteral routes of immunization, QS-21 has also been used successfully in intranasal immunization with HIV envelope DNA *(11)*, and oral administration with tetanus toxoid in mice *(19)*. Figure 1 shows the use of QS-21 in an intranasal flu vaccine in mice. An intranasal vaccine comprised of a trivalent flu vaccine was ineffective in raising a systemic antibody response when compared to the same vaccine administered by subcutaneous route. When QS-21 was added to the intranasal vaccine, serum IgG1 and IgG2a antibody titers were substantially improved although not to the same extent as the subcutaneously administered vaccine with or without QS-21. However, the use of intranasal flu vaccine with QS-21 was critical for the observation of a secretory IgA response (determined in nasal wash). The action of QS-21 to aid intranasal immunization has not been elucidated. One potential mechanism is that it aids the delivery of macromolecules by acting as a permeation enhancer. QS-21 and derivatives enable the delivery of insulin through the ocular or intranasal route *(22,23)*. A deacylated form of QS-21 (DS-1) was shown to reduce the tightness of a CACO-2 monolayer (measured as transepithelial electric resistance) *(24)* and was associated with both enhanced mannitol and decapeptide transport across the monolayers. Analysis using a fluorescent probe suggested that DS-1 primarily aided transcellular transport. The effect of QS-21 on the tightness of epithelial barriers was not measured. However, in studies of efficacy of enhancing nasal transport of insulin, QS-21 was shown to be more effective than DS-1, suggesting that it might also reduce the tightness of epithelial barriers *(23)*.

In oral immunization studies with QS-21 and tetanus toxoid, it was noted that interleukin (IL)-4 appeared to be critical for secretory IgA responses in fecal and vaginal washes *(19)*. Interestingly, it was noted that the stimulation of Th1- and Th2-type immune responses was strongly dependent on adjuvant dose when the vaccine was given orally. Low doses of QS-21 (50 µg) led to Th2-type responses (IgG1, IgA, IgE, IL-4, IL-5, IL-6, and IL-10 cytokines) whereas higher doses of QS-21 (>100 µg) led to Th1-type responses (IgG2a, interferon [IFN]$\gamma$, IL-2 cytokines) *(19)*. In contrast, the threshold QS-21 dose required for stimulation of IgG1 and IgG2a responses to a subcutaneous ovalbumin vaccine in C57BL/6 mice is apparently equivalent (approx 5–10 µg) *(8)*. QS-21 has not yet been used by either intranasal or oral route in clinical studies.

*Cellular Immune Response*

The generation of cytotoxic T lymphocytes (CD8[+]) typically requires the expression of endogenous antigen so that the antigen can enter the cytosol and associate with class I MHC. Subunit antigens, in absence of adjuvant, are "exog-

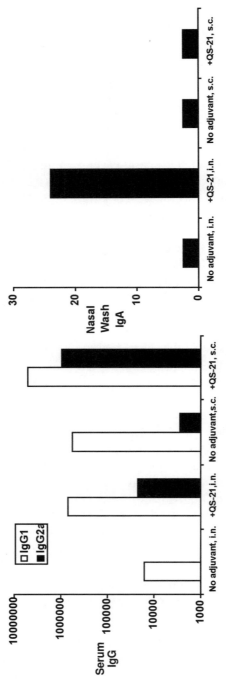

**Fig. 1.** Intranasal immunization of mice with trivalent flu vaccine. Balb/c mice (female, 8 weeks of age, 5 per group) were immunized with a commercial trivalent influenza vaccine ('97/'98 formulation) by either subcutaneous or intranasal route with or without 10 μg QS-21. Each dose contained 0.45 μg hemagglutinin of each of three flu strains (A/Johannesburg/82/96 (H1N1), A/Nanchang/933/95 (H3N2), and B/Harbin/7/94) in a volume of 0.2 mL for subcutaneous immunizations or 10 μL for intranasal immunizations. Immunizations were given on days 0, 14, and 28. Sera and nasal washes collected on day 42 were evaluated for IgG or IgA responses against the immunogen by EIA.

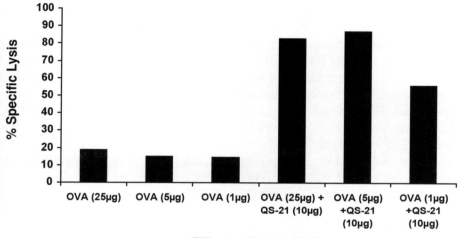

**Effector:Target Ratio**

**Fig. 2.** Generation of CTL responses to ovalbumin as a function of antigen dose. C57BL/6 mice (female, 8 weeks of age, five per group) were immunized twice by the subcutaneous route at 2-week intervals with a vaccine consisting of 1, 5, or 25 µg ovalbumin with or without 10 µg QS-21. At 2 weeks postimmunization, splenocytes (a pool from each group) were used for determination of cytotoxic T-lymphocyte killing of E.G7-OVA. Splenocytes were stimulated for 6 days with irradiated E.G7-OVA and then used as effector cells in a standard $^{51}$Cr-release assay against E.G7-OVA target cells. The background lysis of EL4 cells was subtracted to determine specific lysis. The percentage of specific lysis at a 3:1 effector:target ratio is shown.

enous" antigens that typically do not enter the class I antigen processing/presentation pathway *(25)*. However, certain strategies can be utilized to alter the pathway for exogenous antigens, including the use of liposomal formulations or the use of particulate antigen. QS-21 also enables exogenous antigen to be presented by the class I pathway. It stimulates CTL responses to subunit vaccines in mice. Examples include ovalbumin *(26)*, HIV gp120 *(27)*, RSV fusion protein *(10)*, and soluble, mutant RAS protein *(28)*. Figure 2 shows the CTL response induced by two immunizations of C57BL/6 mice with ovalbumin with or without QS-21 at various antigen doses; the CTL response is stronger with a 1 µg ovalbumin (OVA) vaccine with QS-21 than to a nonadjuvanted vaccine containing 25 µg OVA.

There are fewer examples of CD8[+] CTL responses from human clinical studies, but some recent studies have shown that QS-21 adjuvanted vaccines can stimulate CD8[+] CTL responses. CTL responses were observed to a QS-21 adjuvanted HIV lipopeptide vaccine evaluated in volunteers in France although responses were also observed in volunteers receiving a nonadjuvanted vaccine *(29)*. This was measured by a classic bulk CTL assay based on $^{51}$Cr release. QS-21 was shown to contribute to sustained CD4$^+$ T-cell responses in a followup of the same study *(30)*. Enzyme-linked immunospot (ELISPOT) assays enabled a more sensitive measurement of human CD8$^+$ T-cell responses in a melanoma vaccine study. Tyrosinase peptide adjuvanted with QS-21 was shown to induce peptide-specific CD8$^+$ cells (measured by IFN$\gamma$ ELISPOT) *(31)*. A further study of melanoma peptides compared adjuvant formulations. A melanoma vaccine consisting of tyrosinase and gp100 peptides and QS-21 was shown to induce tyrosinase-specific CD8$^+$ responses in approximately half of the volunteers; this was higher than for a group receiving peptide in incomplete Freund's adjuvant and equivalent to a group receiving GM-CSF *(32)*.

## Influence of QS-21 on Innate Immune Response

Many immunomodulators are now known to influence the innate immune response. The innate immune system is the body's first defense against pathogens. The host recognizes pathogen-associated molecular patterns (PAMP) via various receptors (termed pathogen recognition receptor [PRR]) on exposure to a pathogen *(33)*. The PAMPs are distinct from the host and activate various host defense pathways. Various immunomodulators are recognized by the host as PAMPs. For example, dendritic cells are activated via interaction of the Toll-like receptors (TLR)4 or TLR9 with LPS or CpG, respectively *(2)*. This activation can lead to secretion of antimicrobial cytokines and subsequent priming of T- and B-cell responses.

Does QS-21 mimic a PAMP? It is now known to stimulate innate immune responses. It stimulates the secretion of cytokines tumor necrosis factor-$\alpha$ and IL-6 from murine macrophages in in vitro culture *(34)*. It is also a stimulator of natural killer cell activity *(34)*. Administration of mice with a single dose of QS-21, in absence of adjuvant, appears to protect mice from a subsequent challenge with *Listeria monocytogenes* 3 days later (Fig. 3). These are suggestive of QS-21 stimulation of innate immune responses. However, a specific PRR for QS-21 has not been identified. It is not likely to be TLR4 because QS-21 was shown to be a strong adjuvant for a *Borrelia burgdorferi* subunit vaccine in LPS hyporesponsive mice, which have a defect in TLR4 (C3H/Hej) *(35)*. The search for a receptor for QS-21 is complicated by the physicochemical nature of this molecule. It is amphipathic and associates with cell membranes. In fact, saponins from *Quillaja* are often used to permeabilize cholesterol-containing cell membranes for flow cytometry staining of intracellular membrane antigens *(36)*. Hence, the question remains regarding whether there is a specific receptor for QS-21 or whether QS-21 interaction with immune cells is mediated entirely through nonspecific membrane permeabilization.

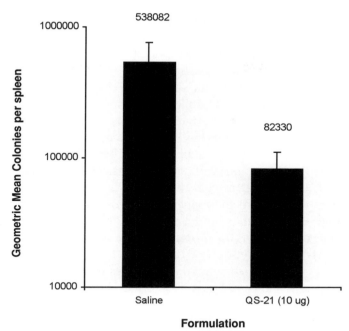

**Fig. 3.** QS-21 protects against *Listeria monocytogenes* in a model of innate immunity. QS-21 (10 µg) or saline was administered by subcutaneous route to Balb/c mice (10 per group) on day 1. On day 4, the mice received an intraperitoneal administration of $10^5$ CFU *Listeria monocytogenes*. On day 7, the *Listeria* burden in the spleens of the mice was determined. The QS-21 group was shown to be significantly different from the saline group by the Mann-Whitney U test ($p < 0.05$).

## MECHANISMS

### Structure/Function Studies

The chemical structure of QS-21 was established by carbohydrate linkage analysis *(7)*, fast atom bombardment mass spectroscopy *(37)*, $^1$H-NMR, and $^{13}$C-NMR methods *(38)*. As mentioned in the introduction, QS-21 is an acylated triterpene glycoside. The triterpene quillaic acid is heavily glycosylated at its carbon 3 and carbon 28. QS-21 has two distinctive structure features compared to other natural nonquillaja saponins. One of them is an aldehyde group on the triterpene moiety and the other one is a glycosylated acyl domain. The acyl domain of QS-21 can be easily removed under mild alkaline hydrolysis. The predominant site of acylation was shown to be the 4-hydroxyl of the fucose although an intramolecular acyl migration between the hydroxyls on C3 and C4 of the fucose occurs in aqueous solution. This acyl migration does not appear to affect adjuvant activity *(39)*.

The triterpene aldehyde group of QS-21 is critical to its adjuvant activity for antibody and CTL responses *(37)*. Modifications at the aldehyde group severely diminish the adjuvant effect associated with QS-21 (the highest dose tested was 40 µg). One possible mechanism involving the aldehyde might be the formation of an Schiff base with a free amino group on a cellular target to stabilize a cellular interaction. Stabilization of interaction of MHC class II⁺ APCs and Th cells via Schiff base interaction between free amino groups on APCs and aldehyde on the T cells has been noted as a possible mechanism for adjuvant function *(40)*. However, a direct Schiff base stabilized interaction of QS-21 with a particular immune cell population has not yet been demonstrated. It should be noted that QS-21 is highly effective adjuvant with hydrophilic polysaccharides that do not have amino groups, suggesting that the formation of a saponin–antigen complex may not be essential for strong immune responses.

A broad dose range study (0 to 240 µg) in mice showed that the acyl domain is critical to Th1-type responses (IgG2a and CTL), but less critical to Th2 type responses (IgG1) *(41)*. The structure of two analogs prepared to assess the effect of the acyl domain is shown in Fig. 4. DS-1 (deacylated QS-21) can stimulate a similar maximum IgG1 response as an optimal dose of QS-21 (10 µg) although the minimum dose of DS-1 required is several fold higher. However, DS-1 does not induce IgG2a and CTL responses to co-administered antigens at DS-1 doses up to 240 µg. The acyl domain itself was also evaluated as an adjuvant at doses that covered the adjuvant-effective range of QS-21 to determine if the adjuvant activity of QS-21 resided entirely or mostly within the fatty acid domain. The results showed that the fatty acid domain of QS-21 was inactive as an adjuvant for both humoral and cell-mediated immune responses.

Reacylation of DS-1 (deacylated QS-21) with a fatty acid at a different site, the glucuronic acid carboxyl group, cannot restore the diminished adjuvant activity associated with QS-21 *(41)*. A QS-21 analogue known as RDS-1 (DS-1, which was reacylated at the glucuronic acid carboxyl group with dodecylamine) does not produce CTL responses to OVA even at doses above 200 µg. RDS-1 showed some stimulation of IgG2a responses, but only at doses above 200 µg. These results suggest that the acylation site of QS-21 is critical to QS-21 adjuvant activity. Interestingly, the migration of QS-21 acyl domain between the 4-hydroxyl and the 3-hydroxyl of the fucose apparently does not affect the adjuvant activity of QS-21 although it could not be ruled out that the activity was because of a single isomer formed through re-equilibration in vivo *(39)*.

QS-21 is anionic at neutral pH because of a glucuronic acid carboxyl group. This anionic moiety may not play a critical role in the adjuvant activity of QS-21. Analogs in which the glucuronic acid carboxyl group was conjugated to ethylamine, ethylenediamine, or glycine through an amide bond (creating neutral, cationic, and anionic analogues at physiologic pH, respectively) retained

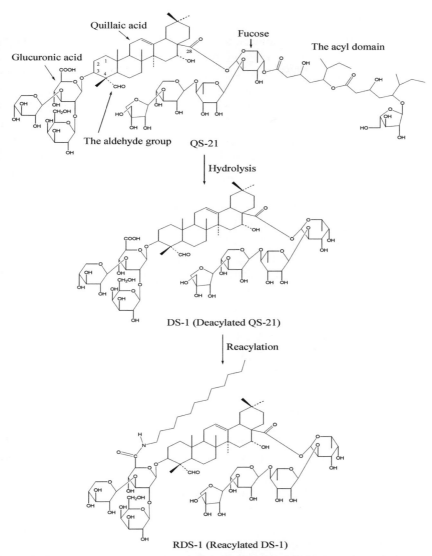

**Fig. 4.** Structure of QS-21 and preparation of QS-21 analogs. DS-1 (deacylated QS-21) and RDS-1 (deacylated QS-21 reacylated at the glucuronic acid carboxyl via conjugation to dodecylamine) were prepared from QS-21.

adjuvant activity for antibody and CTL responses to OVA. However, the threshold dose for modified derivatives was shifted two- to sixfold higher than for native QS-21, suggesting that the modification may have sterically interfered with a critical site *(37)*.

## Accessory Cell Studies

APCs, particularly macrophages, are essential for inducing CTL responses to viruses, soluble protein, and protein associated with cellular membranes. Other types of APC, particularly dendritic cells (DCs), are also capable of processing and presenting some antigens to CD8[+] T lymphocytes, however, their ability to replace macrophages in vivo has not been proven. When QS-21 adjuvant was included in immunizations with alum-absorbed OVA, in vivo and in vitro depletion studies of macrophages indicated how significant these accessory cells are for induction of CD8[+] CTL *(42)*. C57BL/6 mice were given 1 mg of silica or 1 mg of carrageenan-λ daily by the intraperitoneal route starting 2 days before the first immunization with alum-absorbed OVA plus QS-21 to immobilize macrophages. A third group of mice were treated by a similar regimen; however, these mice were given GK1.5 rat monoclonal antibody to deplete mice of CD4[+] T lymphocytes. Control mice received sterile saline only. Although these treatments did not significantly deplete total mononuclear cells in the silica and carrageenan-λ treated mice, there was depletion in the anti-CD4-treated mice of primarily CD4[+] cells. When precursor CTLs were induced to mature into functional effector CTLs by culture with mitomycin-C-treated E.G7-OVA expressing target cells, CD4[+] depletion had no effect on CTL activity. However, mice treated with either silica or carrageenan-λ were equivalent to genetically CD8[+]-deficient mice that did not receive any treatments *(42)*. This data suggests that phagocytic APC, most likely macrophages, are essential for the in vivo induction of CD8[+] CTL responses whereas CD4[+] T lymphocytes (assessed in mice depleted by antibody treatment or genetic manipulation) are not required. Although this issue is somewhat controversial, CD8[+] T lymphocytes can produce many of the same cytokines that are typically produced by CD4[+] T-lymphocytes so there may be sufficient help to induce maturation of precursor CTL.

When antigen-specific proliferative and antibody responses were evaluated in these immunized/treated mice, depletion of CD4[+] T lymphocytes significantly reduced the proliferative response to denatured OVA and mitomycin-C-treated E.G7-OVA cells. Serum analysis by enzyme-linked immunoabsorbent assay (ELISA) for total IgG antibody to OVA was totally abrogated in the CD4-depleted mice. This demonstrates the differential helper T-lymphocyte requirements for antibody and CTL responses.

Because in vivo treatment of mice probably blocks the primary induction of CTL, the role of APC in vitro on induction of precursor CTL to mature was evaluated. Splenocytes from mice that were immunized with alum-absorbed OVA plus QS-21 were cultured with denatured OVA to induce maturation of precursor CTL. Metrizamide gradient-based depletion of macrophages or dendritic cells revealed that only macrophage-depletion but not DC-depletion, affected specific lysis of E.G7-OVA target cells to background levels. Because DC are not phagocytic, they would not have been affected by the in vivo treatments with silica or carrageenan-λ. Although this activity could be restored with splenic mononuclear cells obtained from immunized mice with or without QS-21 adjuvant in the formulation, it suggests that QS-21 can increase the function of APC in processing and presentation of protein antigens to CD8$^+$ T lymphocytes. This difference in APC function was further revealed when different OVA antigens were used to induce precursor CTL maturation. Soluble OVA requires the presence of macrophages to induce maturation of CTL; however, neither E.G7-OVA cells or OVA$_{258-276}$ synthetic peptide require macrophages. Because these findings are similar to what has been reported using virus to induce CTL responses, QS-21 adjuvant may be useful as a tool to evaluate the cellular components involved in the induction of CD8$^+$ CTL to various antigens.

## SUMMARY

Saponins affect both innate and adaptive immunity. Certain structural features have been identified as important for the activity, including the acyl domain and the aldehyde residue on the triterpene. Additionally, QS-21 is membrane-active suggesting that nonspecific membrane interactions may be involved in the mechanism. However, there remain many unanswered questions about the mechanism of action of QS-21 and other saponin adjuvants. For example, a specific pattern recognition receptor has not been identified. Further studies focusing both on identification of specific and nonspecific interactions of QS-21 with immune cells will be required to elucidate the mechanism of action of this important class of adjuvants.

## REFERENCES

1. Allison AC. The mode of action of immunological adjuvants. In: Brown F, Haaheim LR, eds. Modulation of the Immune Response to Vaccine Antigens. Basel: Karger, 1998; 3–11.
2. Bendelac A, Medzhitov R. Adjuvants of immunity: harnessing innate immunity to promote adaptive immunity. J Exp Med 2002;195:F19–F23.
3. Hostettman K, Marston A. Saponins. Cambridge: Cambridge University Press, 1995.
4. Espinet RG. Nouveau vaccin antiaphteux a complexe glucoviral. Gac vet (B Aires) 1951;13:268–273.
5. Dalsgaard K. Isolation of a substance from *Quillaja saponaria* Molina with adjuvant activity in foot-and-mouth disease vaccines. Arch Gesamte Virusforsch 1974; 44:243–254.
6. van Setten DC, van de Werken G, Zomer G, Kersten GFA. Glycosyl compositions and structural characteristics of the potential immuno-adjuvant active saponins in the *Quillaja* saponaria Molina extract Quil A. Rapid Communications in Mass Spectrometry 1995;9:660–666.

7. Kensil CR, Patel U, Lennick M, Marciani D. Separation and characterization of saponins with adjuvant activity from Quillaja saponaria Molina cortex. J Immunol 1991;146:431–437.
8. Kensil CR, Newman MJ, Coughlin RT, et al. The use of Stimulon adjuvant to boost vaccine response. Vaccine Research 1993;2:273–281.
9. Coughlin RT, Fattom A, Chu C, White AC, Winston S. Adjuvant activity of QS-21 for experimental *E. coli* 018 polysaccharide vaccines. Vaccine 1995;13:17–21.
10. Hancock GE, Speelman DJ, Frenchick PJ, Mineo-Kuhn MM, Baggs RB, Hahn DJ. Formulation of the purified fusion protein of respiratory syncytial virus with the saponin QS-21 induces protective immune responses in Balb/c mice that are similar to those generated by experimental infection. Vaccine 1995;13:391–400.
11. Sasaki S, Sumino K, Hamajima K, et al. Induction of systemic and mucosal immune responses to human immunodeficiency virus type 1 by a DNA vaccine formulated with QS-21 saponin adjuvant via intramuscular and intranasal routes. J Virol 1998; 72:4931–4939.
12. Kim SK, Ragupathi G, Musselli C, Choi SJ, Park YS, Livingston PO. Comparison of the effect of different immunological adjuvants on the antibody and T-cell response to immunization with MUC1-KLH and GD3-KLH conjugate cancer vaccines. Vaccine 1999;18:597–603.
13. Chen D, Endres R, Maa YF, et al. Epidermal powder immunization of mice and monkeys with an influenza vaccine. Vaccine 2003;21:2830–2836.
14. Evans TG, McElrath MJ, Matthews T, et al. QS-21 promotes an adjuvant effect allowing for reduced antigen dose during HIV-1 envelope subunit immunization in humans. Vaccine 2001;19:2080–2091.
15. Nardin EH, Oliveira GA, Calvo-Calle JM, et al. Synthetic malaria peptide vaccine elicits high levels of antibodies in vaccinees of defined HLA genotypes. J Infect Dis 2000;182:1486–1496.
16. Livingston PO, Adluri S, Helling F, et al. Phase 1 trial of immunological adjuvant QS-21 with a GM2 ganglioside-keyhole limpet haemocyanin conjugate vaccine in patients with malignant melanoma. Vaccine 1994;12:1275–1280.
17. Helling F, Zhang S, Shang A, et al. GM2-KLH conjugate vaccine: increased immunogenicity in melanoma patients after administration with immunological adjuvant QS-21. Cancer Res 1995;55:2783–2788.
18. Wyde PR, Guzman E, Gilbert BE, Couch RB. Immunogenicity and protection in mice given inactivated influenza vaccine. In: Osterhaus ADME, Cox N, Hampson AW, eds. Options for the Control of Influenza. New York: Excerpta Medica, 2001, pp. 999–1005.
19. Boyaka PN, Marinaro M, Jackson RJ, et al. Oral QS-21 requires early IL-4 help for induction of mucosal and systemic immunity. J Immunol 2001;166:2283–2290.
20. Chen D, McMichael JC, VanDerMeid KR, et al. Evaluation of purified UspA from Moraxella catarrhalis as a vaccine in a murine model after active immunization. Infect Immun 1996;64:1900–1905.
21. Wang ZG, Williams LJ, Zhang XF, et al. Polyclonal antibodies from patients immunized with a globo H-keyhole limpet hemocyanin vaccine: isolation, quantification, and characterization of immune responses by using totally synthetic immobilized tumor antigens. Proc Natl Acad Sci USA 2000;97:2719–2724.

22. Pillion DJ, Recchia J, Wang P, Marciani DJ, Kensil CR. DS-1, a modified Quillaja saponin, enhances ocular and nasal absorption of insulin. J Pharm Sci 1995;84: 1276–1279.

23. Pillion DJ, Amsden JA, Kensil CR, Recchia J. Structure-function relationship among Quillaja saponins serving as excipients for nasal and ocular delivery of insulin. J Pharm Sci 1996;85:518–524.

24. Chao AC, Nguyen JV, Broughall M, et al. Enhancement of intestinal model compound transport by DS-1, a modified Quillaja saponin. J Pharm Sci 1998;87:1395–1399.

25. Yewdell JW, Bennink JR. The binary logic of antigen processing and presentation to T cells. Cell 1990;62:203–206.

26. Newman MJ, Wu JY, Gardner BH, et al. Saponin adjuvant induction of ovalbumin-specific CD8+ cytotoxic T lymphocyte responses. J Immunol 1992;148:2357–2362.

27. Wu JY, Gardner BH, Murphy CI, et al. Saponin adjuvant enhancement of antigen-specific immune responses to an experimental HIV-1 vaccine. J Immunol 1992;148: 1519–1525.

28. Fenton RG, Keller CJ, Hanna N, Taub DD. Induction of T-cell immunity against Ras oncoproteins by soluble protein or Ras-expressing Escherichia coli. J Natl Cancer Inst 1995;87:1853–1861.

29. Gahery-Segard H, Pialoux G, Charmeteau B, et al. Multiepitopic B- and T-cell responses induced in humans by a human immunodeficiency virus type 1 lipopeptide vaccine. J Virol 2000;74:1694–1703.

30. Gahery-Segard H, Pialoux G, Figueiredo S, et al. Long-term specific immune responses induced in humans by a human immunodeficiency virus type 1 lipopeptide vaccine: characterization of CD8+-T-cell epitopes recognized. J Virol 2003; 77:11220–11231.

31. Lewis JJ, Janetzki S, Schaed S, et al. Evaluation of CD8(+) T-cell frequencies by the Elispot assay in healthy individuals and in patients with metastatic melanoma immunized with tyrosinase peptide. Int J Cancer 2000;87:391–398.

32. Schaed SG, Klimek VM, Panageas KS, et al. T-cell responses against tyrosinase 368-376(370D) peptide in HLA*A0201+ melanoma patients: randomized trial comparing incomplete Freund's adjuvant, granulocyte macrophage colony-stimulating factor, and QS-21 as immunological adjuvants. Clin Cancer Res 2002;8:967–972.

33. Medzhitov R, Janeway CA Jr. Decoding the patterns of self and nonself by the innate immune system. Science 2002;296:298–300.

34. Kensil C, Mo A, Truneh A. Current vaccine adjuvants: An overview of a diverse class. Frontiers in Bioscience 2004;9:2972–2988.

35. Ma J, Bulger PA, Davis DR, et al. Impact of the saponin adjuvant QS-21 and aluminium hydroxide on the immunogenicity of recombinant OspA and OspB of Borrelia burgdorferi. Vaccine 1994;12:925–932.

36. Goldenthal KL, Hedman K, Chen JW, August JT, Willingham MC. Postfixation detergent treatment for immunofluorescence suppresses localization of some integral membrane proteins. J Histochem Cytochem 1985;33:813–820.

37. Soltysik S, Wu JY, Recchia J, et al. Structure/function studies of QS-21 adjuvant: assessment of triterpene aldehyde and glucuronic acid roles in adjuvant function. Vaccine 1995;13:1403–1410.

38. Jacobsen NE, Fairbrother WJ, Kensil CR, Lim A, Wheeler DA, Powell MF. Structure of the saponin adjuvant QS-21 and its base-catalyzed isomerization product by 1H and natural abundance 13C NMR spectroscopy. Carbohydr Res 1996;280: 1–14.
39. Cleland JL, Kensil CR, Lim A, et al. Isomerization and formulation stability of the vaccine adjuvant QS-21. J Pharm Sci 1996;85:22–28.
40. Rhodes J. Evidence for an intercellular covalent reaction essential in antigen-specific T cell activation. J Immunol 1989;143:1482–1489.
41. Liu G, Anderson C, Scaltreto H, Barbon J, Kensil CR. QS-21 structure/function studies: effect of acylation on adjuvant activity. Vaccine 2002;20:2808–2815.
42. Wu JY, Gardner BH, Kushner NN, et al. Accessory cell requirements for saponin adjuvant-induced class I MHC antigen-restricted cytotoxic T-lymphocytes. Cell Immunol 1994;154:393–406.

# 12

# Monophosphoryl Lipid A and Synthetic Lipid A Mimetics As TLR4-Based Adjuvants and Immunomodulators

## Jory Baldridge, Kent Myers, David Johnson, David Persing, Christopher Cluff, and Robert Hershberg

## INTRODUCTION TO AND HISTORY OF MPL® ADJUVANT

MPL adjuvant, a monophosphoryl lipid A (MLA) derivative of the lipopolysaccharide (LPS) from *Salmonella minnesota* R595, and RC-529, a synthetic lipid A mimetic, are promising adjuvant candidates for a number of human vaccines and have been shown to be safe, well-tolerated, and to effectively enhance immune responses to co-administered vaccine antigens. Preliminary evidence suggests that, like LPS, MLA and RC-529 activate cells via the pattern recognition receptor, Toll-like receptor 4 (TLR4).

As TLR4 agonists, these adjuvants induce the production and secretion of inflammatory chemokines and cytokines effectively recruiting a variety of cells to the site of inflammation and mediating their activation. Among the cells recruited and activated are macrophages and dendritic cells (DCs) with enhanced capacities to process and present antigens to responding T and B lymphocytes. Within this milieu, TLR-induced cytokines direct the maturation of the lymphocytes into antigen-specific effector and memory cells. Although the earliest actions in this innate response are geared to providing the host immediate protection against invading microbes, it has become increasingly clear that the culmination of these orchestrated events is the development of antigen-specific, adaptive immunity. For today's recombinant vaccine antigens, MLA and RC-529 provide the critical function of engaging the cells of the innate immune system via TLR4 and setting off the cascade of events that amplify and transition the response to vaccine antigens into long-term, antigen-specific immunity.

LPS, the major component of Gram-negative bacterial cell walls, has long been known as a powerful immunomodulator. Over a century ago, a New York

From: *Vaccine Adjuvants: Immunological and Clinical Principles*
Edited by: C. J. Hackett and D. A. Harn, Jr. © Humana Press Inc., Totowa, NJ

physician, William B. Coley, noted that some cancer patients experienced spontaneous tumor regression following episodes of acute bacterial illness. Hypothesizing a correlation between the bacterial infection and tumor regression, Dr. Coley went on to successfully treat hundreds of tumor-bearing patients with heat-killed bacterial cultures known as Coley's Toxins *(1,2)*. We now realize that Coley's Toxins contained a number of TLR agonists including LPS, which undoubtedly stimulated innate immunity in Coley's cancer patients leading to nonspecific tumor regression. Meanwhile other investigators were demonstrating that antibody responses to exogenous antigens could be enhanced by co-administration of bacteria *(3)*, and Arthur Johnson eventually determined the adjuvant-active component of Gram-negative bacteria is LPS *(4)*. Despite its ability to enhance clinically relevant immune responses, LPS would be considered too toxic by current standards to be utilized clinically because of the induction of excessive amounts of inflammatory cytokines that provoke a sepsis-like syndrome. In efforts to unlink this extreme toxicity and the beneficial immune enhancing characteristics, Edgar Ribi and colleagues systematically evaluated modifications to LPS. Through sequential steps of acid and base hydrolysis, an immunoactive lipid A fraction containing a single phosphate group was eventually isolated. This monophosphoryl lipid A or MLA preparation exhibited significantly reduced toxicity and pyrogenicity compared to the parent LPS *(5)*, but retained much of the immunostimulatory activity, leading to the development of MPL adjuvant for use in human vaccines.

Drawing from our experience with MLA, a collection of novel synthetic lipid A mimetics was recently developed that contains chemically unique, acylated monosaccharides called amino alkyl glucosaminide 4-phosphates (AGPs) *(6)*. In preclinical studies the lead AGP, RC-529, demonstrated adjuvant activity very similar to that induced with MLA. Clinical experience with RC-529 (clinical GMP product is called Ribi.529) indicates it is a safe and effective vaccine adjuvant *(6,7)*. In this review, we provide an update of the pre-clinical and clinical experiences with MLA and the lipid A mimetic RC-529.

## *Chemistry, Manufacturing, Control, and Use of MPL Adjuvant*

MPL adjuvant is being developed by Corixa Corporation as an adjuvant for use in human vaccines. MPL adjuvant has been tested in numerous clinical trials and has been shown to be safe and effective as a vaccine adjuvant. In this section, the chemistry, manufacturing, and control aspects of MPL adjuvant are reviewed briefly. Considerations for the formulation of MPL adjuvant into final vaccine products are also discussed. For clarity, we refer to MPL adjuvant when discussing the specific Food and Drug Administration (FDA)-regulated clini-

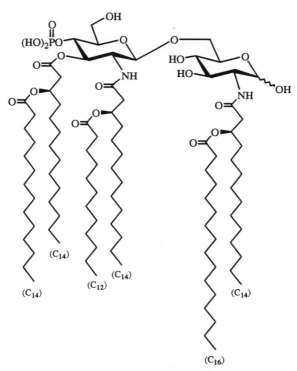

**Fig. 1.** The structure of the major hexaacyl3 D-MLA component in MPL adjuvant.

cal product, whereas we use MLA when considering the generic compound or its chemical constituents.

## Chemistry

MPL adjuvant is obtained by sequential acid and base hydrolyses of the LPS obtained from S. *minnesota* R595, a deep rough mutant strain. The resulting product is a complex mixture of closely related 3-0-desacyl-4'-MLA (3D-MLA) species that all share the same disaccharide backbone structure but that differ with respect to the number and distribution of fatty acids. 3D-MLA species with the same number of fatty acids are referred to as congeners, and MPL adjuvant contains congener groups with between three and six fatty acids (i.e., triacyl through hexaacyl). The most abundant hexaacyl 3D-MLA component in MPL adjuvant is shown in Fig. 1.

The backbone in all 3D-MLA species in MPL adjuvant consists of a disaccharide of β-1',6-linked 2-deoxy-2-aminoglucose that is substituted with a phosphate at the 4' position and with C14 fatty acids at the 2, 2', and 3' positions. These fatty acids may be tetradecenoic, 3-(R)-hydroxytetradecanoic, or 3-(R)-

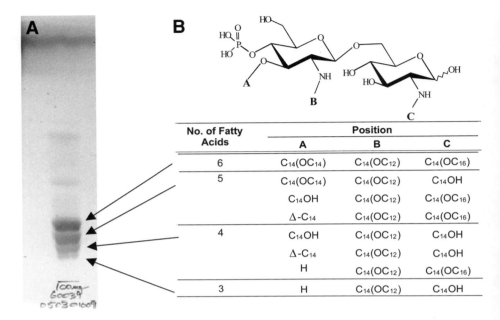

Fig. 2. The composition for MPL adjuvant by thin layer chromatography (TLC). (A) The TLC profile on silica gel of MPL adjuvant. (B) The MLA species corresponding to each TLC band, based on mass spectrometry data. Abbreviations are as follows: $C_{14}(OC_{16})$, 3-(R)-hexadecanoyloxytetradecanoic acid (similar meaning applies to $C_{14}$ [$OC_{14}$] and $C_{14}$ [$OC_{12}$]); $C_{14}OH$, 3-(R)-hydroxytetradecanoic acid; $\Delta$-$C_{14}$, tetradecenoic acid.

acyloxytetradecanoic acid, and in the latter case the acyloxy residue may be dodecanoyloxy, tetradecanoyloxy, or hexadecanoyloxy, depending on the backbone position. The 1,3,4, and 6' hydroxyls of the disaccharide backbone are unsubstituted in all MLA species present in MPL adjuvant. The heterogeneity inherent in MPL adjuvant is readily apparent by, for example, thin layer chromatography (TLC; see Fig. 2). The TLC pattern obtained on silica gel has a ladder-like appearance in which each band corresponds to a specific congener group from triacyl (lowest Rf) to hexaacyl (highest Rf). Structural assignments for the major 3D-MLA species within each band (congener group) have been made by mass spectrometry (see Fig. 2B) (8).

The congener composition of MPL adjuvant is also readily apparent by reverse-phase high performance liquid chromatography (HPLC) and electrospray mass spectrometry (ES-MS; see Fig. 3). The chromatogram and ES-MS spectrum closely resemble each other because of clustering of peaks for each 3D-MLA congener group. Reverse-phase HPLC is used as a quality control test to

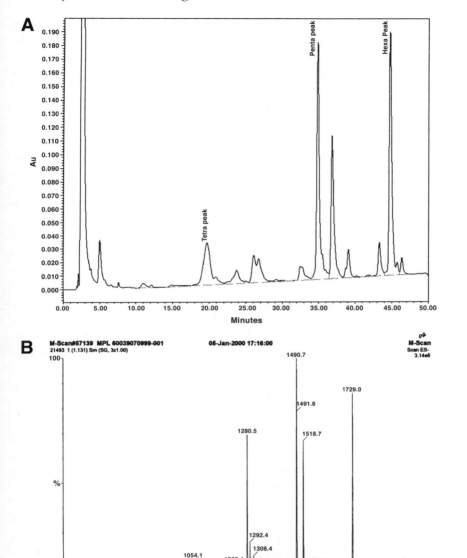

**Fig. 3.** Reverse-phase HPLC and electrospray mass spectrometry of MPL adjuvant. The profiles observed by HPLC (**A**) and ES-MS (**B**) resemble each other because of the clustering of 3D-MLA species (congeners) with the same number of fatty acids. Acylation increases as one moves from left to right in both the chromatogram (increased retention time) and the mass spectrum (increased mass/charge). The major hexaacyl congener occurs at the far right in both panels.

ensure the consistency of each lot of MPL adjuvant with respect to congener composition (*see* the section titled Control). The individual congener groups in MPL adjuvant (triacyl through hexaacyl) have been isolated and evaluated for adjuvant activity. We have found that these groups exhibit similar adjuvant activity (antibody, cytotoxic T lymphocytes [CTL]) and that they all contribute to the activity of MPL adjuvant.

## Manufacturing

As summarized in Fig. 4, the unit processes involved in the production of MPL adjuvant are (a) cell growth and harvest, (b) extraction of LPS from the cells, (c) conversion to crude product by sequential acid and base hydrolyses, (d) purification by ion-exchange chromatography (IEC), (e) final purification and conversion to the acid form, and (f) formation of the TEA salt, fill, and lyophilization. This manufacturing process is conducted in accordance with the FDA Good Manufacturing Practices (GMP) regulations at Corixa's facility in Hamilton, MT.

The presence of multiple 3D-MLA species in MPL adjuvant is attributable both to biosynthetic effects and to changes that occur during manufacture. The biosynthetic contributions arise from variability in the acylation of the lipid A by the parent organism. Bacterial endotoxins (LPS) in general tend to be highly heterogeneous, with variable structures in the O-antigen, core, and lipid A regions present in the LPS from a given organism *(9)*. The LPS obtained from *S. minnesota* R595, although much simpler than wild-type (smooth) LPS, exhibits considerable heterogeneity in the lipid A structure, both in terms of polar substituents that occur in non-stoichiometric levels on the phosphates and, significantly, in the fatty acid distribution (*see* Fig. 4) *(10)*. This variability in lipid A acylation arises both from adaptations by the parent organism in response to environmental conditions and from substrate promiscuity by the acyl transferase enzymes involved in biosynthesis *(11,12)*. Variability in acylation of lipid A is, of course, reflected in the 3D-MLA composition of the final MPL adjuvant.

The manufacturing process for MPL adjuvant also contributes to the heterogeneity of this product. This occurs primarily because of loss of ester-linked fatty acids during the acid hydrolysis step, leading to the generation of congeners with lower acylation levels (e.g., triacyl and tetraacyl) and with non-native fatty acids (i.e., tetradecenoic acid). The contribution of the acid hydrolysis step to heterogeneity was demonstrated by subjecting a synthetic 3D-MLA analog to acid hydrolysis conditions similar to those used in the manufacturing process, which yielded a product with an HPLC profile similar to that of MPL adjuvant.

## Control and Release of MPL Product

Each lot of MPL adjuvant must undergo quality control (QC) testing and release before it can be used in human vaccines. These QC tests are intended to

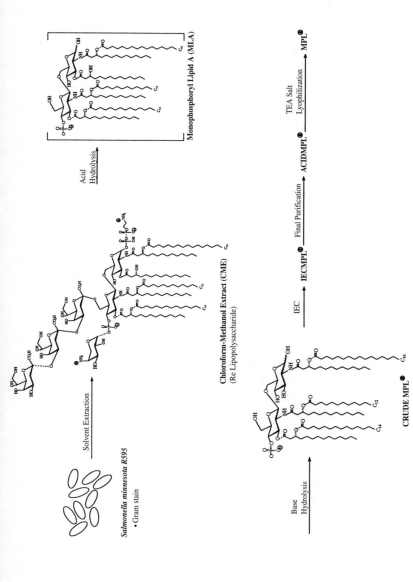

**Fig. 4.** The unit processes involved in the manufacture of MPL adjuvant. Each unit process in the above scheme, with the exception of the acid hydrolysis step, results in a stored in-process intermediate. The acid hydrolysis product, MLA, is not isolated and is therefore shown in brackets. Chemical moieties that are present in non-stoichiometric amounts are indicated with dashed lines for bonds.

241

demonstrate the safety, identity, and purity of each lot of bulk adjuvant before it is released for further processing into the final vaccine.

The safety and potency of the incorporated MPL adjuvant are further evaluated by QC testing performed on the final vaccine product. The safety of each lot of MPL adjuvant is evaluated using the chick embryo 50% lethal dose ($CELD_{50}$) assay and the USP rabbit pyrogen test. Both of these biological test methods are very sensitive to the presence of bacterial endotoxins and therefore provide assurance that there is no contamination by residual parent *S. minnesota* R595 LPS, diphosphoryl lipid A, or other bacterial endotoxin. Note that it is not possible to use the limulus amebocyte lysate assay with MPL adjuvant because of strong cross reactivity with 3D-MLA. Identity is confirmed by a reverse phase HPLC method in which the relative percentages of the individual congener groups are quantitated (*see* Fig. 3A). Additionally, the levels of phosphorus and glucosamine are measured to confirm the expected structure of the 3D-MLA, and the TEA content is measured to establish the identity as the TEA salt. The purity of each lot is assessed by measuring the levels of potential product impurities. These impurities can be regarded as either process- or product-related. Process-related impurities include proteins and peptides from the culture medium, residual solvents, and residual moisture. Product-related impurities include bacterial proteins, nucleic acids, KDO, and free fatty acids.

## Formulation of MPL Adjuvant

MPL adjuvant is an amphipathic compound that is characterized by well-defined polar and nonpolar domains. As such, it does not dissolve in water to yield a solution of fully solvated single molecules, but instead forms aggregated structures (e.g., micelles, liposomes) in which the hydrophobic regions are sequestered away from the aqueous milieu. The solubility characteristics of MPL adjuvant must therefore be considered carefully when developing vaccine formulations that contain this adjuvant. Formulations that provide an interfacial surface in contact with bulk water are particularly well-suited for use with MPL adjuvant, with examples including oil-in-water emulsions, alum, and liposomes. MPL can also be stabilized in a micellar form by admixture with surfactants at an appropriate molar ratio. The choice of adjuvant formulation is dependent on several factors, including compatibility with the vaccine antigen, the route of administration, the immune response desired, and the degree of reactogenicity that can be tolerated. Aqueous formulations of MPL adjuvant have been studied extensively in clinical trials and possess excellent safety profiles. Aqueous MPL adjuvant is readily compatible with alum-adsorbed antigens and is suitable for administration to mucosal surfaces, where it shows promise for mediating mucosal immunity. Stable oil-in-water emulsions containing MPL adjuvant (MPL-SE) provide another formulation option, in which the lipophilic

MPL adjuvant readily dissolves in the oil phase of the emulsion. MPL-SE or other MPL adjuvant-containing emulsions generally induce more vigorous immune responses, which are accompanied by a higher degree of reactogenicity.

## DESIGN AND SYNTHESIS OF THE AGP CLASS OF LIPID A MIMETICS

As discussed in the section titled Chemistry, MPL adjuvant is a chemically modified form of lipid A comprised of several components, which differ principally with respect to the degree and type of fatty acid acylation and to a lesser extent with respect to microheterogeneity in fatty acid chain length. Purification and structural analysis of this heterogeneous product is also complicated by the fact that the individual MLA components are reducing sugars and exist as a mixture of two anomeric forms.

Chemical synthesis and biological evaluation of the major components present in MPL adjuvant have shown that the biological activity of these molecules depends on both the degree and type of fatty acid acylation; many of the beneficial immune stimulating properties of MPL adjuvant have been attributed to the major hexaacyl component 1 (Fig. 5) *(13,14)*. This finding corroborates other studies showing that a β-(1–6) diglucosamine moiety possessing six fatty acids is prerequisite to the full expression of immunostimulant activities *(15)*.

Because of the heterogeneity of MPL adjuvant and difficulty in performing structure–activity relationship (SAR) studies with such natural products via chemical modification, we chose to pursue the design and synthesis of a structurally simpler mimetic of component 1 that was amenable both to systematic SAR studies and to chemical synthesis on a large scale in highly purified form. A synthetic mimetic of component 1 would make it possible to carry out precise investigations on the relationship between chemical structure and biological activity without ambiguity because of heterogeneity in the naturally derived product and/or contamination by other bioactive substances.

Accordingly, we designed a new class of synthetic lipid A mimetics structurally related to major MLA component 1 *(6,16)*. Known chemically as ω-aminoalkyl 2-amino-2-deoxy-4-phosphono-β-D-glucopyranosides (aminoalkyl glucosaminide phosphates, AGPs) and possessing general structure 2 (Fig. 5), the AGPs are synthetic mimetics of compound 1 in which the reducing sugar has been replaced with an *N*-[(R)-3-*n*-alkanoyloxytetradecanoyl]aminoalkanyl (aglycon) unit. We speculated that a conformationally flexible aglycon unit would permit energetically favored close packing of the six fatty acyl chains; tight packing of six fatty acids in a hexagonal array is believed to play an essential role in the bioactivity of lipid A-like molecules *(17)*. Further, recent evidence suggests that the interaction of lipid A and its analogs with the pattern recognition receptor TLR4 is determined in part by the conformational shape and supra-

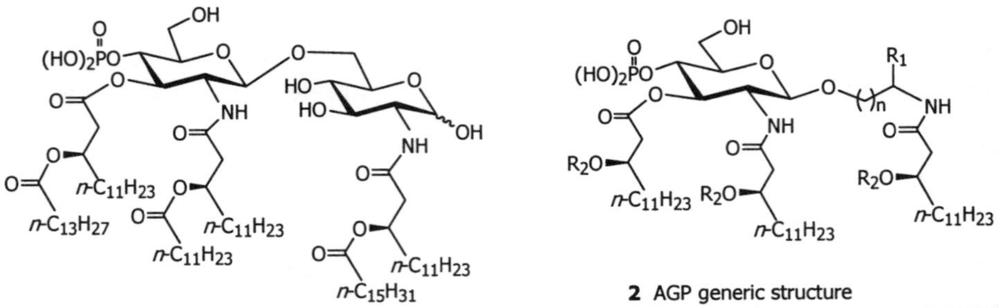

**1** major component in MPL adjuvant

**2** AGP generic structure
**3** $R_1$=H, $R_2$=$n$-$C_{13}H_{27}CO$, n=1 (RC-529)

**Fig. 5.** Synthetic and naturally derived lipid A derivatives.

molecular assembly of the compounds in solution, which in turn is dependent on fatty acid chain length and their three-dimensional arrangement in space *(18–20)*. Structural parameters such as acyl chain length and spacing and physico-chemical properties important to adjuvant activity can be manipulated readily in the AGP series.

Our initial SAR studies on the AGP class of lipid A mimetics have shown that the spacial arrangement of the three acyloxyacyl residues (i.e., as determined by the aglycon chain length or "n" in formula 2 (Fig. 5), the length of the fatty acid chains $R_2$ and the nature of the $R_1$ substituent can profoundly affect biological activity *(6,21)*. On the other hand, subtle differences in fatty acid chain length such as the fatty acid dissimilitude present in MLA component 1 is not essential for immune stimulation or favorable activity/toxicity profiles *(22)*. These observations led to the development of the RC-529 (structure 3; Fig. 5) as a synthetic mimetic of compound 1. RC-529, which possesses three (R)-3-tetra-decanoyloxytetradecanoyl residues, contains the same absolute number of fatty acid carbon atoms as compound 1 and similar physicochemical properties.

Owing in part to the close structural similarity between compound 1 and RC-529, MPL adjuvant and RC-529 exhibit similar biological properties *(23)*. Both markedly enhance humoral and cell-mediated immune responses to protein antigens in murine models *(6,14)*. Of particular note, RC-529 and MPL adjuvant augment the expression of complement-fixing IgG subclasses and vaccine-induced cytotoxic T lymphocytes (CTLs), reflecting their ability to potentiate T-helper (Th)l type responses with protein antigens. Although both MPL adjuvant and RC-529 exhibit low pyrogenicity when compared to lipid A preparations, RC-529 appears to be less pyrogenic than MPL adjuvant and its major component 1 in rabbits. The potent adjuvanticity and low toxicity of RC-529, combined with its ability to be produced consistently by chemical synthesis (*see* Fig. 6) on a large scale and in high purity, suggests that RC-529 has certain

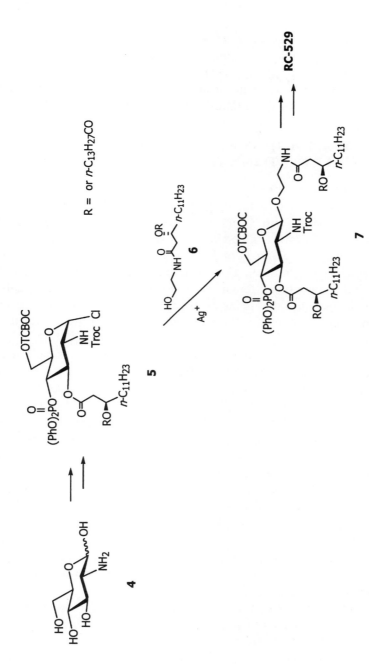

**Fig. 6.** Synthesis of RC-529.

advantages over MLA as a vaccine adjuvant, particularly in pediatric vaccines where adjuvant pyrogenicity and biological contamination must be minimized. As a result, RC-529 has become Corixa's lead synthetic vaccine adjuvant. The clinical utility of Ribi.529 as a vaccine adjuvant was recently demonstrated in a phase III pivotal trial with a recombinant hepatitis B antigen *(7,16)*.

## BIOLOGY OF MPL ADJUVANT
## INCLUDING TLR4 AND INNATE IMMUNITY

### Molecular Characterization

The capacity of MLA to enhance protective immunity to co-administered vaccine antigens results from its interactions with cells of the immune system that express TLR4. Defining the precise biological activities of MLA is difficult, in part because of the variety of TLR4 positive target cells, the complexity of the mediators associated with TLR4 activation, and the specific anatomical features associated with the different routes and formulations used for delivery. Nonetheless, insight into the mechanisms of action can be inferred from the results of an extensive number of studies performed with MLA over the past two decades.

The ability of MLA to stimulate "innate" immune responses has been well documented. Originally, the activity of MLA was related in part to its ability to nonspecifically induce tumor regression in mice *(25)*. Subsequent studies demonstrated mice treated with MLA given without exogenous antigen or microbe were able to resist lethal microbial challenge by Gram-positive and Gram-negative bacteria, including *Staphylococcus, Listeria, E. coli,* and *Salmonella* and influenza virus challenge *(14,26)*. The duration of this nonspecific protection lasts up to 14 days depending on the dose and formulation administered. Resistance imparted by aqueous formulations lasts approx 4 to 7 days following administration but if the MLA is sequestered for slow release in an oil-in-water emulsion, the protection can last up to 14 days and repeat administrations can extend the period of protection. The kinetics of this so-called "nonspecific protection" (because it does not require co-administration with antigen) is consistent with the activation of phagocytic cells and the rapid induction of pro-inflammatory cytokines and chemokines.

These hypotheses above that relate to the ability of MPL (and, more recently the synthetic TLR4 agonists) to induce nonspecific protection against a variety of infectious agents have been supported by numerous experimental studies. In vitro studies with mouse-derived cells document that monocytes and macrophages have increased respiratory bursts and phagocytic indices following stimulation with MLA *(27,28)*. Saha and associates reported similar findings, showing that human monocytes become activated to produce reactive oxygen intermediates in the presence of MLA *(29)*. Not only do cells of the monocyte/ macrophage lineage provide nonspecific protection through degradative phago- cytosis of pathogens, they can also function as antigen-presenting cells (APCs) critical for the induction of antigen-specific antibody and T-cell responses. The critical importance of macrophages in this respect was demonstrated by Wijburg and associates, who showed ovalbumin formulated with MLA as an oil-in-water emulsion-induced ovalbumin specific CTLs, while mice depleted of macrophages prior to vaccination were unable to produce CTL *(30)*. In vitro studies by De Becker and colleagues confirmed the importance of macrophages, which were able to prime naïve T cells to secrete interferon (IFN)$\gamma$, interleukin (IL)-4, and IL-5 following MLA stimulation *(31)*. The discovery of TLR4 as the LPS/Lipid A receptor *(32,33)* and the abundant expression of TLR4 on cells of the macrophage/monocytes lineage supports the findings that MLA acts directly on these cell types. Taken together these results indicate the importance of monocytes and macrophages in mediating the biological effects of MLA for inducing nonspecific resistance and priming lymphocytes for antigen-specific immunity.

DCs are also critical APCs that express TLR4 on their surface and respond to MLA stimulation. De Becker et al. found that MLA administered to mice by iv injection induced splenic DCs to migrate from the marginal zones to the T-cell areas of the spleen *(31)*. Following migration the majority of the DCs expressed maturation markers including increased expression of class II MHC molecules and B7 costimulatory molecules. Ismaili and associates found simi- lar results using human monocyte-derived DCs *(34)*. MLA stimulation of the DCs induced upregulation of MHC class II molecules (HLA-DR) and both B7.1 and B7.2 costimulatory molecules. In both studies, MLA stimulated DCs became competent to mediate activation of T cells. These results suggest that MLA activates dendritic cells allowing for enhanced interactions with T lym- phocytes following vaccination.

In addition to cell activation, MLA triggers the production and secretion of a number of cytokines. Human whole blood or PBMC cultures stimulated with MLA produce a wide variety of cytokines and chemokines, including IL-8 and MIP-1$\beta$ *(21)* (M. Lacy, personal conversation, 2002). The early production of these chemokines may help shape the immune response to co-administered antigens. IL-8 is important for the recruitment of neutrophils whereas MIP-1$\beta$ can cause the influx of macrophages, DC, and natural killer (NK) cells *(35)*. Additionally, macrophages exposed to MLA elaborate tumor necrosis factor (TNF)-$\alpha$ and IL-1$\beta$, both of which induce activation and maturation of DCs *(36)*. DCs exposed to MLA produced IL-12, IFN$\gamma$, and IL-5, cytokines that direct development of Th1 and Th2 adaptive responses *(34)*. These results sup- port findings from vaccine studies that indicate MLA stimulates both Th1 and

Th2 responses. MLA injected into mice resulted in the induction of IFNγ and its production was increased in the presence of TNF-α *(37)*. NK cells, possibly recruited by MIP-1β are a likely source of the IFNγ. The local production of these chemokines and cytokines conceivably leads to the enhanced recruitment, interaction and communication of immunocompetent cells, thus linking and enhancing acquired immunity to co-administered vaccine antigens. To date, strong evidence indicates that the activity of MLA is mediated via interactions with TLR4. C3H/HEJ mice harbor a single point mutation resulting in an amino acid change in TLR4 and because of this mutation the mice are hyporesponsive to LPS and lipid A *(33)*. In contrast to wild-type mice, C3H/HEJ mice treated with MLA produced no IFNγ. Similarly, B cells from wild-type but not C3H/HEJ mice proliferate in response to MLA exposure *(14)*. More recently, we have used an in vitro system in which HeLa cells (which do not express TLRs on their surface) are transfected with expression constructs that direct the expression of specific TLRs on their surface *(38)*. Using this approach, we have been able to demonstrate both the requirement for and specificity of TLR4 (and the associated MD-2 molecule), *(39)* in the response to MLA. Using antibodies specific for TLR4 or TLR2, we have observed that the response to MLA in human monocytes and human monocytic cells lines is dependent on TLR4, but not TLR2. Our latter findings are not completely consistent with the results from a recent report suggesting that MPL adjuvant can signal via TLR4 and TLR2 *(40)*. The basis for this apparent discrepancy is not currently clear.

## *Preclinical Adjuvant Studies*

MLA has been studied extensively in preclinical animal studies as a vaccine adjuvant. In this respect it has been shown to be a potent adjuvant capable of enhancing both humoral and cell-mediated immunity to a wide variety of vaccine antigens *(13)*. In these studies, MLA mediated an overall increase in antibody titers to polysaccharide, protein, and peptide antigens. In most cases, the response to antigen alone induces predominantly antibodies of IgG1 isotype, indicating a Th2 type of response. The inclusion of MLA as an adjuvant generally induced a qualitative shift in the response, such that IgG2a titers are boosted significantly, providing a more balanced Th1/Th2 response to the vaccine antigen. These studies indicate MLA has the capacity to up-regulate Th1 responses, which is consistent with strong cell-mediated immune responses. Additional studies confirmed this concept, demonstrating the ability of MPL adjuvant to mediate cell-mediated immunity in the form of Th cells and CTLs *(30,41)*.

The ability of MLA to serve as a Th1-promoting adjuvant in the context of an established Th2 immune response was recently tested in an allergy model by Wheeler and associates *(42)*. IgE responses were induced in Brown Norway rats (high IgE responders) by immunization with KLH/alum adsorbates plus

*Bordetella pertussis* bacteria. The rise in IgE titers following subsequent vaccinations with KLH was blocked by the addition of MLA to the vaccines. In a related experiment, the ratio of ragweed-specific Th2 to Th1 antibody isotypes was dramatically decreased from 16:1 to 2:1 in the sera of mice vaccinated with a ragweed vaccine (Pollinex R; Allergy Therapeutics, Ltd, UK) formulated with MLA compared to sera from mice receiving only the Pollinex vaccine *(42)*. Taken together, these results suggest that MLA preferentially enhances a Th1-biased response that can attenuate an existing Th2 response.

Interestingly, MLA and some of the synthetic TLR4 agonists also have adjuvant activity when administered to mucosal surfaces. When applied with vaccines to intranasal *(41,43)* or oral *(44)* mucosal surfaces, MLA promotes antigen-specific immune responses at local and distal mucosal sites and systemic immunity. These responses are characterized by enhanced antigen-specific IgA both locally and at distal mucosal sites. Importantly, the mucosal vaccination strategy with MLA also induced systemic humoral and cell-mediated immune responses, including CTL induction, and mediated protection against lethal challenge *(14,41)*. The ability of MLA to actively mediate mucosal and systemic immunity is important for the development of protective vaccine immunity against a wide range of infectious diseases where infectious challenge occurs at mucosal sites.

The synthetic AGP adjuvant, RC-529, has demonstrated comparable adjuvant activity to MLA in preclinical studies. When RC-529 is formulated with hepatitis B surface antigen (HBsAg) significant improvement in both antibody titers and CTL responses were observed *(23)*. Similar to the effects seen with MLA, the incorporation of RC-529 into the hepatitis vaccine significantly shifted the response from one dominated by antibodies of the IgG1 isotype to a response that also contained high levels of complement-fixing IgG2a antibodies. As a result of its desirable safety profile and effective adjuvant activity, RC-529 (now called Ribi.529) has emerged as one of Corixa's lead synthetic vaccine adjuvant for clinical evaluation.

## Clinical Adjuvant Studies

MPL adjuvant has been evaluated extensively in human clinical trials with infectious disease, cancer and allergy vaccines. In these studies, vaccines contained MPL adjuvant alone or a combination of MPL adjuvant and other adjuvants, including alum, cell wall skeleton of *Mycobacterium phlei* or QS21. Through these trials greater than 12,000 volunteers have received MPL adjuvant and acceptable safety and efficacy profiles have been established (Table 1). Results of clinical trials conducted before 1994 were reviewed previously *(13)*.

Several clinical trials demonstrated that the inclusion of MPL adjuvant in a hepatitis B vaccine increases the rate of seroprotection *(45,46)*. Healthy normal

**Table 1**
**Clinical Trials With MLA and Ribi.529**

| Clinical indication | Adjuvant system | Trial highlights and/or immune parameters | Ref. |
|---|---|---|---|
| Hepatitis B | MPL + alum (SBAS-4) | Enhanced seroconversion; higher GMT; enhanced cell-mediated immunity | *45* |
| Hepatitis B | MPL + alum (SBAS-4) | Enhanced seroconversion; higher GMT; enhanced cell-mediated immunity | *46* |
| Hepatitis B | MPL + alum (SBAS-4) | Enhanced seroconversion; higher GMT; enhanced cell-mediated immunity | *50* |
| Hepatitis B | MPL + alum (SBAS-4) | Enhanced seroconversion; higher GMT; enhanced cell-mediated immunity | *51* |
| Malaria | MPL + QS21 oil-in-water emulsion (SBAS-2) | Resistance to parasitemia | *52* |
| Herpes type 2 | MPL + Alum (SBAS-4) | Enhanced binding and neutralizing antibody; enhanced cell proliferation; enhanced IFNγ | *47* |
| Streptococcus pneumoniae | MPL + Alum | Neonate patient population; enhanced cell proliferation; enhanced IFNγ | *48* |
| Melanoma | MPL + CWS (Detox) | Extended survival | *53* |
| Grass pollen allergy | MPL + Tyrosine | Reduced nasal and ocular symptoms; reduced skin-prick sensitivity | *49* |
| Hepatitis B | Ribi.529 | Enhanced seroconversion; higher GMT | *7* |

volunteers were seroprotected after only two doses of a hepatitis B vaccine formulated with MPL adjuvant, in contrast to volunteers requiring three doses of the Hepatitis B vaccine without MPL adjuvant. Assessment of the immune parameters indicated that the vaccine containing MPL adjuvant elicited higher geometric mean titers and enhanced cell-mediated immunity compared to the non-MPL-adjuvanted hepatitis B vaccine alone.

A herpes vaccine formulated with MPL adjuvant was demonstrated to provide significant protection against genital herpes in women who were seronegative for both herpes simplex virus (HSV)-1 and HSV-2 before vaccination *(47)*. The vaccine elicited both binding and neutralizing antibodies against HSV, and cellular responses as indicated by lymphoproliferation and IFNγ secretion.

The results of these trials are potentially significant, because no other vaccine has been demonstrated to prevent genital infection with HSV. The effectiveness of the vaccine is hypothesized to be because of the Th1-biasing activity of MPL adjuvant.

The safety and efficacy of an investigational nine-valent pneumococcal-CRM197 protein conjugate vaccine (PCV9) combined with 10, 25, or 50 μg MPL adjuvant in the presence or absence of alum was recently evaluated in 129 healthy children *(48)*. A dose-dependent effect of MPL adjuvant on antigen-specific cellular immune responses was reported. Addition of 10 μg MPL adjuvant to the antigen in the absence of alum significantly enhanced CRM197-specific T-cell proliferation and IFNγ production compared to the antigen plus alum. The results demonstrate that MPL adjuvant-stimulated Th1 responses to the carrier protein in a dose-dependent fashion, and supported the idea that MPL adjuvant is sufficiently safe for use in children.

To test the possibility that MPL adjuvant, a Th1-inducing adjuvant, has potential utility in vaccines designed to treat allergies in humans, a placebo-controlled, randomized, double-blind clinical study was conducted with a standardized allergy vaccine comprising a tyrosine-adsorbed glutaraldehyde-modified grass pollen extract containing MPL adjuvant *(49)*. The MPL adjuvant containing vaccine was significantly better than placebo at reducing nasal and ocular symptoms, and a significant reduction in sensitivity to skin prick testing. This vaccine is now available in a number of countries as Pollinex Quattro®.

## CONCLUSION

MPL adjuvant has been administered to more than 12,000 humans and has proven to be both safe and effective in a variety of clinical contexts. Used in combination with antigen, MPL adjuvant alone, or combined with other adjuvants has been shown to augment humoral and cell-mediated immune responses. The corresponding increase in geometric mean titers and rate of seroconversion/seroprotection in the hepatitis B vaccine augmented with MPL adjuvant has reduced the dosing requirement compared to the alum-based vaccine. The ability of MPL adjuvant to enhance cellular immune responses including CTL responses highlight the utility of this adjuvant in cancer vaccines. Recent mechanistic data suggest that MPL augments immune responsiveness via the production of a wide array of pro-inflammatory cytokines and chemokines via signaling through TLR4. A new class of wholly synthetic lipid A mimetic molecules have been developed with TLR4 agonist activity. The lead compound in this group of compounds within this family of AGPs is RC-529. This compound has already proven to be a safe and effective adjuvant in a human clinical study. Studies from a variety of animal models suggest that MPL adjuvant and members of the synthetic AGP family are highly active when delivered to mucosal surfaces and can enhance mucosal immune responses. Taken together, TLR4 based adjuvants represent an efficient means to augment humoral and cellular responses following systemic or mucosal delivery. The excellent safety profile and extensive clinical experience with these adjuvants in humans highlight broad applicability for MPL adjuvant and RC-529 in a wide variety of vaccine strategies.

## REFERENCES

1. Nauts HC, Swift WE, Corley BL. Treatment of malignant tumors by bacterial toxins as developed by the late William B. Coley, M.D., reviewed in light of modern research. Cancer Res 1946;6:205–216.
2. Hall SS. A Commotion in the Blood. New York: Henry Holt and Company, Inc., 1997.
3. Munoz J. Effects of bacteria and bacteria products on antibody response. In: Dixon FJ, Kunkel HG, eds. Advances in Immunology. New York: Academic Press, 1964, pp. 397–440.
4. Johnson AG, Gaines S, Landy M. Studies of the O antigen of *Salmonella typhosa* V. Enhancement of antibody response to protein antigens by the purified lipopolysaccharide. J Exp Med 1956;103:225–246.
5. Ribi EE, Strain SM, Mizuno Y, et al. Peptides as requirement for immunotherapy of the guinea-pig line-10 tumor with endotoxins. Cancer Immunol Immunother 1979;7:43–58.
6. Johnson DA, Sowell CG, Johnson CL, et al. Synthesis and biological evaluation of a new class of vaccine adjuvants: Aminoalkyl glucosaminide 4-phosphates (AGPs). Biog Med Chem Lett 1999;9:2273–2278.
7. Dupont J-C, Altclas J, Sigelchifer M, Von Eschen EB, Timmermans I, Wagener A. Efficacy and safety of AgB/RC529: A novel two dose adjuvant vaccine against hepatitis B. 2002; 42nd Interscience Conference on Antimicrobial Agents and Chemotherapy, San Diego, CA.
8. Hagen SR, Thompson JD, Snyder DS, Myers KR. Analysis of a monophosphoryl lipid A immunostimulant preparation from *Salmonella minnesota* R595 by high-performance liquid chromatography. J Chromatogr A 1997;767:53–61.
9. Nowotny A. Heterogeneity in endotoxins. In: Rietschel E, ed. Handbook of Endotoxin Vol. 1: Chemistry of Endotoxin. Philadelphia: Elsevier, 1984, pp. 308–338.
10. Caroff M, Deprun C, Karibian D, Szabo L. Analysis of unmodified endotoxin preparations by 252Cf plasma desorption mass spectrometry. Determination of molecular masses of the constituent native lipopolysaccharides. J Biol Chem 1991; 266:18543–18549.
11. Trent MS, Pabich W, Raetz CR, Miller SI. A PhoP/PhoQ-induced Lipase (PagL) that catalyzes 3-0-deacylation of lipid A precursors in membranes of *Salmonella typhimurium*. J Biol Chem 2001;276:9083–9092.
12. Brozek KA, Raetz CRH. Biosynthesis of Lipid A in *Escherichia coli.* J Biol Chem 1990;265:15410–15417.
13. Ulrich JT, Myers KR. Monophosphoryllipid A as an Adjuvant. Past experiences and new directions. In: Powell MF, Newman MJ, eds. Vaccine Design: The Subunit and Adjuvant Approach. New York: Plenum Press, 1995, pp. 495–524.
14. Persing DH, Coler RN, Lacy MJ, et al. Taking toll: Lipid A mimetics as adjuvants and immunomodulators. Trends Microbiol 2002;10:S32–S37.

15. Qureshi N, Takayama K. Structure and function of lipid A. In: Iglewski BH, Clark VL, eds. The Bacteria, Vol. XI. Madison, WI: Academic Press, Inc., 1990, pp. 319–338.

16. Baldridge JR. A synthetic adjuvant, RC-529, moves into the clinic. 3rd Meeting on Novel Adjuvants Currently in/Close to Human Clinical Testing, Foundation Merieux, Annecy, France, January 7–9, 2002.

17. Seydel U, Labischinski H, Kastowsky M, Brandenburg K. Phase behavior, supramolecular structure, and molecular conformation of lipopolysaccharide. Immunobiol 1993;187:191-211.

18. Fukuoka S, Brandenburg K, Muller M, Lindner B, Koch MH, Seydel U. Physicochemical analysis of lipid A fractions of lipopolysaccharide from Erwinia carotovora in relation to bioactivity. Biochim Biophys Acta 2001;1510:185–197.

19. Fukase K, Oikawa M, Suda Y, et al. New synthesis and conformational analysis of lipid A: biological activity and supramolecular assembly. J Endotoxin Res 1999; 5:46–51.

20. Brandenburg K, Matsuura M, Heine H, et al. Biophysical characterization of triacyl monosaccharide lipid a partial structures in relation to bioactivity. Biophys J 2002; 83:322–333.

21. Baldridge JR, Cluff CW, Evans JT, et al. Immunostimulatory activity of amino alkyl glucosaminide 4-phosphates (AGPs): induction of protective innate immune responses by RC-524 and RC-529. J Endotoxin Res 2002;8:453–458.

22. Johnson DA, Keegan DS, Sowell CG, et al. 3-O-Desacyl monophosphoryl lipid A derivatives: synthesis and immunostimulant activities. J Med Chem 1999;42: 4640–4649.

23. Evans JT, Cluff CW, Johnson DA, Lacy MJ, Persing DH, Baldridge JR. Enhancement of antigen-specific immunity via the TLR4 ligands MPL adjuvant and Ribi. 529. Expert Review Vaccines 2003;2:89–99.

24. Keegan DS, Johnson DA, Hagen SR. Efficient asymmetric synthesis of *(R)*-hydroxy- and alkanoyloxytetradecanoic acids and method for the determination of enantiomeric purity. Tetrahedron: Asymmetry 1996;7:3559–3564.

25. Ribi EE, Granger DL, Milner KC, Strain SM. Tumor regression caused by endotoxins and mycobacterial fractions. J Natl Cancer Inst 1975;55:1253–1257.

26. Ulrich JT, Masihi KN, Lange W. Mechanisms of nonspecific resistance to microbial infections induced by trehalose dimycolate (TDM) and monophosphoryl lipid A (MPL). In: Masihi KN, Lange W, eds. Advances in the Biosciences. London: Pergamon Journals Ltd., 1988, pp. 167–178.

27. Masihi KN, Lange W, Johnson AG, Ribi E. Enhancement of chemiluminescence and phagocytic activities by nontoxic and toxic forms of lipid A. J Biol Response Mod 1986;5:462–469.

28. Pohle C, Rohde-Schulz B, Masihi KN. Effects of synthetic HIV peptides, cytokines and monophosphoryl lipid A on chemiluminescence response. In: Masihi KN, Lange W, eds. Immunotherapeutic Prospects of Infectious Diseases. Heidelberg: Springer-Verlag Berlin, 1990, pp. 143–149.

29. Saha DC, Barua RS, Astiz ME, Rackow EC, Eales-Reynolds U. Monophosphoryl lipid A stimulated up-regulation of reactive oxygen intermediates in human monocytes in vitro. J Leukoc Biol 2001;70:381–385.

30. Wijburg OL, van den Dobbelsteen GP, Vadolas J, Sanders A, Strugnell RA, van Rooijen N. The role of macrophages in the induction and regulation of immunity elicited by exogenous antigens. Eur J Immunol 1998;28:479–487.

31. De Becker G, Moulin V, Pajak B, et al. The adjuvant monophosphoryl lipid A increases the function of antigen-presenting cells. Int Immuno 2000;12:807–815.

32. Poltorak A, Ricciardi-Castagnoli P, Citterio S, Beutler B. Physical contact between lipopolysaccharide and toll-like receptor 4 revealed by genetic complementation. Proc Natl Acad Sci USA 2000;97:2163–2167.

33. Poltorak A, He X, Smimova I, et al. Defective LPS signaling in C3H/HeJ and C57BL/10ScCr mice: mutations in Tlr4 gene. Science 1998;282:2085–2088.

34. Ismaili J, Rennesson J, Aksoy E, et al. Monophosphoryl lipid A activates both human dendritic cells and T cells. J Immunol 2002;168:926–932.

35. Luster AD. The role of chemokines in linking innate and adaptive immunity. Curr Opin Immunol 2002;14:129–135.

36. Belardelli F, Ferrantini M. Cytokines as a link between innate and adaptive antitumor immunity. Trends Immunol 2002;23:201–208.

37. Gustafson GL, Rhodes MI. Effects of tumor necrosis factor and dexamethasone on the regulation of interferon-γ induction by monophosphoryl lipid A. J Immunother Emphasis Tumor Immunol 1994;15:129–133.

38. da Silva CJ, Soldau K, Christen U, Tobias PS, Ulevitch RJ. Lipopolysaccharide is in close proximity to each of the proteins in its membrane receptor complex. transfer from CD14 to TLR4 and MD-2. J Biol Chem 2001;276:21129–21135.

39. da Silva CJ, Ulevitch RJ. MD-2 and TLR4 N-linked glycosylations are important for a functional lipopolysaccharide receptor. J Biol Chem 2002;277:1845–1854.

40. Martin M, Michalek SM, Katz J. Role of innate immune factors in the adjuvant activity of monophosphoryl lipid A. Infect Immun 2003;71:2498–2507.

41. Baldridge JR, Yorgensen Y, Ward JR, Ulrich JT. Monophosphoryllipid A enhances mucosal and systemic immunity to vaccine antigens following intranasal administration. Vaccine 2000;18:2416–2425.

42. Wheeler AW, Marshall JS, Ulrich JT. A Thl-inducing adjuvant, MPL, enhances antibody profiles in experimental animals suggesting it has the potential to improve the efficacy of allergy vaccines. Int Arch Allergy Immunol 2001;126:135–139.

43. VanCott TC, Kaminski RW, Mascola JR, et al. HIV-1 neutralizing antibodies in the genital and respiratory tracts of mice intranasally immunized with oligomeric gp160. J Immunol 1998;160:2000–2012.

44. Doherty TM, Olsen AW, van Pinxteren L, Andersen P. Oral vaccination with subunit vaccines protects animals against aerosol infection with *Mycobacterium tuberculosis*. Infect Immun 2002;70:3111–3121.

45. Thoelen S, Van Damme P, Mathei C, et al. Safety and immunogenicity of a hepatitis B vaccine formulated with a novel adjuvant system. Vaccine 1998;16:708–714.

46. Thoelen S, De Clercq N, Tornieporth N. A prophylactic hepatitis B vaccine with a novel adjuvant system. Vaccine 2001;19:2400–2403.

47. Stanberry LR, Spruance SL, Cunningham AL, et al. Glycoprotein-D-adjuvant vaccine to prevent genital herpes. N Engl J Med 2002;347:1652–1661.

48. Vernacchio L, Bernstein H, Pelton S, et al. Effect of monophosphoryl lipid A (MPL((R)) on T-helper cells when administered as an adjuvant with pneumocococcal-CRM(197) conjugate vaccine in healthy toddlers. Vaccine 2002;20:3658–3667.

49. Drachenberg KJ, Wheeler AW, Stuebner P, Horak F. A well-tolerated grass pollen-specific allergy vaccine containing a novel adjuvant, monophosphoryl lipid A, reduces allergic symptoms after only four preseasonal injection. Allergy 2001;56: 498–505.
50. Desombere I, Van der WM, Van Damme P, et al. Immune response of HLA DQ2 positive subjects, vaccinated with HBsAg/AS04, a hepatitis B vaccine with a novel adjuvant. Vaccine 2002;20:2597–2602.
51. Jacques P, Moens G, Desombere I, et al. The immunogenicity and reactogenicity profile of a candidate hepatitis B vaccine in an adult vaccine non-responder population. Vaccine 2002;20:3644–3649.
52. Stoute JA, Slaoui M, Heppner DG, et al. A preliminary evaluation of a recombinant circumsporozoite protein vaccine against *plasmodium falciparum* malaria. N Engl J Med 1997;336:86–91.
53. Sosman JA, Unger JM, Liu PY, et al. Adjuvant immunotherapy of resected, intermediate-thickness, node-negative melanoma with an allogeneic tumor vaccine: impact of HLA class I antigen expression on outcome. J Clin Oncol 2002;20:2067–2075.

# 13

# Microparticles and DNA Vaccines

## Kimberly Denis-Mize, Manmohan Singh, Derek T. O'Hagan, Jeffrey B. Ulmer, and John J. Donnelly

## INTRODUCTION

Developing deoxyribonucleic acid (DNA) vaccines potent enough to be clinically useful will likely require an understanding of the mechanism of action both of naked DNA vaccines themselves, and of adjuvant formulations that may be combined with DNA. Mechanisms of action attributed to naked DNA vaccines described thus far include transfection of keratinocytes *(1)*, muscle cells *(2)*, and dendritic cells (DCs) *(3)*, and activation of innate immunity by pathogen-associated molecular patterns (PAMPs) such as unmethylated CpG-containing immunostimulatory sequences *(4)*. Improving the immunogenicity of DNA vaccines has focused on four areas of investigation: increasing stability and efficiency of transfection, maximizing the ability of the antigen to be presented by DCs, and stimulating the immune response to the target antigen. A collective body of work demonstrating the versatility and mechanism of action of microparticle/DNA vaccine formulations supports promise of developing effective DNA vaccines utilizing this potent adjuvant/delivery system. Understanding the mechanism of action of DNA/microparticles provides both a basis for rational optimization of the formulation and basic insights into efficient induction of immunity.

Particulate adjuvant/delivery systems have been reported to enhance vaccine immunogenicity by several mechanisms. The activity of aluminum salt adjuvants is most widely described in terms of a repository effect *(5)*, and poly(DL-lactide-co-glycolide) (PLG) has been used to prepare vaccine formulations that provide a depot of vaccine with controlled release properties *(6)*. Recently Dupuis and associates have shown that submicron emulsion droplets affect the trafficking of antigen presenting cells to the site of injection and the draining lymph node *(7,8)*. A series of sub-10 μm particulates including liposomes *(9)*, ISCOMS *(10)*, emulsions, and PLG microspheres *(11)*, have been reported to

From: *Vaccine Adjuvants: Immunological and Clinical Principles*
Edited by: C. J. Hackett and D. A. Harn, Jr. © Humana Press Inc., Totowa, NJ

deliver either antigen or PAMP/"danger signal" to antigen-presenting cells (APCs) *(12,13)*. Particulate transfection-enhancing formulations based on cationic liposomes *(14)* and cationic emulsions *(15)*, have been described for non-viral gene therapy. Similar approaches have been applied to DNA vaccines *(16)* and technology platforms with plasmid DNA either encapsulated within, or adsorbed onto the surface of PLG microparticles show significant promise in improving the immunogenicity of DNA vaccines.

## PREPARATION OF PLG/DNA MICROPARTICLE FORMULATIONS

### Microparticles With Entrapped DNA

Numerous reports have demonstrated the utility of biodegradable polymer, PLG, for controlled release of encapsulated plasmid DNA. The principle method employed in the preparation of microparticles with encapsulated DNA is similar to one used extensively for encapsulating proteins, namely the multiple emulsion technique. Microparticles can be prepared by homogenizing a 6% w/v polymer solution (RG 505) in methylene chloride, with DNA in Tris-EDTA buffer (2 mg/mL) using an IKA homogenizer with a 3 mm probe at 23K. This results in an oil-in-water emulsion, which is added to a 10% PVA solution and homogenized using an Omni homogenizer with a 10 mm probe at 10K. The resulting oil in water in oil emulsion is stirred at 1000 rpm for 12 hours, the methylene chloride is allowed to evaporate, and resulting particles are washed, lyophilized and analyzed for DNA load by hydrolysis.

### Microparticles With Adsorbed DNA

A second technology platform utilizes biodegradable PLG microparticles with a cationic surface to adsorb negatively charged plasmid DNA. Microparticles with adsorbed DNA are prepared differently from the encapsulated ones. Here, a blank cationic PLG microparticle preparation is used to surface adsorb the plasmid DNA *(17)* (Fig. 1). One method to prepare the microparticles is to emulsify a 5% w/v polymer (RG 504) solution in methylene chloride with buffer at high speed using a homogenizer. This results in a primary emulsion, which is added to distilled water containing 0.5% cetyltrimethylammonium bromide, (CTAB) (0.5% w/v) to impart a surface positive charge to the preparation. The secondary water/oil/water emulsion is then stirred at 6000 rpm for 12 hours at room temperature, allowing the methylene chloride to evaporate completely, followed by washing and lyophilization. The blank cationic microparticle preparation is used to adsorb the DNA of choice by incubating 100 mg of microparticles in 1 mg/mL solution of DNA at 4°C for 6 hours. The microparticles are then separated by centrifugation, washed, and freeze-dried.

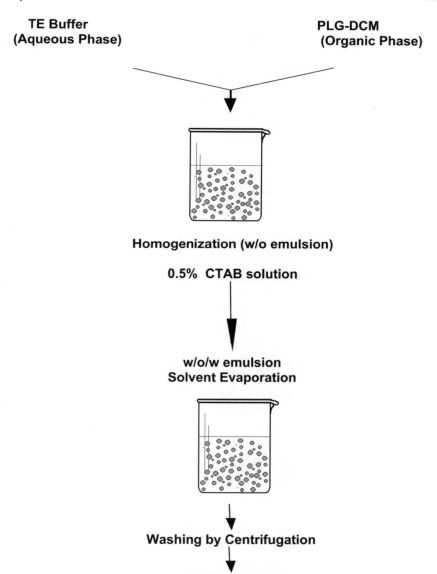

**TE Buffer**
**(Aqueous Phase)**

**PLG-DCM**
**(Organic Phase)**

**Homogenization (w/o emulsion)**

**0.5% CTAB solution**

**w/o/w emulsion**
**Solvent Evaporation**

**Washing by Centrifugation**

**PLG-CTAB Microparticles**

**Fig. 1.** Preparation of PLG-CTAB microparticles.

## Characterization of Cationic PLG Microparticles With Adsorbed DNA

The size distribution of the resulting microparticles are determined using a particle size analyzer (Master Sizer, Malvern Instruments, UK). The zeta potential is measured using a Malvern Zeta analyzer (Malvern Instruments, UK). Some

**Table 1**
**Physical Characterization of PLG-CTAB Microparticles**

| Process | Surfactant | Size (pre-adsorption) | Size (post-adsorption) | Zeta potential | Targeted load | Day 1 release |
|---------|-----------|----------------------|----------------------|----------------|---------------|---------------|
| W/O/W Evap | 0.5% CTAB | 1.2 μm | 6.5–8.2 μm | −18 mV | 0.96% w/w | 42% |

CTAB, cetyltrimethylammonium bromide.

of the routine characterization of cationic PLG microparticles with adsorbed plasmid DNA are summarized in Table 1.

## DELIVERY AND INTERNALIZATION

One approach to increasing the immunogenicity of DNA vaccines is to improve delivery and internalization of the gene of interest to ultimately increase expression and antigen presentation. Possible mechanisms include targeted uptake by either phagocytic or non-phagocytic APCs, or localization at the site of injection or draining lymph node. The hypotheses have been addressed using either fluorescence-labeled formulations or gene detection methods in both in vitro cell culture systems and in vivo models.

Biodegradable polymer microspheres such as PLG are readily internalized by phagocytic cells up to a diameter of 5 μm *(18)* and have been utilized as carriers for drug delivery systems. The application of synthetic biopolymers for nucleic acid delivery has proven advantageous for both protecting DNA against nuclease activity *(17)*, and increasing the efficiency of cellular uptake *(19)*. Although poly-alkylcyanoacrylate nanoparticles have been used to bind cetyltrimethylammonium bromide (CTAB)-oligonucleotide complexes to deliver antisense oligonucleotides to macrophage cell lines in vitro *(19,20)*, these vehicles have not been shown to transfect APC with plasmids carrying recombinant genes.

To test the hypothesis that microparticle/DNA formulations targeted APCs, Denis-Mize and associates used murine bone marrow-derived DCs as an in vitro model system to examine internalization of PLG/CTAB/DNA complexes *(21)*. DCs can capture antigen at peripheral sites via micropinocytosis using membrane ruffling, or may also internalize antigen by receptor-mediated processes involving Fcγ III, the mannose receptor, or the C-type lectin DEC-205 *(22)*. Thus, DCs may be targeted by the capture of larger (>250 nm) particulate antigens by phagocytosis. Phagocytic cells including macrophages and DC internalized rhodamine-labeled plasmid DNA formulated on PLG/CTAB microparticles. The intracellular distribution of rhodamine signal was primarily localized to endosomal compartments, which is similar to cellular uptake patterns of naked fluorescent-labeled plasmid in vitro, and what has been reported for plasmid taken up by Mac-1⁺ cells in vivo *(23)*.

The presence of the cationic surfactant on the surface of microparticles may contribute to endosomal disruption and increased cytoplasmic or nuclear localization, although the mechanism of endosomal escape remains unclear. Newman and associates reported cytoplasmic localization of Texas red labeled dextran encapsulated in PLGA microspheres following phagocytosis by mouse peritoneal macrophages *(24)*. Furthermore, Benoit and colleagues have postulated that microparticles entrapping poly-lysine pDNA may escape lysosomal degradation resulting in observed GFP reporter gene expression in a bovine macrophage cell line *(25)*.

An alternate formulation of plasmid DNA adsorbed onto the surface of cationic microparticles composed of DAEM (Poly butylmethacrylate, (2-dimethyl-aminoethyl) methacrylate, methylmethacrylate) or PEI (polyethyleneimine) has been described by Walter and associates *(26)*. In contrast to PLG/CTAB formulations, the microparticles (size range 2.68–7.81 μm) did not release free DNA. The cationic polymer DAEM is soluble at low pH, and postulated to dissociate in acidic phagosomal compartments. DAEM microparticles formulated with ethidium bromide homodimer-1-labeled DNA have been detected in primary human macrophages, but signal was not localized to the nucleus *(26)*.

Two studies to date have examined the in vivo tissue distribution and persistence of PLG/DNA microparticles. The first, by Lunsford and associates examined microparticle-encapsulated DNA and demonstrated primary localization to the injection site and lymphoid organs following intramuscular (im) or subcutaneous (sc) administration *(27)*. Analysis of phagocytic cells by flow cytometry following iv or sc injection of microparticles containing YOYO-labeled DNA suggested internalization by DCs and macrophages in the spleen. Furthermore, plasmid DNA was detected at the site of injection for up to 60 days following im injection, and up to 120 days following sc injection using a sensitive polymerase chain reaction (PCR) method developed by Nichols and associates *(28)*.

A recent report described in vivo effects of im administration of PLG/CTAB/DNA on DNA and PLG microparticle distribution, DNA persistence, and gene expression, by microscopic tracking of both fluorescence-labeled DNA (rhodamine-PNA) and PLG particles (DiI), and PCR analysis of both plasmid DNA and mRNA sequences *(29)*. At 3 hours postinjection, DiI-labeled microparticles are found primarily at the periphery of the tibialis anterior muscle with perceptible penetration into the interstitial space between fibrillar bundles. Fluorescent signal is also detected at the draining lymph node by the 3-hour time point. This distribution is similar to that observed on im administration of 50 μL naked DNA vaccine *(23)*. Observations at 7 days postinjection of PLG/CTAB/DNA clearly show the presence of a depot of particles at the injection site in which rhodamine fluorescence persists. The absence of this depot at 17 days postinjection is consistent with the degradation time of the PLG polymer *(29)*.

Coincident with the presence of the depot of PLG/CTAB/DNA microparticles at the periphery of the injected anterior tibialis muscle, an influx of mononuclear cells was observed concentrated at the muscular sheath. These cells are strongly labeled with the DNA-bound rhodamine-PNA tag and the population displays macrophage (CD11b$^+$) and myeloid DCs (CD11c$^+$) markers. Fractions of the population displayed elevated class I major histocompatability complex (MHC) and class II MHC levels, and the activation markers CD80 and CD86 *(29)*. Although Dupuis and associates have previously observed uptake of fluorescence-labeled naked DNA by a small population of mononuclear cells at the injection site and transport of the fluorescent signal to the draining lymph node *(23)*, PLG/CTAB/DNA formulations magnify the influx of phagocytic APC to the injection site providing a repository for internalization, antigen expression and presentation.

## EXPRESSION AND ANTIGEN PRESENTATION

The pattern of gene expression, and ultimately the efficiency of antigen presentation, dictates the efficacy of DNA-based vaccines. Formulation of DNA with microparticles may affect both, by increasing the amount and duration of antigen expression, as demonstrated by nearly five times greater luciferase expression levels following PLG/CTAB/DNA immunization as compared to naked DNA *(17)*, and by directing gene expression in APC following phagocytosis.

Two basic hypotheses developed to explain the immunogenicity of naked DNA vaccines have resulted in development of new formulations, particularly microparticle-DNA formulations, to increase the efficiency of DNA vaccines. The first hypothesis is that direct priming occurs, in which microparticle-formulated DNA is internalized by APC, released from microparticles following escape from endosomal degradation, and localized to the nucleus for expression and subsequent antigen presentation. An alternative hypothesis, termed cross-priming, suggests that the immunologically important event is the release of DNA from nonphagocytosed microparticles, and transfection of nonlymphoid cells in somatic tissues, resulting in expression of the antigen of interest and its subsequent processing by APC in the form of free antigen or apoptotic bodies.

Cross-priming is thought to be an important mechanism of immunogenicity of naked DNA vaccines. Fu and associates showed that in semi-allogeneic bone marrow chimeras injected intramuscularly with naked DNA encoding influenza NP, CD8$^+$ T cells recognized the antigen only in the context of the MHC molecules present on their bone marrow derived APC. These studies also showed that implantation of C2C12 myoblasts transfected with the gene for influenza

NP into semi-allogeneic bone marrow chimeras likewise recognized NP only in the context of H2 molecules present on bone marrow-derived APC *(30)*. In support of cross-priming as a mechanism of antigen expression and presentation, Dupuis and associates examined the distribution of unformulated plasmid DNA labeled with rhodamine-PNA clamps. Following im administration, the detectable intracellular fluorescence was limited to endocytic vesicles and target gene expression could not be demonstrated in the draining lymph node *(23)*. These results led to the conclusion that gene expression in the muscle was the principal source of antigen, and that cross-priming was a significant mechanism of immune induction following im administration of naked DNA vaccines *(23)*. Using DNA-loaded PEI and DAEM microparticles as described above, Walter and associates *(26)* have reported direct transfection of both a phagocytic macrophage cell line, and nonphagocytic 293 cells as detected by fluorescence microscopy from a green fluorescent protein-expressing plasmid. The DNA-loaded PEI and DAEM microparticles exhibited significant toxicity toward primary macrophages in vitro. Further evidence supporting direct transfection of cells by PLG formulations was reported by Ciftci and Su who found PLG microparticles containing a DNA:polycation complex provided controlled release of DNA and enhanced uptake and gene expression in 293 and MCF-7 cells *(31)*.

Using the bone marrow-derived DC described above as a model in vitro system, Denis-Mize and associates detected plasmid-encoded gene expression by reverse transcriptase-PCR, indicating PLG/CTAB-mediated transfection of DC in vitro *(21)*. Furthermore, PLG/CTAB-transfected DC efficiently presented the antigen of interest to T cells. The in vitro model system used an H-2K$^d$-restricted T-cell hybridoma to detect presentation of the human immunodeficiency virus (HIV)-1 gag- p7g epitope by APCs. DC pulsed with PLG/CTAB microparticles formulated with the pCMVKm2.GagMod.SF2 plasmid encoding the HIV gag protein could specifically stimulate the antigen-specific T-cell hybridoma to produce IL-2, although equivalent doses of the naked plasmid could not. The presentation of epitope was dose-dependent and sustained up to 5 days following transfection *(21)*. These data led the authors to conclude that direct transfection of DC may contribute to the increased immunogenicity observed following immunization with PLG/CTAB-formulated DNA vaccines *(17)*.

A follow-up study similar in design to that described above by Dupuis and associates was conducted with plasmid DNA adsorbed onto cationic PLG/CTAB microparticles *(29)*. The observation that administration of PLG/CTAB/DNA results in expression of the gene encoding the antigen in the draining lymph node is consistent with the interpretation that the particulate formulation enhances transfection of APCs, which may migrate to the draining lymph node. It is also possible that the direct transfection of muscle cells contributes to the immunogenicity of formulated DNA vaccines, because all active formulations have been shown to rapidly release a significant fraction of DNA within 1 to 24 hours under in vitro conditions *(17)*. Taken together with the observed transfection of mouse bone marrow-derived DCs by PLG/CTAB/DNA in vitro, and specific class I MHC-mediated presentation of epitope to a T-cell hybridoma *(21)*, the data suggest that enhanced immunogenicity obtained with the PLG/CTAB formulation results, in part, from a more efficient direct-priming mechanism.

Nonparenteral modes of administration, such as mucosal delivery of microparticle/DNA formulations may also provide a source of antigen for cross-priming or direct priming via transfection of APC. Several studies have examined the utility of plasmid DNA encapsulated within, or adsorbed onto, PLG microparticles for immunization by mucosal routes. Kaneko and associates examined weekly oral or im delivery of a plasmid encoding the HIV *env* gene encapsulated in 1.1 to 10 µm PLG microparticles (mean size 6.7 µm) *(32)*. One day after the final immunization, gene expression was detected by RT-PCR in small and large intestines of Balb/c mice (oral dose only, not im), suggesting the potential for nonphagocytic cells as the source of antigen.

Further evidence for enhancement of mucosal priming by formulation of DNA on microparticles has been presented in two studies employing intranasal (IN) delivery of PLG/CTAB/DNA formulations. Following IN immunization, immunofluorescent staining of cervical lymph nodes and spleen detected HIV-gag protein in phagocytic APC (CD11b[+]), suggesting either direct uptake and expression or cross priming by APC internalization of expressed protein *(33)*. Singh and colleagues have also reported an increase in the duration of persistence of antigen 7 days following IN administration of PLG/CTAB/DNA microparticles, compared with naked DNA immunization *(34)*.

## CHARACTERIZATION OF IMMUNE RESPONSE

The primary goal of formulating DNA with microparticles is to enhance the immunogenicity and effectiveness of DNA-based vaccination. Many reports demonstrate substantial augmentation of both humoral and cellular responses and protection in preclinical models of infection. Early reports described formulations of plasmid DNA encapsulated in 2 µm PLG microparticles. The plasmid DNA was characterized primarily as open circular form, and following release from microparticles, its competence to transform bacteria by electroporation was reduced by 25%. However, the formulation elicited serum immunoglobin (Ig)G, IgA, and IgM responses, and stool IgA responses in mice following a single dose administered intraperitoneally or by the oral route *(35)*. Additionally, PLG-encapsulated DNA vaccines designed to transfect APC were shown to elicit cytotoxic T-lymphocyte (CTL) responses *(36)*.

Subsequent studies demonstrated the ability of microparticle/DNA formulations to elicit protective immune responses in preclinical models of infection.

Chen and associates described protective immunity in an epizootic diarrhea of infant mice (EDIM) infection model obtained following a single oral immunization with rotavirus VP6 DNA encapsulated in PLG microparticles *(37)*. A subsequent report demonstrated a combination vaccine with VP4 and VP7 EDIM DNA encapsulated in PLG microparticles was also effective *(38)*.

Formulations of DNA and microparticles may improve the immune responses to DNA vaccination by decreasing the required dose of DNA, increasing the rate of seroconversion, resulting in an overall increase in antibody titers and CTL responses as compared to naked DNA vaccines. Using DNA encapsulated in PLG, Kaneko and associates reported comparable antibody titers following immunization with 10 μg PLG/DNA or 100 μg naked DNA *(32)*. Singh and associates reported detectable lysis of target cells by CTL following im administration of a single dose of 1 μg plasmid DNA adsorbed onto the surface of either PLG/CTAB or PLG/DDA microparticles. These data are comparable to response observed with $2 \times 10^7$ plaque forming units of vaccinia virus, and in contrast to the absence of detectable CTL activity at equivalent 1 μg doses of plasmid DNA alone *(17)*. Furthermore, one study comparing immune responses to naked DNA vaccines demonstrated a 100-fold increase in CTL response and a 1000-fold increase in antibody titers *(39)*. Although results may vary with formulation and antigen of interest, it is clear that DNA/PLG microparticle formulations significantly augment immune responses, potentially requiring less DNA and fewer doses.

The relationship between structural properties of PLG/CTAB/DNA formulations and immunological outcomes provides additional insights into the mechanism of action. Immunization with PLG/CTAB/DNA formulated with 30 μm particles induces no greater antibody titer than DNA alone *(17)*. The expected depot formation has been observed with this formulation, however neither uptake by APC nor influx of cells to the injection site has been observed *(29)*. A requirement for association of DNA with the PLG/CTAB formulation has also been observed. Administration of DNA with noninteractive polyvinylalcohol-stabilized PLG microparticles has been shown to be no more effective than administration of DNA alone even in the presence of exogenously added CTAB *(17,40)*. A recent report has also shown that independent administration of DNA and PLG/CTAB microparticles to the same site at separate times is also ineffective for enhancement of antibody titer though cellular influx is enhanced by administration of 1 μm PLG microparticles *(29)*. Thus, uptake of a PLG/CTAB/DNA complex by APC plays an essential role in the enhanced immunogenicity induced by the formulated DNA vaccine.

Formulation of plasmid DNA with microparticles also offers the potential for mucosal delivery of DNA vaccines. Plasmid DNA encapsulated in PLG microparticles has been administered by both the oral or im routes, eliciting both systemic and mucosal immune responses. Kaneko and associates correlated systemic and mucosal cellular immune responses in mice by detecting interferon (IFN)γ following in vitro restimulation of splenocytes, Peyer's patches and lamina propria and CTL lysis of labeled antigen-presenting target cells *(32)*. Additionally, mucosal responses were detected in the form of IgA from fecal wash samples and a reduction in vaccinia virus titer in the ovaries following intrarectal challenge with a recombinant vaccinia virus expressing the antigen of interest *(32)*. Studies with plasmid DNA adsorbed onto cationic PLG microparticles demonstrate the utility of IN immunization for induction of both local and systemic cell-mediated immune responses as detected by IFNγ enzyme-linked immunospot (ELISPOT) from cervical lymph nodes and spleen, and CTL activity in the spleen. Corresponding immunization with naked DNA resulted in only splenic responses, suggesting an increase in the breadth of the immune response imparted by the PLG/CTAB/DNA formulation *(33,34)*.

Murine systems are the primary model for evaluating the potential of PLG/ DNA microparticle formulations, and tend to exhibit broad, substantial immune responses to the antigen of interest. Additional species such as rabbits, guinea pigs, and non-human primates have also been examined. O'Hagan and associates have reported a rapid onset of antibody response in guinea pigs, and demonstrating higher neutralizing titers over DNA/alum formulations, and serum antibody titers equivalent to protein formulated with the water/oil emulsion adjuvant MF59 *(39)*. Furthermore, rhesus macaques immunized with a 0.5 mg PLG/DNA dose induced rapid seroconversion as early as 2 weeks after first immunization and three out of five had detectable CTL activity at this time point *(39)*. Such promising immune responses have led to rapid development of the technology platform and progression to clinical trials.

## TECHNOLOGY DEVELOPMENT/FUTURE DIRECTIONS

Formulations of DNA and microparticles exhibit great promise in the search for effective DNA vaccines. A body of evidence demonstrating internalization by phagocytic APCs, antigen expression and presentation, and enhanced humoral and cellular immune responses in multiple animal models, opens the door for continued development of this exciting technology platform. Furthermore, the demonstration of neutralizing antibody titers *(39)*, and protection from infectious disease *(37,38)*, and modified syngeneic tumor models *(41)* clearly warrants further clinical development. An encouraging preclinical safety profile was reported by Lunsford and colleagues whereby tissue distribution was extensively examined following im, sc, or iv administration of plasmid DNA encapsulated in PLG microparticles. Detection of DNA was durable in some cases out to day 120 following im or sc administration at the injection site or draining lymph node, whereas PCR signal was notably absent in the brain and gonads.

However, iv administration resulted in a more systemic distribution with plasmid found in the muscle, spleen, lung, kidney, liver, brain, heart– and persistent at most sites 14 days postadministration *(27)*.

Recently, results of a phase I clinical trial were reported, exploring the safety profile, in addition to evaluating the histological, immune, and clinical responses elicited by ZYC101, an encapsulated PLG/DNA microparticle formulation encoding the COOH-terminal end of the HPV-16 E7 protein *(42)*. Twelve HLA-A2 and HPV-16-positive males diagnosed with high-grade dysplasia of the anal mucosa received four im injections of 50 to 400 µg of the PLG/DNA formulation at 3-week intervals. The formulation was well-tolerated with the majority of toxicities reported as mild to moderate injection site pain. Ten of the 12 subjects elicited positive IFNγ ELISPOT results, and a 25% partial response rate was observed, generally at the higher dose levels. Following these encouraging results, subsequent studies are planned to evaluate second-generation products designed to target a wider range of HPV and HLA haplotypes *(42)*.

Although PLG/DNA formulations are rapidly moving through nonhuman primate models into development of new vaccines for both human and veterinary applications *(43)*, novel DNA/microparticle formulations may well lead to even more effective vaccine candidates. Several recent reports have described potential improvements in the formulation of DNA microparticles, such as the addition of lipophilic additives (monomethoxy polyethylene-glycol-distearoyl-phosphatidylethanolamine [PEG-DSPE] and taurocholic acid [TA]) during DNA encapsulation process resulting in increased incidence of responders and a trend toward increased antibody titers *(41)*. Others are reporting alternative immunization strategies, such as an oral administration of an encapsulated DNA prime followed by a recombinant vaccinia virus boost to augment systemic and mucosal immunity *(44)*. Yet another interesting approach is to further utilize the adjuvant properties of the PLG microparticle platform to include additional immunomodulators such as CpG oligonucleotides *(45)*, or plasmid DNA encoding an Interleukin-2/Ig fusion *(44)* further influence the breadth and strength of the desired immune response.

## CONCLUSIONS

A systematic approach to optimization of DNA vaccines for induction of both humoral and cellular responses remains a long-term goal. The distribution and magnitude of protein expression had been found to correlate with immunogenicity of DNA vaccines in preclinical models. We propose that these factors also influence the immunogenicity of DNA vaccines in humans. Although a spectrum of delivery and adjuvant approaches will be tested empirically, approaches targeting specific immune function may lead to more rapid progress. Both contin-

268                                                                                        *Denis-Mize et al.*

ued investigation into the mechanism of action of microparticle/DNA formulations and further development of APC-targeted DNA vaccine formulations are
warranted. Ongoing human trials of formulated DNA vaccines will provide
essential information to bridge the existing body of animal and in vitro data to
human immune responses. The success of these clinical studies will help determine whether DNA vaccines can achieve the potential that was proposed for
them more than a decade ago.

## REFERENCES

1. Porgador A, Irvine KR, Iwasaki A, Barber BH, Restifo NP, Germain RN. Predominant role for directly transfected dendritic cells in antigen presentation to
   CD81 T cells after gene gun immunization. J Exp Med 1998;188:1075–1082.
2. Manthorpe M, Cornefertjensen F, Hartikka J, et al. Gene-therapy by intramuscular injection of plasmid DNA—studies on firefly luciferase gene-expression in
   mice. Hum Gene Ther 1993;4:419–431.
3. Akbari O, Panjwani N, Garcia S, Tascon R, Lowrie D, Stockinger B. DNA vaccination: transfection and activation of dendritic cells as key events for immunity.
   J Exp Med 1999;189:169–178.
4. Sato Y, Roman M, Tighe H, et al. Immunostimulatory DNA sequences necessary
   for effective intradermal gene immunization. Science 1996;273:352–354.
5. Gupta RK, Rost BE, Relyveld E, Siber GR. Adjuvant properties of aluminum and
   calcium compounds. Pharm Biotechnol 1995;6:229–248.
6. Gupta RK, Singh M, O'Hagan DT. Poly(lactide-co-glycolide) microparticles for
   the development of single-dose controlled-release vaccines. Adv Drug Deliv Rev
   1998;32:225–246.
7. Dupuis M, McDonald DM, Ott G. Distribution of adjuvant MF59 and antigen
   gD2 after intramuscular injection in mice. Vaccine 1999;18:434–439.
8. Dupuis M, Denis-Mize K, LaBarbara A, et al. Immunization with the adjuvant
   MF59 induces macrophage trafficking and apoptosis. Eur J Immunol 2001;31:
   2910–2918.
9. Ignatius R, Mahnke K, Rivera M, et al. Presentation of proteins encapsulated in
   sterically stabilized liposomes by dendritic cells initiates CD8(+) T-cell responses
   in vivo. Blood 2000;96:3505–3513.
10. Morein B, Bengtsson KL. Immunomodulation by ISCOMS, immune stimulating
    complexes. Methods 1999;19:94–102.
11. Johansen P, Men Y, Merkle HP, Gander B. Revisiting PLA/PLGA microspheres:
    an analysis of their potential in parenteral vaccination. Eur J Pharm Biopharm 2000;
    50:129–146.
12. Matzinger P. Tolerance, danger, and the extended family. Annu Rev Immunol 1994;
    12:991–1045.
13. Janeway CA Jr. The immune system evolved to discriminate infectious nonself
    from noninfectious self. Immunol Today 1992;130:11–16.
14. Liu Y, Mounkes LC, Liggitt HD, et al. Factors influencing the efficiency of cationic
    liposome-mediated intravenous gene delivery. Nat Biotechnol 1997;15:167–173.

15. Yi SW, Yune TY, Kim TW, et al. A cationic lipid emulsion/DNA complex as a physically stable and serum-resistant gene delivery system. Pharm Res 2000;17: 314–320.
16. Ishii N, Fukushima J, Kaneko T, et al. Cationic liposomes are a strong adjuvant for a DNA vaccine of human immunodeficiency virus type 1. AIDS Res Hum Retroviruses 1997;13:1421–1428.
17. Singh M, Briones M, Ott G, O'Hagan D. Cationic microparticles: A potent delivery system for DNA vaccines. Proc Natl Acad Sci USA 2000;97:811–816.
18. Tabata Y, Ikada Y. Phagocytosis of polymer microspheres by macrophages. Adv Polymer Sci 1990;94:107–141.
19. Chavany C, Saison-Behmoaras T, Le Doan T, Puisieux F, Couvreur P, Helene C. Adsorption of oligonucleotides onto polyisohexylcyanoacrylate nanoparticles protects them against nucleases and increases their cellular uptake. Pharm Res 1994; 11:1370–1378.
20. Fattal E, Vauthier C, Aynie I, et al. Biodegradable polyalkylcyanoacrylate nanoparticles for the delivery of oligonucleotides. J Control Release 1998;53:137–143.
21. Denis-Mize KS, Dupuis M, MacKichan ML, et al. Plasmid DNA adsorbed onto cationic microparticles mediates target gene expression and antigen presentation by dendritic cells. Gene Ther 2000;7:2105–2112.
22. Lanzavecchia A. Mechanisms of antigen uptake for presentation. Curr Opin Immunol 1996;8:348–354.
23. Dupuis M, Denis-Mize K, Woo C, et al. Distribution of DNA vaccines determines their immunogenicity after intramuscular injection in mice. J Immunol 2000;165: 2850–2858.
24. Newman KD, Kwon GS, Miller GG, Chlumecky V, Samuel J. Cytoplasmic delivery of a macromolecular fluorescent probe by poly(d, l-lactic-co-glycolic acid) microspheres. J Biomed Mater Res 2000;50:591–597.
25. Benoit MA, Ribet C, Distexhe J, et al. Studies on the potential of microparticles entrapping pDNA-poly(aminoacids) complexes as vaccine delivery systems. J Drug Target 2001;9:253–266.
26. Walter E, Merkle HP. Microparticle-mediated transfection of non-phagocytic cells in vitro. J Drug Target 2002;10:11–21.
27. Lunsford L, McKeever U, Eckstein V, Hedley ML. Tissue distribution and persistence in mice of plasmid DNA encapsulated in a PLGA-based microsphere delivery vehicle. J Drug Target 2000;8:39–50.
28. Nichols WW, Ledwith BJ, Manam SV, Troilo PJ. Potential DNA vaccine integration into host cell genome. Ann NY Acad Sci 1995;772:30–39.
29. Denis-Mize K, Dupuis M, Singh M, et al. Mechanisms of increased immunogenicity for DNA-based vaccines absorbed onto cationic microparticles. Cell Immunol 2003;225:12–20.
30. Fu TM, Ulmer JB, Caulfield MJ, et al. Priming of cytotoxic T lymphocytes by DNA vaccines: requirement for professional antigen presenting cells and evidence for antigen transfer from myocytes. Mol Med 1997;3:362–371.
31. Ciftci K, Su J. DNA-PLGA Microparticles: A promising delivery system for cancer gene therapy. In: 1999 AAPS Annual Meeting Abstracts Online; 1999. Available from: http://www.aapspharmsci.org/abstracts/AM_1999/2214.htm

32. Kaneko H, Bednarek I, Wierzbicki A, et al. Oral DNA vaccination promotes muco-
    sal and systemic immune responses to HIV envelope glycoprotein. Virology 2000;
    267:8–16.
33. Vajdy M, O'Hagan DT. Microparticles for intranasal immunization. Adv Drug
    Deliv Rev 2001;51:127–141.
34. Singh M, Vajdy M, Gardner J, Briones M, O'Hagan D. Mucosal immunization
    with HIV-1 gag DNA on cationic microparticles prolongs gene expression and
    enhances local and systemic immunity. Vaccine 2001;20:594–602.
35. Jones DH, Corris S, McDonald S, Clegg JC, Farrar GH. Poly(DL-lactide-co-gly-
    colide)-encapsulated plasmid DNA elicits systemic and mucosal antibody responses
    to encoded protein after oral administration. Vaccine 1997;15:814–817.
36. Hedley ML, Curley J, Urban R. Microspheres containing plasmid-encoded anti-
    gens elicit cytotoxic T-cell responses. Nat Med 1998;4:365–368.
37. Chen sc, Jones DH, Fynan EF, et al. Protective immunity induced by oral immu-
    nization with a rotavirus DNA vaccine encapsulated in microparticles. J Virol 1998;
    72:5757–5761.
38. Herrmann JE, Chen SC, Jones DH, et al. Immune responses and protection obtained
    by oral immunization with rotavirus VP4 and VP7 DNA vaccines encapsulated in
    microparticles. Virology 1999;259:148–153.
39. O'Hagan D, Singh M, Ugozzoli M, et al. Induction of potent immune responses
    by cationic microparticles with adsorbed HIV DNA vaccines. J Virol 2001;75:
    9037–9043.
40. Briones M, Singh M, Ugozzoli M, et al. The preparation, characterization, and
    evaluation of cationic microparticles for DNA vaccine delivery. Pharm Res 2001;
    18:709–711.
41. McKeever U, Barman S, Hao T, et al. Protective immune responses elicited in
    mice by immunization with formulations of poly(lactide-co-glycolide) micropar-
    ticles. Vaccine 2002;20:1524–1531.
42. Klencke B, Matijevic M, Urban RG, et al. Encapsulated plasmid DNA treatment
    for human papillomavirus 16-associated anal dysplasia: a Phase I study of ZYC101.
    Clin Cancer Res 2002;8:1028–1037.
43. Bowersock TL, Martin S. Vaccine delivery to animals. Adv Drug Deliv Rev 1999;
    38:167–194.
44. Wierzbicki A, Kiszka I, Kaneko H, et al. Immunization strategies to augment oral
    vaccination with DNA and viral vectors expressing HIV envelope glycoprotein.
    Vaccine 2002;20:1295–1307.
45. Singh M, Ott G, Kazzaz J, et al. Cationic microparticles are an effective delivery
    system for immune stimulatory CpG DNA. Pharm Res 2001;18:1476–1479.

# Index

## A

Ab
  DC binding, 62
Adaptive immune responses
  QS-21, 222–226
Adaptive immunity, 87
  dendritic cells, 28–31
Adaptive T-cell responses
  bacterial products, 62
Adenylate cyclase toxin (CyaA), 112, 133, 134
Adjuvants, 56, 57
  bacterial toxins, 118
  bypassing conventional, 62
  in early life
  cytosine phosphate guanine
    oligodeoxynucleotides, 94
  LNFPIII/Lewis X, 184, 185
  LT, 122t, 123t
  pertussis toxin, 129
  QS-21, 222–227
Adoptive transfer, 51
Adsorbed cationic PLG
    microparticles
  deoxyribonucleic acid (DNA), 259, 260
Adsorbed deoxyribonucleic acid
    cationic PLG microparticles, 259, 260
Ag
  challenge, 51, 52
  DC migration to lymph nodes, 57, 58
Allergic rhinitis, 197
Allergies
  grass pollen
    MPL adjuvant, 250t
  MPL adjuvant, 251

Allergy vaccine adjuvant
  cytosine phosphate guanine
    oligodeoxynucleotides, 99, 100
  cytosine phosphate guanine
    oligodeoxynucleotides (CpG ODN), 99, 100
Alum, 89
Aluminum-hydroxide adjuvanted
    vaccine
  QS-21, 222
Antigen(s)
  major histocompatibility
    complex, 11
  peptide, 62
  schistosome egg, 99
Antigen-presenting cells (APC), 49
  LNFPIII/Lewis X, 185, 186
  murabutide, 203
  QS-21, 230
Antigen-specific T-cell responses
  in vivo, 51f
Anti-human serum antigen classes
  endpoint titers
    in immunized mice, 182t
Anti-human serum antigen IgE
    antibodies
  endpoint titers
    in immunized mice, 183t
Anti-human serum antigen IgG
  endpoint titers
    in immunized mice, 182t
Anti-inflammatory cytokines
  murabutide, 204, 205
Antiretrovirals (ARV)
  murabutide potentiation, 207
AP-1
  murabutide, 203
APC, see Antigen-presenting cells
  (APC)